Liver Biopsy
Interpretation

PETER J. SCHEUER, M.D., D.Sc.(Med.), F.R.C.Path.

Professor Emeritus (Histopathology)
University of London
Royal Free Hospital School of Medicine
London

JAY H. LEFKOWITCH, M.D.

Professor of Clinical Pathology
College of Physicians and Surgeons of Columbia University
New York

With a Foreword by
Professor Dame Sheila Sherlock

Liver Biopsy Interpretation

Fifth Edition

Volume 31 in the Series
MAJOR PROBLEMS IN PATHOLOGY

W.B. Saunders Company Ltd
LONDON PHILADELPHIA TORONTO SYDNEY TOKYO

This book is printed on acid-free paper

W. B. Saunders   24–28 Oval Road
Company Ltd   London, NW1 7DX

The Curtis Center
Independence Square West
Philadelphia, PA 19106-3399, USA

55 Horner Avenue
Toronto, Ontario, M8Z 4X6, Canada

Harcourt Brace & Company (Australia) Pty Ltd
30–52 Smidmore Street
Marrickville
NSW 2204, Australia

Harcourt Brace Japan Inc.
Ichibancho Central Building, 22-1 Ichibancho
Chiyoda-ku, Tokyo 102, Japan

A catalogue record for this book is available from the British Library

ISBN 0-7020-1594-6

Typeset by Latimer Trend & Company Ltd, Plymouth
Printed and bound in Hong Kong by Dah Hua

Foreword

The fifth edition of this bible of liver biopsy interpretation, first published in 1968, has undergone a radical transformation – a new young co-author from the United States, a new publisher, an abundance of descriptions of new techniques and many more figures in colour.

Traditionally, liver biopsy histology was interpreted on a single haematoxylin and eosin-stained section, perhaps with a couple of extra stains. Now the techniques of molecular biology have arrived. They include such methods as the polymerase chain reaction (PCR), *in situ* hybridization and flow cytometry. Jay Lefkowitch from New York discusses these clearly. They allow liver biopsy interpretation to take on a new, functional, dynamic role.

Chronic hepatitis is one of the most difficult conditions to understand. Classifications have come and gone. Peter Scheuer replaces them by a histological division into portal and parenchymal lesions, and bases classification mainly on aetiology.

World-wide, liver transplantation is now a routine procedure. The histopathologist has become an integral member of the liver transplant team. Every recipient of a liver transplant can anticipate four to six liver biopsies, whether protocol or because of complications. The pathologist uses this material to help in the decision on how to manage the patient, by identification of complications such as rejection, infection, biliary problems or indeed a combination. These aspects are fully covered in this new edition.

The authors have wisely kept the size of the book manageable. It is intended to be a work-manual but with the added advantage of an up-to-date, even up to 1994, selective reference list. Histopathologists, clinicians and all those interested in the liver can continue to rely on this book. It will not fail them as a guide in their day-to-day work. It will continue to keep them up to date on advances in modern hepatology.

Sheila Sherlock

v

Preface to the Fifth Edition

The fifth edition of *Liver Biopsy Interpretation* makes two notable departures from its predecessors. First, it has two authors in the place of one. Jay Lefkowitch joins as co-author, and has participated in the planning of the whole book as well as being responsible for the detailed content of Chapters 7, 11, 13, 15, 16 and 17. One of these is a newly separated chapter on the pathology of transplantation as applied to the liver, an area in which pathologists increasingly need training and advice. In acquiring a second author the book now spans the Atlantic Ocean. The second innovation is the transfer to W.B. Saunders, and specifically to the Major Problems in Pathology series. The authors welcome this change, while wishing to pay tribute to Baillière Tindall, a member of the same publishing group, who have published the four previous editions and with whom Peter Scheuer has had a most fruitful and pleasant relationship since the mid-1960s.

The purpose of the book once more remains unchanged. It is intended as a bench book to which the practising pathologist or clinical hepatologist can turn when confronted with a diagnostic problem. The medical student and research worker may also find it helpful as a compact guide to liver disease. It is not intended to compete with larger textbooks of medicine or pathology, to which the reader should turn for more detailed discussion of pathogenesis. The bibliography of each chapter has been chosen as a combination of recent relevant papers and reviews, important historical papers and, where appropriate, suitable background reading. The emphasis throughout is on biopsy rather than autopsy pathology, although some reference to the latter is inevitable.

Despite many developments in liver disease and pathology we have resisted the temptation to enlarge the book substantially. Notable developments since the last edition, published in 1988, have been the rapid increase in liver transplantation throughout the world, the discovery of the hepatitis C virus, and the growth of immunocytochemical and molecular biological methods in diagnostic pathology. Because of this growth, the chapter originally devoted to electron microscopy now encompasses some of the many newer techniques with which the pathologist should be familiar.

PETER J. SCHEUER
JAY H. LEFKOWITCH

Acknowledgements

We are greatly indebted to the many pathologists and clinicians who have provided us with liver biopsies and who have discussed with us the problems of their interpretation. This book is particularly addressed to them. The technical staff of the laboratories of the Royal Free Hospital and of the College of Physicians and Surgeons of Columbia University made the illustrations possible by providing high-quality sections for photography. In New York, Mr Alfred Lamme produced the photographs, while in London Mr Francis Moll and Miss Jackie Lewin gave valuable help and advice. Several generous donors of figures are acknowledged in the appropriate captions.

Our colleagues on both sides of the Atlantic contributed by checking and criticizing drafts of the manuscript; as future users of the book, their advice carried much weight. They included Dr Siddharta Datta Gupta, Dr Mohamed El Batanony, Dr Amany El Refaie, Dr Luca Mondazzi, Dr Heidrun Rotterdam and Dr Neil Theise. We are especially grateful to our teachers, notably Professor Dame Sheila Sherlock and Dr Hans Popper. The latter sadly died in 1988, but his influence is very much with us. Finally, Seán Duggan, Nigel Eyre and Rachael Stock of W.B. Saunders have made our contacts with the world of publishing an education and a pleasure.

P.J.S.
J.H.L.

Contents

GENERAL CONSIDERATIONS 1

The diagnosis and management of patients with liver disease depend on many sophisticated investigations, ranging from imaging methods to molecular biological techniques. In spite of the rapid development of these diagnostic tools, liver biopsy has retained its central place. This is partly because the concepts and classifications of liver disease are to a large extent based on morphology, but also because looking at a liver biopsy specimen under the microscope is a very direct way of visualizing disease processes. Liver biopsy is an invasive technique which requires a skilled operator, and all possible safeguards to minimize the risk of complications.

The specimen of liver tissue can be obtained by a variety of routes and methods. Blind percutaneous transthoracic biopsy, the classical method, is still used but ultrasound- or CT-guided biopsy has become increasingly popular in recent years.[1] Guided biopsy is particularly helpful when a focal lesion needs to be sampled or when the liver is unusually small.[2–4] The needle track may be plugged with gelatin sponge (Fig. 1.1) or other materials[5] (Fig. 1.2) to prevent bleeding.[6–8] Alternatively the specimen can be obtained by the transvenous route, via the jugular vein[7,9–11] or even via the femoral vein. Fine-needle aspiration is helpful in the diagnosis of liver tumours,[4,12–15] though its use in medical liver disease is much more restricted. A combination of histological and cytological examination of tumour material is often helpful. Specimens may also be taken under direct vision at laparotomy or laparoscopy.[16] Operative wedge biopsies are usually taken from the inferior margin of the right lobe. The procedure is followed by necrosis of adjacent liver cells and healing by granulation tissue within a few weeks.[17] For the techniques of liver biopsy and discussion of the various needles available, the reader is referred to clinical texts.[3,18] Whatever method is chosen, the operator should carefully consider whether the specimen obtained is likely to be adequate for the intended purpose. For example, a small needle specimen obtained with a small-bore needle guided by ultrasound may be adequate for the diagnosis of hepatocellular carcinoma, but quite unsuitable for the diagnosis and histological evaluation of chronic hepatitis. With needles of the Menghini type the biopsy core is aspirated and may fragment if the liver is cirrhotic. This is discussed further in Chapter 10.

Biopsy pathology differs from autopsy pathology in that there are pitfalls peculiar to small samples. A needle biopsy specimen of liver represents perhaps one fifty-thousandth of the whole organ and there is therefore an obvious possibility of sampling error. Some diseases of the liver are diffuse and involve every acinus, so that sampling error is unlikely; these can be diagnosed with confidence even in small specimens. Thus, for example, a diagnosis of acute viral hepatitis can be established in a needle specimen only some 5 mm long,[19] whereas a specimen of similar size may not be adequate for the accurate diagnosis of chronic liver disease,[20] or for the detection of focal lesions such as tumour deposits.

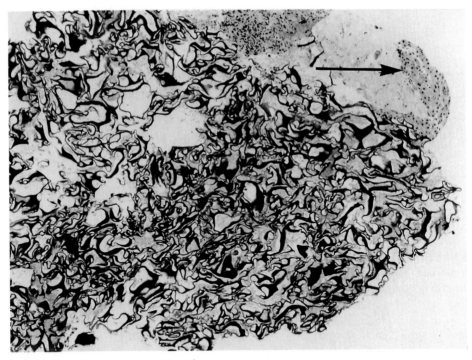

Figure 1.1. *Foreign material*. This is absorbable gelatin which was used to plug a needle track. A small amount of liver tissue is seen at the point of the arrow. Needle biopsy, haematoxylin and eosin (H & E).

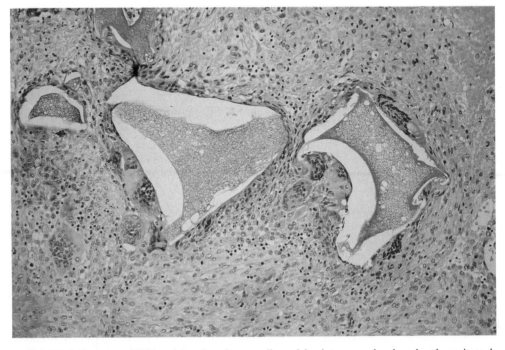

Figure 1.2. *Foreign material*. Material used to plug a needle track has here escaped and produced a peritoneal foreign-body giant cell reaction.[5] H & E.

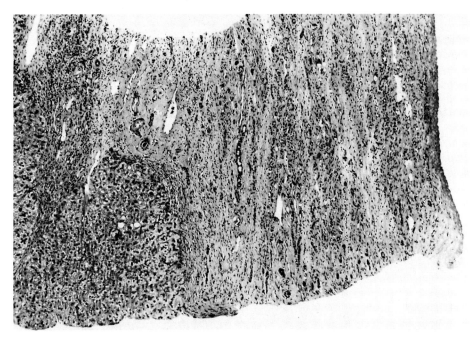

Figure 1.3. *Subcapsular necrosis.* There is a zone of multiacinar necrosis immediately deep to the liver capsule (right) in this patient with chronic hepatitis. The changes are less severe in the deeper tissue to the left. A small superficial sample would have presented problems of interpretation. Needle biopsy, H & E.

Granulomas may be found in one sample but not in another from the same liver.[21] Focal or unevenly distributed lesions cannot therefore be entirely excluded on the basis of their absence from an unguided needle biopsy specimen. When focal lesions are suspected, multiple biopsies may help to reduce sampling error.[22,23]

Chronic hepatitis and cirrhosis present particular sampling problems. In some patients with hepatitis there is a zone of extensive necrosis deep to the capsule, whereas the deeper parenchyma is less severely affected. A small specimen consisting of tissue from the subcapsular zone of the liver would then give a misleadingly pessimistic impression (Fig. 1.3). In cirrhosis the structure of a nodule is sometimes very similar to that of normal liver, so that a sample consisting almost entirely of the parenchyma from within a nodule may present serious diagnostic difficulties (Fig. 1.4). These are accentuated by the resistance of dense fibrous tissue; in a patient with cirrhosis an aspiration biopsy needle may glance off fibrous septa and selectively sample the softer nodular parenchyma. For this reason some clinicians prefer to use cutting needles in patients with suspected cirrhosis.[24,25]

Abnormalities in a liver biopsy may represent changes remote from a pathological lesion rather than the lesion itself. In large bile duct obstruction, for example, the results of the obstruction are clearly seen in the biopsy sample whereas the cause of the obstruction is usually not visible. The biopsy may be taken from the vicinity of a focal liver lesion such as metastatic carcinoma, and present one or more of a range of pathological features often puzzling to the interpreter (Fig. 1.5). Similarly disease elsewhere in the body may give rise to reactive changes in the liver; biopsy appearances are not normal, but at the same time do not indicate primary liver disease.

Biopsies reveal lesions or diseases rarely seen at autopsy because of their relatively benign course, such as sarcoidosis. In other conditions the evolution of a disease to an end-stage means that the earlier and more characteristic pathological features are rarely seen at autopsy or even at liver transplantation. In such cases liver biopsies provide valuable insights into the pathology of the disease.

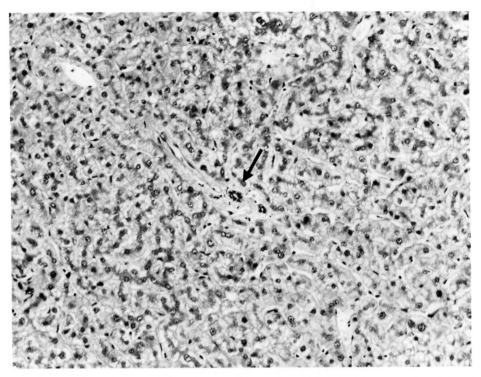

Figure 1.4. *Cirrhosis.* Appearances are nearly normal because the sample is from the centre of a nodule and does not include septa. A portal tract (arrow) is small and poorly formed. Needle biopsy, H & E.

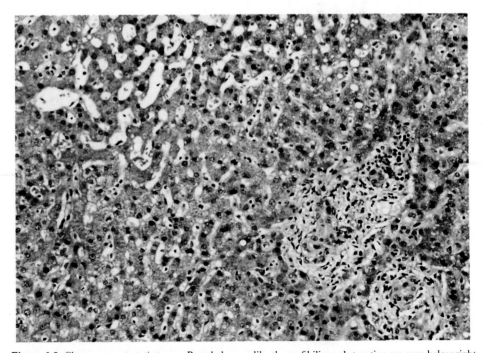

Figure 1.5. *Changes near metastatic tumour.* Portal changes like those of biliary obstruction are seen below right, and there is sinusoidal dilatation in the perivenular area above left. Needle biopsy, H & E.

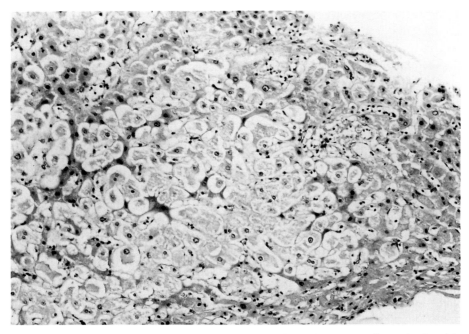

Figure 1.6. *Fixation artefact.* Hepatocytes in the central part of the specimen are swollen and pale-staining because of poor fixation. Needle biopsy, H & E.

Liver biopsy does not always provide a final or complete diagnosis. Sometimes it even fails to give helpful information. In most cases, however, an adequate and properly processed biopsy is an important item among the diagnostic tests to which the patient is subjected. Its limitations, together with the fact that the morphological reactions of the liver are limited in number, determine the need for full clinical, biochemical, immunological and imaging data to complement the biopsy findings. Pathologists need this information in order to minimize unnecessary errors, even if they may prefer to read the slides before the clinical data to avoid bias.[26]

Accurate assessment of the often subtle changes in a liver biopsy requires sections of high quality. The pathologist is usually aware of possible artefacts in liver biopsy material, as in any histological specimen. It is clearly desirable that artefacts should be avoided whenever possible and recognized as such when they do occur. A biopsy of adequate size may be rendered undiagnosable by rough handling, poor fixation, overheating, poor microtome technique and bad staining, all of which can obscure the criteria on which histological diagnoses are based. Poor fixation sometimes leads to potentially confusing liver-cell swelling, recognizable as artefact by its location away from the edges of the specimen (Fig. 1.6). False-positive staining for iron is unrelated to particular cells or structures, or is in a different focal plane from the tissue.

This book deals mainly with changes seen in conventionally stained paraffin sections. However, other techniques can be applied, many of which are discussed in Chapter 17. Some of them are of help in routine diagnosis while others remain research tools for the time being but may become routine tests in the future. Fine-needle aspiration of liver, the details of which are beyond the scope of this book, has a well-established place in the diagnosis of liver tumours. Microbiopsy fragments obtained by aspiration may require conventional paraffin embedding to supplement information from cytological preparations.

Immunocytochemical staining of tissue sections is particularly helpful in the detection of components of the hepatitis B virus (Figs 1.7 and 1.8), the hepatitis D virus,

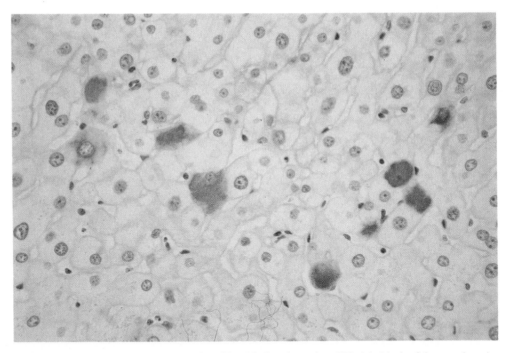

Figure 1.7. *Immunocytochemical demonstration of hepatitis B surface antigen (HBsAg).* Much of the cytoplasm is intensely stained in a minority of hepatocytes. These correspond to the ground-glass cells seen with other stains. Needle biopsy, specific immunoperoxidase.

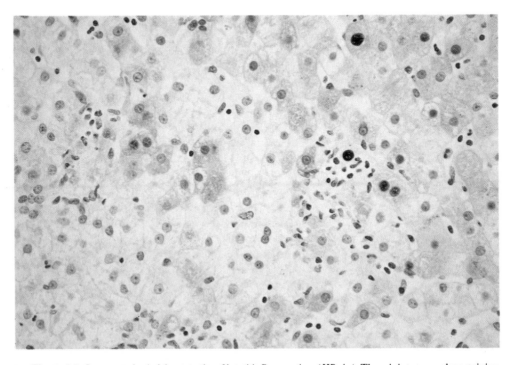

Figure 1.8. *Immunocytochemical demonstration of hepatitis B core antigen (HBcAg).* There is intense nuclear staining in several hepatocytes, as well as weaker cytoplasmic positivity. Needle biopsy, specific immunoperoxidase.

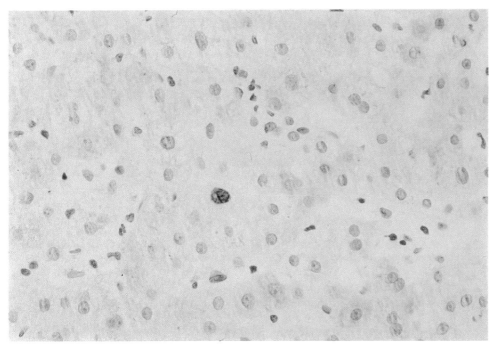

Figure 1.9. *In situ hybridization for cytomegalovirus DNA.* Positive staining of a hepatocyte nucleus (centre) indicates presence of viral DNA. Illustration kindly provided by Dr Neil Theise, New York.

cytomegalovirus and other infective agents. It is the most accurate way of diagnosing α_1-antitrypsin deficiency morphologically. It sometimes helps in the diagnosis of neoplasms of doubtful histogenesis or differentiation, though in this respect it is less useful than in many other areas of tumour work. Specific uses of immunocytochemistry are quoted in the appropriate chapters.

In situ hybridization has been applied to liver tissue for the identification or assessment of replication of infective agents including hepatitis A virus,[27] hepatitis B virus,[28,29] hepatitis C virus,[30–32] the delta agent[33,34] and cytomegalovirus[29] (Fig. 1.9). Its uses will undoubtedly increase, although identification of viruses is sometimes more easily achieved by immunocytochemical methods. The polymerase chain reaction (PCR) can be applied to liver tissue, and provides more direct evidence of virus infection than serum PCR. It has been used for the detection of the hepatitis C virus.[35–37] A combination of PCR with *in situ* hybridization[38,39] has proved successful and may provide pathologists with a particularly sensitive tool.

Part of the biopsy specimen can be analysed for copper, iron or abnormally stored substances, and enzyme activities can be assayed by micromethods. In the case of copper and iron, these measurements can if necessary be made after paraffin embedding, as discussed in Chapter 14. Elution of Sirius red from sections after staining provides an accurate method for the measurement of tissue collagen.[40] *In situ* demonstration of enzymes can be achieved by immunocytochemical methods or by means of enzyme histochemistry and has provided convincing evidence of metabolic zonation in human liver.[41,42]

Well-established techniques of morphometry, applied to tissue sections, have been used to obtain baseline data for relative volumes of tissue components in normal human liver[43,44] and in disease.[45] Three-dimensional reconstruction using a computer has helped in the understanding of disease processes and of the relationship between anatomical structures,[46,47] but is unlikely to have routine application at present.

Finally, semiquantitative assessment of pathological features is increasingly used for monitoring the effects of therapeutic drugs, especially in chronic viral hepatitis. This is further discussed in Chapter 9. Different systems of quantification are currently in use and in some instances the pathologist must devise a new system of grading appropriate for a particular purpose.

REFERENCES

1. Papini E, Pacella CM, Rossi Z et al. A randomized trial of ultrasound-guided anterior subcostal liver biopsy versus the conventional Menghini technique. *J Hepatol* 1991; **13**: 291–297.
2. Limberg B, Höpker WW, Kommerell B. Histologic differential diagnosis of focal liver lesions by ultrasonically guided fine needle biopsy. *Gut* 1987; **28**: 237–241.
3. Degos F, Degott C, Benhamou JP. Liver biopsy. In McIntyre N, Benhamou J-P, Bircher J, Rizzetto M, Rodes J (eds): Oxford Textbook of Clinical Hepatology. Oxford: Oxford University Press, 1991, pp 320–324.
4. Buscarini L, Fornari F, Bolondi L et al. Ultrasound-guided fine-needle biopsy of focal liver lesions: techniques, diagnostic accuracy and complications. A retrospective study on 2091 biopsies. *J Hepatol* 1990; **11**: 344–348.
5. Thompson NP, Scheuer PJ, Dick R, Hamilton G, Burroughs AK. Intraperitoneal ivalon mimicking peritoneal malignancy following plugged percutaneous liver biopsy. *Gut* 1993; **34**: 1635.
6. Tobin MV, Gilmore IT. Plugged liver biopsy in patients with impaired coagulation. *Dig Dis Sci* 1989; **34**: 13–15.
7. Sawyerr AM, McCormick PA, Tennyson GS et al. A comparison of transjugular and plugged-percutaneous liver biopsy in patients with impaired coagulation. *J Hepatol* 1993; **17**: 81–85.
8. Zins M, Vilgrain V, Gayno S et al. US-guided percutaneous liver biopsy with plugging of the needle track: a prospective study in 72 high-risk patients. *Radiology* 1992; **184**: 841–843.
9. McAfee JH, Keeffe EB, Lee RG, Rösch J. Transjugular liver biopsy. *Hepatology* 1992; **15**: 726–732.
10. Furuya KN, Burrows PE, Phillips MJ, Roberts EA. Transjugular liver biopsy in children. *Hepatology* 1992; **15**: 1036–1042.
11. Corr P, Beningfield SJ, Davey N. Transjugular liver biopsy: a review of 200 biopsies. *Clin Radiol* 1992; **45**: 238–239.
12. Glenthøj A, Sehested M, Torp-Pedersen S. Diagnostic reliability of histological and cytological fine needle biopsies from focal liver lesions. *Histopathology* 1989; **15**: 375–383.
13. Farnum JB, Patel PH, Thomas E. The value of Chiba fine-needle aspiration biopsy in the diagnosis of hepatic malignancy: a comparison with Menghini needle biopsy. *J Clin Gastroenterol* 1989; **11**: 101–109.
14. Fornari F, Civardi G, Cavanna L et al. Ultrasonically guided fine-needle aspiration biopsy: a highly diagnostic procedure for hepatic tumors. *Am J Gastroenterol* 1990; **85**: 1009–1013.
15. Edoute Y, Tibon-Fisher O, Ben Haim S, Malberger E. Ultrasonically guided fine-needle aspiration of liver lesions. *Am J Gastroenterol* 1992; **87**: 1138–1141.
16. Orlando R, Lirussi F, Okolicsanyi L. Laparoscopy and liver biopsy: further evidence that the two procedures improve the diagnosis of liver cirrhosis. A retrospective study of 1,003 consecutive examinations. *J Clin Gastroenterol* 1990; **12**: 47–52.
17. Helpap B. Pathologisch-anatomische Folgen der Leberkeilexcision. *Dtsch Med Wochenschr* 1973; **98**: 81–85.
18. Sherlock S, Dooley J. Needle biopsy of the liver. In: Diseases of the Liver and Biliary System, 9th edn. Oxford: Blackwell, 1993, pp 33–43.
19. Hølund B, Poulsen H, Schlichting P. Reproducibility of liver biopsy diagnosis in relation to the size of the specimen. *Scand J Gastroenterol* 1980; **15**: 329–335.
20. Schlichting P, Hølund B, Poulsen H. Liver biopsy in chronic aggressive hepatitis. Diagnostic reproducibility in relation to size of specimen. *Scand J Gastroenterol* 1983; **18**: 27–32.
21. Dutt MK, Davies DR, Grace RH, Thompson RP. Sampling variability of liver biopsy in inflammatory bowel disease. *Arch Pathol Lab Med* 1983; **107**: 451–452.
22. Abdi W, Millan JC, Mezey E. Sampling variability in percutaneous liver biopsy. *Arch Intern Med* 1979; **139**: 667–669.
23. Maharaj B, Maharaj RJ, Leary WP et al. Sampling variability and its influence on the diagnostic yield of percutaneous needle biopsy of the liver. *Lancet* 1986; **1**: 523–525.
24. Vargas-Tank L, Martínez V, Jirón MI, Soto JR, Armas-Merino R. Tru-cut and Menghini needles: different yield in the histological diagnosis of liver disease. *Liver* 1985; **5**: 178–181.
25. Colombo M, Del Ninno E, de Francis R et al. Ultrasound-assisted percutaneous liver biopsy: superiority of the Tru-Cut over the Menghini needle for diagnosis of cirrhosis. *Gastroenterology* 1988; **95**: 487–489.
26. Ludwig J. A review of lobular, portal, and periportal hepatitis. Interpretation of biopsy specimens without clinical data. *Hum Pathol* 1977; **8**: 269–276.
27. Taylor M, Goldin RD, Ladva S, Scheuer PJ, Thomas HC. In situ hybridization studies of hepatitis A viral RNA in patients with acute hepatitis A. *J Hepatol* 1994; **20**: 380–387.
28. Burrell CJ, Gowans EJ, Rowland R, Hall P, Jilbert AR, Marmion BP. Correlation between liver histology

and markers of hepatitis B virus replication in infected patients: a study by in situ hybridization. *Hepatology* 1984; **4**: 20–24.

29. Naoumov NV, Alexander GJM, Eddleston ALWF, Williams R. In situ hybridisation in formalin fixed, paraffin wax embedded liver specimens: method for detecting human and viral DNA using biotinylated probes. *J Clin Pathol* 1988; **41**: 793–798.

30. Haruna Y, Hayashi N, Hiramatsu N et al. Detection of hepatitis C virus RNA in liver tissues by an in situ hybridization technique. *J Hepatol* 1993; **18**: 96–100.

31. Tanaka Y, Enomoto N, Kojima S et al. Detection of hepatitis C virus RNA in the liver by *in situ* hybridization. *Liver* 1993; **13**: 203–208.

32. Yamada G, Nishimoto H, Endou H et al. Localization of hepatitis C viral RNA and capsid protein in human liver. *Dig Dis Sci* 1993; **38**: 882–887.

33. Pacchioni D, Negro F, Chiaberge E, Rizzetto M, Bonino F, Bussolati G. Detection of hepatitis delta virus RNA by a nonradioactive in situ hybridization procedure. *Hum Pathol* 1992; **23**: 557–561.

34. Lopez-Talavera JC, Buti M, Casacuberta J et al. Detection of hepatitis delta virus RNA in human liver tissue by non-radioactive in situ hybridization. *J Hepatol* 1993; **17**: 199–203.

35. Bresters D, Cuypers HTM, Reesink HW et al. Detection of hepatitis C viral RNA sequences in fresh and paraffin-embedded liver biopsy specimens of non-A, non-B hepatitis patients. *J Hepatol* 1992; **15**: 391–395.

36. Sallie R, Rayner A, Portmann B, Eddleston ALWF, Williams R. Detection of hepatitis 'C' virus in formalin-fixed liver tissue by nested polymerase chain reaction. *J Med Virol* 1992; **37**: 310–314.

37. Savage K, Dhillon AP, Brown D, Dusheiko G, Scheuer PJ. HCV by PCR of liver in autoimmune hepatitis. *Hepatology* 1992; **16**: 590.

38. Komminoth P, Long AA, Ray R, Wolfe HJ. In situ polymerase chain reaction detection of viral DNA, single-copy genes, and gene rearrangements in cell suspensions and cytospins. *Diagn Mol Pathol* 1992; **1**: 85–97.

39. Nuovo GJ, Lidonnici K, MacConnell P, Lane B. Intracellular localization of polymerase chain reaction (PCR)-amplified hepatitis C cDNA. *Am J Surg Pathol* 1993; **17**: 683–690.

40. Jimenez W, Pares A, Caballeria J et al. Measurement of fibrosis in needle liver biopsies: evaluation of a colorimetric method. *Hepatology* 1985; **5**: 815–818.

41. Lamers WH, Hilberts A, Furt E et al. Hepatic enzymic zonation: a reevaluation of the concept of the liver acinus. *Hepatology* 1989; **10**: 72–76.

42. Sokal EM, Trivedi P, Cheeseman P, Portmann B, Mowat AP. The application of quantitative cyto-chemistry to study the acinar distribution of enzymatic activities in human liver biopsy sections. *J Hepatol* 1989; **9**: 42–48.

43. Ranek L, Keiding N, Jensen ST. A morphometric study of normal human liver cell nuclei. *Acta Pathol Microbiol Scand A* 1975; **83**: 467–476.

44. Rohr HP, Luthy J, Gudat F, Oberholzer M, Gysin C, Bianchi L. Stereology of liver biopsies from healthy volunteers. *Virchows Arch Pathol Anat* 1976; **371**: 251–263.

45. Ranek L, Jensen ST, Keiding N. Karyometry of liver biopsies in virus hepatitis. *Acta Pathol Microbiol Scand A* 1975; **83**: 477–486.

46. Yamada S, Howe S, Scheuer PJ. Three-dimensional reconstruction of biliary pathways in primary biliary cirrhosis: a computer-assisted study. *J Pathol* 1987; **152**: 317–323.

47. Nagore N, Howe S, Boxer L, Scheuer PJ. Liver cell rosettes: structural differences in cholestasis and hepatitis. *Liver* 1989; **9**: 43–51.

GENERAL READING

Jackson JE, Adam A, Allison DJ. Transjugular and plugged liver biopsies. *Baillières Clin Gastroenterol* 1992; **6**: 245–258.

Klatskin G, Conn HO. Histopathology of the Liver. New York, Oxford: Oxford University Press, 1993.

Lee RG. Diagnostic Liver Pathology. St. Louis: Mosby-Year Book, Inc., 1994.

Ludwig J. Practical Liver Biopsy Interpretation. Diagnostic Algorithms. Chicago: ASCP Press, 1992.

MacSween RNM, Anthony PP, Scheuer PJ, Portmann B, Burt AD (eds). Pathology of the Liver, 3rd edn. Edinburgh: Churchill Livingstone, 1994.

Ruebner BH, Montgomery CK, French SW. Diagnostic Pathology of the Liver and Biliary Tract, 2nd edn. New York: Hemisphere Publishing Corporation, 1991.

Schaffner F, Thung S. Liver biopsy. In MacSween RNM, Anthony PP, Scheuer PJ, Portmann B, Burt AD (eds): Pathology of the Liver, 3rd edn. Edinburgh: Churchill Livingstone, 1994.

Snover DC. Biopsy Diagnosis of Liver Disease. Baltimore: Williams & Wilkins, 1992.

Wight DGD (ed). Liver, Biliary Tract and Exocrine Pancreas. Systemic Pathology, 3rd edn., Vol. 11. Edinburgh: Churchill Livingstone, 1994.

LABORATORY TECHNIQUES

2

PROCESSING OF THE SPECIMEN

As soon as a needle biopsy specimen is obtained from the patient it should be expelled gently on to a piece of glass, card or wood. Filter paper is less suitable because fibres tend to adhere to the tissue and may interfere with sectioning. The specimen must be treated with great care and excessive manipulation should be rigorously avoided; distortion of the specimen by rough handling at this stage may seriously interfere with accurate diagnosis, because diagnosis often depends on subtle criteria. At this stage minute pieces can be put into an appropriate fixative for electron microscopy (Chapter 17, p. 297), preferably by an operator experienced in this technique, and samples taken for chemical analysis or freezing. Frozen sections may be needed for demonstration of lipids. If porphyria is suspected, a very small amount of the unfixed tissue should be examined under ultraviolet light or with a suitable quartz halogen source, either whole or smeared on to a glass slide.

Tissue for paraffin embedding should be transferred to fixative as soon as possible, still mounted on card or other firm material. This prevents distortion and undue fragmentation of the specimen in transit. When the latter is likely to involve much movement, it is helpful to fill the container to the brim with fixative.

Buffered formalin and formol saline are both suitable for routine fixation, which is accomplished after 3 h at room temperature or less at higher temperatures (Table 2.1). Operative wedge biopsies and larger specimens need longer fixation. Fixatives other than formalin are successfully used in some centres; handbooks of laboratory technique should be consulted for optimum times and conditions for each fixative.

Minute fragments can be hand-processed more quickly than larger pieces, to avoid

Table 2.1. Sample Tissue Schedules for Liver Biopsies

Agent	Manual (h)	Automatic (h)	Automatic (Vacuum) (50°C)
	(room temperature)		
Buffered formalin	3	3	30 min +
Graded alcohols	—	6	8 min
Formalin–ethanol–water (volumes 10:80:10)	Overnight	—	—
Absolute ethanol	2	4	12 min
Xylene	3	3	16 min
Wax	2	2	12 min
Time	**24**	**18**	**1.5 h +**

undue shrinkage and hardening. Automated vacuum embedding allows the time of processing of needle specimens to be drastically reduced, as shown in the table; the production of a paraffin section in a few hours reduces the need for rapid frozen sectioning to circumstances where immediate diagnosis is needed for a decision at surgery. For the latter, sections can be cut by a standard method using a cryostat. Frozen sections are sometimes adequate for diagnosis of obvious lesions such as neoplasms but are unsuitable for recognition of subtle changes, and can even be dangerously misleading. Non-urgent frozen sections may be needed for immunocytochemical studies with antibodies which currently give unsatisfactory results on paraffin sections. Such antibodies are almost always used in research rather than diagnostic practice.

The exact number of sections routinely cut from a block varies widely from laboratory to laboratory. In the author's (PJS) laboratory, ten consecutive sections 3–5 μm thick are cut from each block and alternative sections used for the staining procedures outlined in the next paragraphs. The remaining sections are stored. Step sections are used when discrete lesions such as granulomas or tumour deposits are suspected, and for serial biopsies following liver transplantation. Large numbers of serial or near-serial sections rarely contribute to the diagnosis.

CHOICE OF STAINS

The stains routinely applied to liver biopsies vary according to local custom. The minimum advised is a haematoxylin and eosin, and a reliable method for connective tissue. The author prefers a silver preparation for reticulin as the principal method for showing connective tissue for reasons discussed below, but trichrome stains also have important applications. Routine staining for iron enables the biopsy to be used to screen for iron storage disease, and the periodic acid-Schiff stain after diastase digestion (DPAS or PASD) provides a relatively crude but practicable screening procedure for α_1-antitrypsin deficiency (p. 206). Other methods are used as required for particular purposes. The extent to which "special" stains form part of the routine set must be decided by each pathologist.

A **reticulin** preparation is important for accurate assessment of structural changes. Without it, thin layers of connective tissue and hence cirrhosis may be missed as may foci of well-differentiated hepatocellular carcinoma, in which the reticulin structure is often highly abnormal (p. 160). Counterstaining is sometimes used but is apt to distract rather than help, bearing in mind that the chief function of the reticulin preparation is to provide a sensitive low-power indicator of structural changes.

Stains for **collagen** such as the chromotrope-aniline blue (CAB) are important for the detection of new collagen formation, especially in alcoholic hepatitis and its imitators (p. 86). Collagen staining is therefore advised for any biopsy showing substantial fatty change. It also helps to show blocked veins within scars; these are easily missed on haematoxylin and eosin.

A stain for **elastic fibres** such as the orcein stain or elastic-van Gieson enables the pathologist to distinguish between recent collapse and old fibrosis, since only the latter is positive (p. 70). Again, this distinction may be very difficult to make on haematoxylin and eosin and even with the help of stains for collagen and reticulin. The orcein stain also shows copper-associated protein and hepatitis B surface material. The Victoria blue method[1] is a useful alternative to orcein.

Staining for **iron** by Perls' or other similar method enables not only iron but also bile, lipofuscin and other pigments to be evaluated, as discussed in the next chapter. Counterstaining should be light to avoid obscuring small amounts of pigment.

Staining of **glycogen** by means of the PAS method or Best's carmine demonstrates the extent of any liver-cell loss, and shows focal areas devoid of hepatocytes such as granulomas. **Glycoproteins** may be demonstrated by the PAS method after digestion with diastase to remove glycogen. This stain serves to accentuate hypertrophied macrophages, such as Kupffer cells filled with ceroid pigment after an acute hepatitis or cholestasis. Alpha$_1$-antitrypsin bodies stain strongly, but the stain is not sufficiently sensitive to enable all examples of α_1-antitrypsin deficiency to be detected.

Staining for **copper** is mainly used in suspected Wilson's disease, although, as explained on p. 220, it is not always helpful and may even be negative. The rhodanine method is preferred because it is easy to distinguish the orange–red colour of copper from bile, a distinction which is occasionally difficult with rubeanic acid. In Wilson's disease, there is variable correlation between the presence of stainable copper and staining for **copper-associated protein**. In chronic cholestasis, however, the two usually correspond.

Other non-immunological methods useful on occasion include the Ziehl–Neelsen stain for **mycobacteria** and for the ova of *Schistosoma mansoni*. When relatively large areas of tissue need to be screened for mycobacteria, the fluorescent auramine method (Fig. 15.8, p. 237) may be used. Specific staining for **bilirubin** is rarely necessary but conjugated bilirubin stains a bright green colour by the van Gieson method (Fig. 4.2, p. 33). **Amyloid** is stained by the usual techniques.

For **immunohistochemical staining**, standard techniques are applied. Among antibodies which are helpful in everyday practice are those against components of the hepatitis B virus, the delta agent, cytomegalovirus and α_1-antitrypsin. Neoplasms of doubtful histogenesis or differentiation are investigated by appropriate panels of antibodies, as in any other organ. Assessment of bile duct loss may require staining of cytokeratins 7 and 19, characteristic of bile-duct rather than liver-cell cytoplasm. The application of immunohistochemistry as well as of other modern techniques is discussed in more detail in Chapter 17.

Most of the staining methods mentioned above are used routinely in many laboratories, and can be found in the books listed under General Reading at the end of this chapter. A selection of methods is given below and in Chapter 17.

STAINING METHODS

Haematoxylin and Eosin; Haematoxylin and Van Gieson

Routine laboratory methods are suitable for liver biopsies.

Silver Impregnation for Reticulin Fibres (Gordon and Sweets)

1. Bring section to distilled water.
2. Treat with acidified potassium permanganate for 10 min; wash in distilled water.
3. Leave section in 1% oxalic acid until pale (about 1 min). Wash well in several changes of distilled water.
4. Mordant in 2.5% iron alum for 10 min. Wash in several changes of distilled water.
5. Treat with silver solution until section is transparent (about 10–15 s). Wash in several changes of distilled water.
6. Reduce in 10% formalin (4% aqueous solution of formaldehyde) for 30 s. Wash in tap water followed by distilled water.

7. Tone if desired in 0.2% gold chloride for 1 min. Rinse in distilled water.
8. Fix in 2.5% sodium thiosulphate for 5 min. Wash several times in tap water.
9. Transfer section to ethanol, clear and mount.

Reticulin appears black. The colour of the collagen varies according to whether step 7 is used; in untoned preparations it is yellow–brown.

Silver Solution

To 5 ml of 10% aqueous silver nitrate add strong ammonia (sp. gr. 0.88) drop by drop until the precipitate which forms is just dissolved. Add 5 ml of 3% sodium hydroxide. Add strong ammonia drop by drop until the resulting precipitate dissolves. The solution does not clear completely. Make up to 50 ml with distilled water. Scrupulously clean glassware should be used throughout.

Acidified Potassium Permanganate

To 95 ml of 0.5% potassium permanganate add 5 ml of 3% sulphuric acid.

Chromotrope–Aniline Blue (CAB) Method for Collagen and Mallory Bodies
(As used at Mount Sinai Hospital, New York; modified from Roque[2] and Churg and Prado[3])

1. Bring section to water.
2. Stain nuclei with Weigert's iron haematoxylin. Rinse in distilled water.
3. Immerse in 1% phosphomolybdic acid for 1–3 min. Rinse well in distilled water.
4. Stain with CAB solution for 8 min. Rinse well in distilled water. Blot.
5. Dehydrate quickly, clear and mount.

Collagen is stained blue. Mallory bodies stain blue or sometimes red. Giant mitochondria stain red.

CAB Solution

Aniline blue (1.5 g) is dissolved in 2.5 ml HCl and 200 ml distilled water with gentle heat. To this is added 6 g chromotrope 2R. The pH should be 1.0.

Orcein Stain for Elastic Fibres, Copper-associated Protein and Hepatitis B Surface Material[4]

1. Bring section to water.
2. Treat with acidified potassium permanganate for 15 min.
3. Rinse in water and decolorize in 2% oxalic acid.
4. Rinse in distilled water, then wash in tap water for 3 min.
5. Stain in orcein solution for 1 h or longer, at room temperature.
6. Rinse in water, then differentiate in 1% HCl in 70% ethanol.
7. Dehydrate, clear and mount.

Elastic fibres, copper-associated protein and hepatitis B surface material (HBsAg) stain brown. The method is less sensitive for HBsAg than immunohistochemical techniques. However, of the components listed copper-associated protein is often the most difficult to stain reliably. Different orceins vary in their staining properties.[5] Natural orceins seem to be more satisfactory than synthetic ones. In case of difficulty, doubling the concentration of orcein and the amount of HCl may help (Hans Popper, personal communication).

Acidified Potassium Permanganate

To 95 ml of 0.5% potassium permanganate add 5 ml of 3% sulphuric acid.

Orcein Solution

Orcein	1.0 g
70% ethanol	100 ml
Concentrated HCl	2.0 ml

The pH of the stain should be 1.0–2.0. The solution keeps for 1–4 weeks.

Modified Perls' Prussian Blue Method for Iron

1. Bring section to distilled water.
2. Immerse in a freshly prepared mixture of equal parts of 2% potassium ferrocyanide and 2% hydrochloric acid for 10 min at room temperature. Wash well in distilled water and rinse in tap water.
3. Counterstain with 0.2% aqueous neutral red for 1 min.
4. Dehydrate, clear and mount.

Ferric iron is stained blue.

Periodic Acid-Schiff Method

1. Bring section to water.
2. If desired, digest with 1% amylase ("diastase") at 37°C in a damp atmosphere for 30 min. Wash in tap water for 10 min, then in distilled water.
3. Oxidize in 1% periodic acid for 5 min. Wash in distilled water.
4. Immerse in Schiff reagent for 5–10 min. Wash in running water.
5. Counterstain with haematoxylin (e.g. Carazzi) 1 min. Blue.
6. Dehydrate, clear and mount.

For staining of glycogen, step 2 is omitted. Positive substances stain deep purple.

Schiff Reagent (de Tomasi)

Dissolve 1 g basic fuchsin in 200 ml boiling distilled water in a stoppered 1 litre flask. Shake for 5 min. Cool to exactly 50°C, filter, and add 20 ml N HCl to the filtrate. Cool further to 25°C and add 1 g sodium metabisulphite. Store for 18–24 h in the dark, add 2 g activated charcoal and shake the mixture for 1 min. Filter off the charcoal. Store the reagent in the dark at 0–4°C.

Rhodanine Stain for Copper[6]

1. Bring section to distilled water.
2. Incubate in rhodanine working solution for 18 h at 37°C or 3 h at 56°C.

3. Rinse in several changes of distilled water and stain with Carazzi's haematoxylin for 1 min.
4. Rinse with distilled water and then quickly in borax solution. Rinse well in distilled water.
5. Dehydrate, clear and mount.

Copper deposits stain bright red. Bile stains green. Weakly positive stains tend to fade, but fading can be reduced by staining at the higher temperature and by using certain mounting media (e.g. Ralmount [Raymond A. Lamb], DPX or Diatex).

Rhodanine Stock Solution

p-Dimethylaminobenzylidene rhodanine	0.2 g
Ethanol	100 ml

The working solution is prepared by diluting 3 ml of the well-shaken stock solution with 47 ml distilled water.

Borax Solution

Disodium tetraborate	0.5 g
Distilled water	100 ml

REFERENCES

1. Tanaka K, Mori W, Suwa K. Victoria blue–nuclear fast red stain for HBs antigen detection in paraffin section. *Acta Pathol Jpn* 1981; **31**: 93–98.
2. Roque AL. Chromotrope aniline blue method of staining Mallory bodies of Laennec's cirrhosis. *Lab Invest* 1953; **2**: 15–21.
3. Churg J, Prado A. A rapid Mallory trichrome stain (Chromotrope-aniline blue). *Arch Pathol* 1956; **62**: 505–506.
4. Shikata T, Uzawa T, Yoshiwara N, Akatsuka T, Yamazaki S. Staining methods of Australia antigen in paraffin section–detection of cytoplasmic inclusion bodies. *Jpn J Exp Med* 1974; **44**: 25–36.
5. Kirkpatrick P. Use of orcein in detecting hepatitis B antigen in paraffin sections of liver. *J Clin Pathol* 1982; **35**: 430–433.
6. Lindquist RR. Studies on the pathogenesis of hepatolenticular degeneration. II. Cytochemical methods for the localization of copper. *Arch Pathol* 1969; **87**: 370–379.

GENERAL READING

Bancroft JD, Stevens A (eds). Theory and Practice of Histological Techniques, 3rd edn. Edinburgh: Churchill Livingstone, 1990.
Carson FL. Histotechnology. A Self-instructional Text. Chicago: ASCP Press, 1990.
Elias JM. Immunohistopathology. A Practical Approach to Diagnosis. Chicago: ASCP Press, 1990.
Polak JM, van Noorden S (eds). Immunocytochemistry. Modern Methods and Applications, 2nd edn. Bristol: Wright, 1986.

3

THE NORMAL LIVER

Light microscopy of the normal liver reveals a regular structure based on the afferent and efferent blood vessels and branches of the biliary tree. The terminal portal venules and branches of the hepatic artery, together with small bile ducts, are contained within the portal tracts. Blood from both arteries and portal venous vessels in these tracts traverses the hepatic parenchyma to reach the terminal hepatic venules. The relationship between vasculature and parenchyma has been explained on the basis of several models, of which the most widely used at present is the acinus of Rappaport[1] (Fig. 3.1). The centre of the acinus is occupied by the terminal branches of the portal vein and hepatic artery; successively less well-oxygenated zones of parenchyma are numbered 1, 2 and 3, the latter adjacent to terminal hepatic venules. This model helps to explain the distribution of some pathological lesions; among these is bridging necrosis, which is widely regarded as representing confluent necrosis of acinar zone 3. The acinar model is, however, only one of several which have been proposed. The classical lobule, with the terminal hepatic venule ("centrilobular vein", "central vein") at its centre and portal tracts at the periphery, is somewhat easier to comprehend and describe than the acinus. Furthermore, the original concept of the acinus, based predominantly on studies of blood flow, has been modified in the light of observed enzyme distribution.[2] From a practical point of view the parenchyma immediately adjacent to small portal tracts can be described as "periportal" in either acinar or lobular nomenclature, while parenchymal cells near the efferent venules are called "perivenular" in acinar terminology but "centrilobular" in lobular terms. The thickness of the terminal hepatic venule varies widely but correlates with the diameter of the vessel.[3] There is no obvious relationship between thickness and age or sex.

Each portal tract consists of connective tissue in which are embedded at least one small artery or arteriole, portal-vein branch and bile duct (Fig. 3.2). Lymphatics, nerves and scanty lymphocytes and mast cells may also be seen. Bile ducts in the smallest tracts are called interlobular ducts, larger ones septal or trabecular ducts. Heterotopic exocrine pancreatic tissue is occasionally found near large bile ducts,[4] but is unlikely to be seen in needle biopsy material. Interlobular bile ducts are lined by cuboidal or low columnar epithelium, resting on a basement membrane which is associated with PAS-positive material resistant to diastase digestion. The epithelial cells contain cytokeratins CK7 and CK19 in addition to CK8 and CK18, the latter two being found in hepatocytes also.[5] Septal ducts are lined by tall columnar cells with basal nuclei (Fig. 3.3) and have an internal diameter of more than 100 μm. Interlobular and septal bile ducts occupy a central position in each portal tract, close to a branch of the portal vein and to an artery of approximately the same diameter as the duct. The plane of any one tissue section may fail to pass through a duct, but 70–80% of arteries are normally seen to be accompanied by ducts.[6]

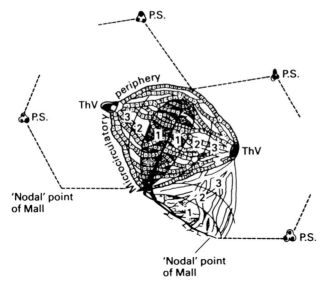

Figure 3.1. *The hepatic acinus.* Diagrammatic representation of the acinar concept in relation to classical lobules, the latter represented by dotted lines. Acinar zone 1 surrounds the terminal portal vessels while zone 3 abuts on the terminal hepatic venules. At the nodal points of Mall, the terminal afferent vessels from neighbouring acini lie close to each other. PS = portal space. Figure adapted from *Pathology of the Liver*, 2nd edn, with permission from Professor R.N.M. MacSween, Professor R.J. Scothorne and Churchill Livingstone.

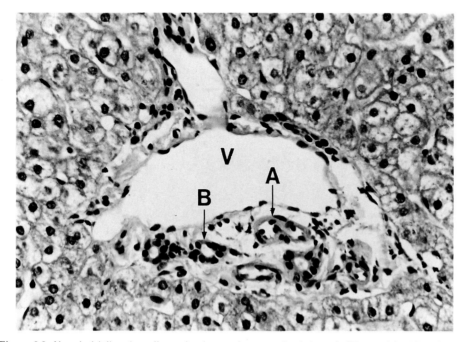

Figure 3.2. *Normal adult liver.* A small portal tract contains a portal-vein branch (V), arterioles (A) and small interlobular bile duct (B) as well as a few lymphocytes. Needle biopsy, H & E.

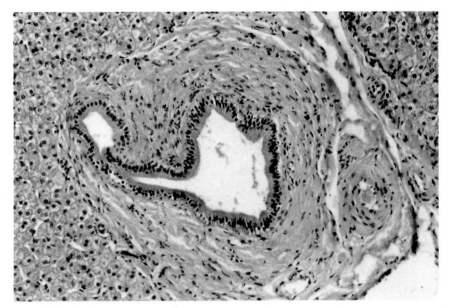

Figure 3.3. *Normal adult liver.* A large interlobular bile duct (left) is seen entering a septal duct (centre). Wedge biopsy, H & E.

Interlobular bile ducts are connected to the bile canalicular network of the hepatic parenchyma by ductules (cholangioles) and canals of Hering. The latter are lined partly by biliary epithelium and partly by hepatocytes, and lie at the edges of the portal tracts. In recent years the canals of Hering have aroused considerable interest because they may represent the site of stem cells capable of differentiating into new hepatocytes or bile ductules under pathological conditions.[7] The putative stem cells express chromogranin-A and on electron microscopy are seen to contain dense-cored secretory granules.[8] Neither ductules nor canals of Hering are often seen in normal liver but they become more conspicuous in some disease states (Fig. 3.4).

The hepatic parenchyma consists of **liver cells** (hepatocytes) which form interconnecting walls or plates separated from each other by the sinusoidal labyrinth (Fig. 3.5). Sinusoids are lined by flattened, fenestrated **endothelial cells** which form an incomplete, porous barrier, allowing easy exchange of materials between blood and hepatocytes. The sinusoidal endothelial cells differ from capillary endothelial cells not only in their morphology but also in their phenotype.[9,10] Within the sinusoidal lumen there is a phenotypically heterogeneous population of macrophages.[11] The principal macrophage is the **Kupffer cell**. This has irregular processes and often straddles the vessel lumen. Kupffer cells are more numerous near the portal tracts and, when active, can be distinguished from endothelial cells by their positive staining for muramidase and with PAS after diastase digestion.

Between the endothelium and the hepatocytes is the **space of Disse**. This is not conspicuous in paraffin sections of biopsy material. It contains **extracellular matrix components, nerves,**[12] **lipocytes** and **pit cells.**[13,14] The latter, probably natural killer (NK) cells, are also found in the sinusoidal lumen. The lipocytes (fat-storing cells, perisinusoidal or parasinusoidal cells, Ito cells, stellate cells) belong to the myofibroblast family and are involved in fibrogenesis[15] and probably also in the control of sinusoidal blood flow.[12] They are slightly more abundant in perivenular than in periportal areas.[16] Difficult to see in conventional paraffin sections, they can be demonstrated in osmium tetroxide-fixed, plastic-embedded material and in oil-red O-stained frozen sections.

The extracellular matrix of the acini, located in the space of Disse, includes collagen

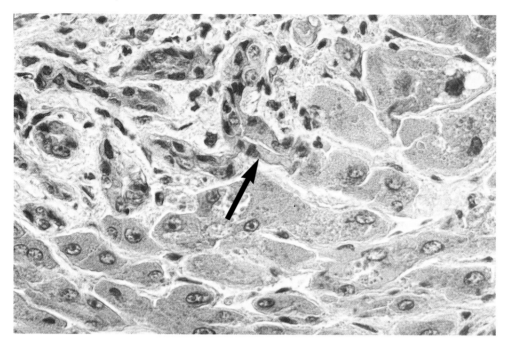

Figure 3.4. *Bile ductules and canals of Hering.* These are unusually prominent in this cirrhotic liver. A liver-cell plate is seen in continuity with a ductular structure (arrow). Needle biopsy, H & E.

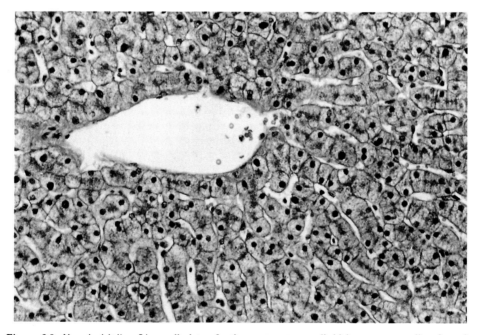

Figure 3.5. *Normal adult liver.* Liver-cell plates, for the most part one cell thick, appear to radiate from the terminal hepatic venule. Wedge biopsy, H & E.

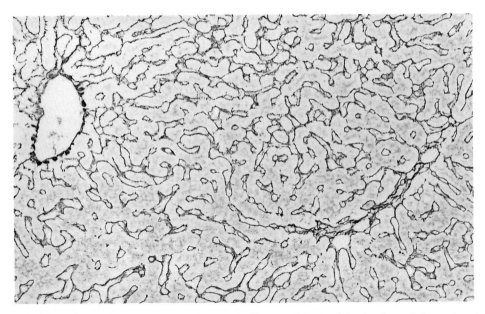

Figure 3.6. *Normal adult liver.* There is a regular reticulin network between the portal tract below and to the right, and the terminal hepatic venule above and to the left. Needle biopsy, reticulin.

types I,III,IV,V and VI, together with proteoglycans and glycoproteins.[17-20] The latter include fibronectin and laminin. Elastic fibres, prominent in the portal tracts, cannot be readily demonstrated in sinusoidal walls by conventional staining. Type I collagen is mainly found in portal tracts and in the walls of efferent veins, while type III is the principal component of collagen fibres in the space of Disse, in fibres of the reticulin type. These fibres form a regular network which sometimes appears to radiate from the terminal hepatic venules (Fig. 3.6).

The hepatocytes are arranged in plates which, in the adult, are normally one cell thick. In any section a few plates will appear thicker as a result of tangential sectioning, but widespread formation of twin-cell plates is regarded as a sign of hyperplasia. The wall of hepatocytes next to a portal tract is known as the limiting plate. Hepatocytes are polygonal cells with well-defined borders. The latter are particularly well seen after staining with diastase-PAS. Each cell contains one or more nuclei; binucleation of a minority of hepatocytes is a normal finding. Nucleoli are often visible. Mitotic figures are rare. Most of the nuclei are diploid,[21,22] but smaller numbers of tetraploid and even larger nuclei are found, especially in older subjects. Polyploidy and a degree of variation in nuclear size are therefore normal characteristics of the adult human liver. A few nuclei may contain abundant glycogen and appear vacuolated, particularly near portal tracts and in children or adolescents.

Healthy hepatocyte cytoplasm is pale-staining, faintly granular and rich in glycogen. Like nuclear glycogen, this does not always survive tissue processing. Large particulate organelles such as mitochondria and lysosomes are sometimes polarized to a particular part of each cell, contrasting with paler-staining areas of endoplasmic reticulum and glycogen (Figs 3.5 and 3.7). A few hepatocytes may contain fat vacuoles in apparently healthy subjects. Rarely, a solitary acidophil body is seen in normal liver tissue. This suggests that apoptosis[23] is a physiological phenomenon in the liver.

Between the hepatocytes, their walls formed by two or three cells, are the bile canaliculi. They are usually too small to be readily visible by light microscopy in routine paraffin sections, or are seen as minute spaces at the biliary poles of the hepatocytes. They can be demonstrated immunocytochemically with polyclonal anti-CEA, which also reacts

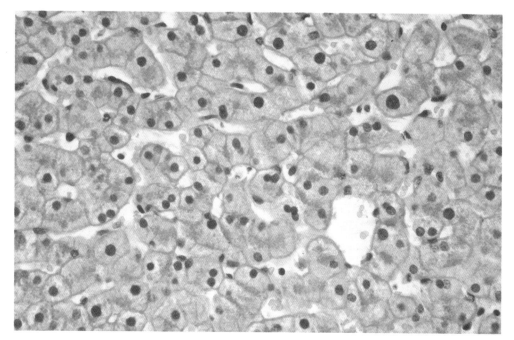

Figure 3.7. *Normal adult liver.* The increased density at the biliary poles of the hepatocytes is partly due to lipofuscin pigment granules. Wedge biopsy, H & E.

with a canalicular antigen. They are CD10-positive in frozen sections.[24] Bile is rarely seen in normal subjects.

HEPATOCELLULAR PIGMENTS (Table 3.1)

Within the cytoplasm of hepatocytes, near the bile canaliculi, there are fine brown–yellow granules of lipofuscin pigment (Figs 3.7 and 3.8). These are a normal constituent of adult liver, and are occasionally seen in children. Most abundant near terminal hepatic venules, lipofuscin granules represent lysosomes filled with undegradable materials. The amount of lipofuscin in normal liver varies greatly, making assessment of increase or decrease in disease subject to error in the absence of well-controlled morphometric data. Lipofuscin also varies in its staining properties according to its constituents and age. It is acid-fast, has reducing properties, and stains variably with diastase-PAS. Perls' stain for iron is negative. Large amounts of lipofuscin may be difficult to distinguish from Dubin–Johnson pigment (p. 211) on light microscopy alone, but the latter is generally coarser and darker. Intracellular bile can usually be distinguished from either by its bright green staining with van Gieson's method (Fig. 4.2, p. 33) and by the presence of bile thrombi in canaliculi. These thrombi are almost always found and intracellular bile pigment should not in general be diagnosed in their absence. An exception to this rule is the situation following liver transplantation, when diffuse intracellular bile accumulation is common.

Staining for iron is usually negative in normal liver but occasionally weakly positive in periportal hepatocytes. Strongly positive staining should lead to a search for a cause such as genetic haemochromatosis (Chapter 14). In young adults even small amounts of stainable iron should be investigated further.

Copper-associated protein is seen in high copper states as grey–brown intracytoplasmic

Table 3.1. Identification of Liver-cell Pigments

	Haemosiderin	Lipofuscin	Dubin–Johnson Pigment	Bile	Copper-associated Protein
Distribution	Periportal	Perivenular	Perivenular: often in Kupffer cells also	Often perivenular: in canaliculi and Kupffer cells also	Periportal in chronic cholestasis
Intracellular site	Pericanalicular	Pericanalicular	Pericanalicular	Pericanalicular or diffuse	Variable
Approximate granule size	1 µm	1 µm	Often more than 1 µm	Very variable	1 µm or less
Colour	Golden brown, refractile	Yellow	Dark brown	Yellow, brown or green	Grey
Perls' stain	Positive	Negative	Negative	Negative	Negative
Diastase-PAS stain	Negative	Variable	Variable	Variable	Positive
Long Ziehl–Neelsen stain	Negative	Positive	Often positive	Negative	Negative
Orcein stain	Negative	Negative	Negative	Negative	Positive

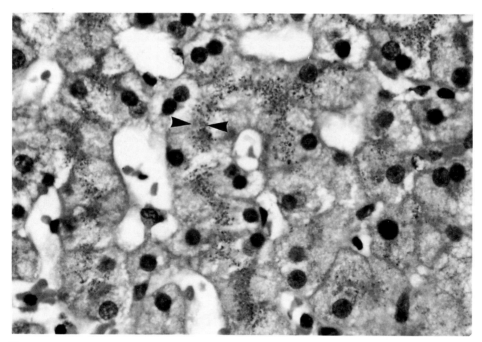

Figure 3.8. *Lipofuscin pigment.* Fine granules of lipofuscin (arrowheads) are seen at the biliary poles of the hepatocytes, away from the sinusoids. Needle biopsy, H & E.

granules, usually periportal in location and, unlike lipofuscin, is stained by the orcein method and with Victoria blue.

NORMAL APPEARANCES IN CHILDHOOD

The regular pattern of portal tracts and terminal venules is already well established by the end of gestation (Fig. 3.9). Foci of haemopoietic cells are seen within portal tracts and sinusoids for a few weeks after birth. Hepatocytes and their nuclei vary much less in size than in the adult, and in younger children the liver-cell plates are for the most part two cells thick. The adult pattern of single-cell plates is usually established at the age of 5 or 6 years. Nuclear vacuolation is common even in the absence of disease. There may be lipofuscin pigment granules in hepatocytes even in young children but in the first decade these are usually scanty.

AGEING

There is more variation in the size of hepatocytes and their nuclei in older subjects than in the young (Fig. 3.10). This is associated with greater numbers of polyploid cells, with increased cell and nuclear volume.[25] Hepatocytes may contain fat vacuoles irrespective of body weight or alcohol intake.[26] Other reported findings in a small proportion of old subjects include isolated hydropic hepatocytes, siderosis, nuclear vacuolation and increased numbers of nucleoli.[27] Lipofuscin pigment becomes more abundant but variation from person to person makes this difficult to interpret. The term "brown atrophy" has been applied to a combination of very abundant lipofuscin with senile or

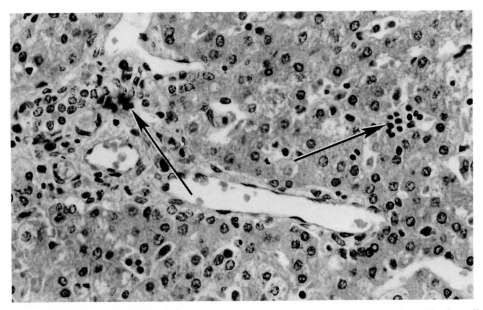

Figure 3.9. *Normal neonatal liver.* There are haemopoietic cells (arrows) in the sinusoids and in the well-developed portal tract. Post-mortem liver, H & E.

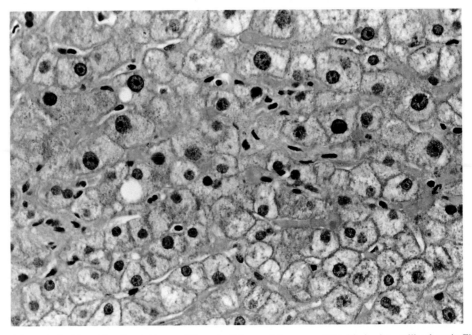

Figure 3.10. *Normal liver in an old person.* Hepatocellular nuclei vary considerably in size, unlike those in Fig. 3.9. Needle biopsy, H & E.

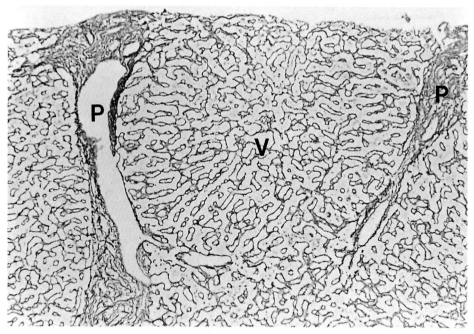

Figure 3.11. *Normal adult liver.* Two normal portal tracts (P), cut longitudinally, mimic septa. Between them is a terminal hepatic venule (V). Needle biopsy, reticulin.

other atrophy of hepatocytes. The connective tissue of the portal tracts becomes more dense with age. Arteries may be thick-walled even in normotensive subjects. These morphological changes are accompanied by alteration of the metabolic function of the liver, including the handling of drugs.[28]

BIOPSY OF THE NORMAL LIVER

The appearances of a biopsy specimen from normal liver are as described above. Care must be taken, however, to distinguish longitudinally cut portal tracts from pathological septa (Fig. 3.11). Percutaneous biopsies are necessarily taken through the liver capsule, and the latter may be seen either at one end of the main specimen or in the form of separate pieces of connective tissue. Capsular connective tissue can be distinguished from most pathological fibrous tissue by its density and maturity. It often contains blood vessels and bile ducts. The thickness of the capsule correlated well in an autopsy study with the amount of connective tissue deeper in the organ, both in normal and fibrotic livers.[29]

Other organs and tissue are sometimes included in a biopsy specimen, in addition to or instead of liver. Skin, pleura and intercostal muscle are common, while other viscera such as colon or kidney are occasionally seen. The close apposition to liver of fibrous tissue or tumour does not necessarily reflect hepatic fibrosis or tumour within the liver.

Transjugular biopsy specimens are obtained by means of a needle which passes through the wall of a hepatic vein into the hepatic parenchyma. While they are often small and fragmented, particularly in patients with cirrhosis, they offer a means of obtaining tissue in patients unsuitable for percutaneous biopsy because of potential bleeding. The material is often adequate for histological diagnosis.[30]

Surgical biopsies are usually taken from the inferior margin of the liver and are in the

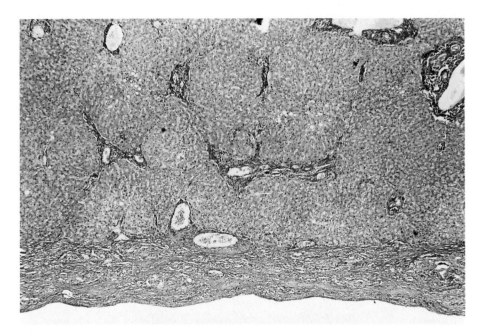

Figure 3.12. *Normal adult liver.* The capsule is thick and portal tracts are prominent. Post-mortem liver, trichrome.

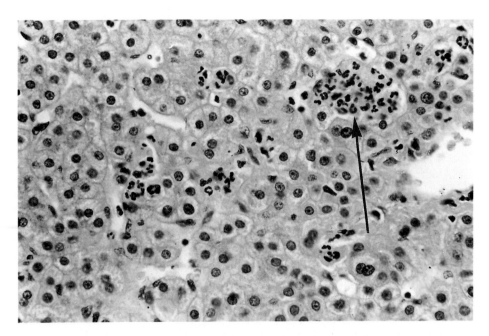

Figure 3.13. *Operative wedge biopsy.* Clumps of neutrophils mark sites of hepatocellular necrosis (arrow), resulting from the procedure. Wedge biopsy, H & E.

form of wedges covered on two aspects by capsule. The structure of this region may differ somewhat from that of the deeper tissue (Fig. 3.12), but as indicated above, there is good correlation between the volume fractions of non-parenchymal components in subcapsular and deeper areas.[29] Appearances mimicking cirrhosis in non-cirrhotic livers do not usually extend for more than 2 mm into the liver.[31] Confusion is therefore unlikely except in very small samples.

In surgical biopsies taken some time after the beginning of an operation, polymorpho-nuclear leucocytes accumulate under the capsule, around terminal hepatic venules and focally within liver-cell plates. Here they are associated with focal loss of hepatocytes (Fig. 3.13). Accompanying portal inflammation must be distinguished from the lesion of cholangitis in which bile ducts are involved and the above focal parenchymal changes are lacking. A similar lesion has been observed after heavy sedation without full anaesthesia.[32] It is also commonly seen in baseline biopsies taken at the time of orthotopic liver transplantation.

REFERENCES

1. Rappaport AM. The microcirculatory acinar concept of normal and pathological hepatic structure. *Beitr Pathol* 1976; **157**: 215–243.
2. Lamers WH, Hilberts A, Furt E et al. Hepatic enzymic zonation: a reevaluation of the concept of the liver acinus. *Hepatology* 1989; **10**: 72–76.
3. Junge J, Vyberg M, Horn T, Christoffersen P. Perivenous and perisinusoidal collagen content in the acinar zone 3 in the "normal" liver. A light microscopical study. *Liver* 1988; **8**: 325–329.
4. Terada T, Nakanuma Y, Kakita A. Pathologic observations of intrahepatic peribiliary glands in 1000 consecutive autopsy livers. Heterotopic pancreas in the liver. *Gastroenterology* 1990; **98**: 1333–1337.
5. van Eyken P, Desmet VJ. Cytokeratins and the liver. *Liver* 1993; **13**: 113–122.
6. Nakanuma Y, Ohta G. Histometric and serial section observations of the intrahepatic bile ducts in primary biliary cirrhosis. *Gastroenterology* 1979; **76**: 1326–1332.
7. De Vos R, Desmet V. Ultrastructural characteristics of novel epithelial cell types identified in human pathologic liver specimens with chronic ductular reaction. *Am J Pathol* 1992; **140**: 1441–1450.
8. Roskams T, De Vos R, van den Oord JJ, Desmet V. Cells with neuroendocrine features in regenerating human liver. *APMIS* 1991; **Suppl. 23**: 32–39.
9. Petrovic LM, Burroughs A, Scheuer PJ. Hepatic sinusoidal endothelium: Ulex lectin binding. *Histopathology* 1989; **14**: 233–243.
10. Scoazec JY, Feldmann G. In situ immunophenotyping study of endothelial cells of the human hepatic sinusoid: results and functional implications. *Hepatology* 1991; **14**: 789–797.
11. Bardadin KA, Scheuer PJ, Peczek A, Wejman J. Immunocytochemical observations on macrophage populations in normal fetal and adult human liver. *J Pathol* 1991; **164**: 253–259.
12. Bioulac-Sage P, Lafon ME, Saric J, Balabaud C. Nerves and perisinusoidal cells in human liver. *J Hepatol* 1990; **10**: 105–112.
13. Bioulac-Sage P, Latry P, Dubroca J, Quinton A, Balabaud C. Pit cells in human liver. In Kirn A, Knook DL, Wisse E (eds): Cells of the Hepatic Sinusoid, Vol. 1. Rijswijk: Kupffer Cell Foundation, 1986, pp 415–420.
14. Bouwens L, Wisse E. Pit cells in the liver. *Liver* 1992; **12**: 3–9.
15. Friedman SL. The cellular basis of hepatic fibrosis. Mechanisms and treatment strategies. *N Engl J Med* 1993; **328**: 1828–1835.
16. Horn T, Junge J, Nielsen O, Christoffersen P. Light microscopical demonstration and zonal distribution of parasinusoidal cells (Ito cells) in normal human liver. *Virchows Arch (A)* 1988; **413**: 147–149.
17. Biagini G, Ballardini G. Liver fibrosis and extracellular matrix. *J Hepatol* 1989; **8**: 115–124.
18. Schuppan D. Structure of the extracellular matrix in normal and fibrotic liver: collagens and glycoproteins. *Semin Liver Dis* 1992; **10**: 1–10.
19. Griffiths MR, Keir S, Burt AD. Basement membrane proteins in the space of Disse: a reappraisal. *J Clin Pathol* 1991; **44**: 646–648.
20. Loréal O, Clément B, Schuppan D, Rescan P-Y, Rissel M, Guillouzo A. Distribution and cellular origins of collagen VI during development and in cirrhosis. *Gastroenterology* 1992; **102**: 980–987.
21. Feldmann G. Liver ploidy. *J Hepatol* 1992; **16**: 7–10.
22. Deprez C, Vangansbeke D, Fastrez R, Pasteels JL, Verhest A, Kiss R. Nuclear DNA content, proliferation index, and nuclear size determination in normal and cirrhotic liver, and in benign and malignant primary and metastatic hepatic tumors. *Am J Clin Pathol* 1993; **99**: 558–565.
23. Wyllie AH. Apoptosis: cell death in tissue regulation. *J Pathol* 1987; **153**: 313–316.
24. Loke SL, Leung CY, Chiu KY, Yau WL, Cheung KN, Ma L. Localisation of CD10 to biliary canaliculi by immunoelectron microscopical examination. *J Clin Pathol* 1990; **43**: 654–656.
25. Watanabe T, Tanaka Y. Age-related alterations in the size of human hepatocytes. A study of mononuclear and binucleate cells. *Virchows Arch (B)* 1982; **39**: 9–20.

26. Hilden M, Christoffersen P, Juhl E, Dalgaard JB. Liver histology in a "normal" population—examinations of 503 consecutive fatal traffic casualties. *Scand J Gastroenterol* 1977; **12**: 593–597.
27. Findor J, Perez V, Iguarta EB, Giovanetti M, Fioravantti N. Structure and ultrastructure of the liver in aged persons. *Acta Hepatogastroenterol Stuttg* 1973; **20**: 200–204.
28. Popper H. Aging and the liver. In Popper H, Schaffner F (eds): Progress in Liver Diseases, Vol. VIII. Orlando: Grune & Stratton, 1986, pp. 659–683.
29. Ryoo JW, Buschmann RJ. Comparison of intralobular non-parenchyma, subcapsular non-parenchyma, and liver capsule thickness. *J Clin Pathol* 1989; **42**: 740–744.
30. Sawyerr AM, McCormick PA, Tennyson GS, et al. A comparison of transjugular and plugged-percutaneous liver biopsy in patients with impaired coagulation. *J Hepatol* 1993; **17**: 81–85.
31. Petrelli M, Scheuer PJ. Variation in subcapsular liver structure and its significance in the interpretation of wedge biopsies. *J Clin Pathol* 1967; **20**: 743–748.
32. McDonald GS, Courtney MG. Operation-associated neutrophils in a percutaneous liver biopsy: effect of prior transjugular procedure. *Histopathology* 1986; **10**: 217–222.

GENERAL READING

Bioulac-Sage P, Saric J, Balabaud C. Microscopic anatomy of the intrahepatic circulatory system. In Okuda K, Benhamou J-P (eds): Portal Hypertension. Clinical and Physiological Aspects. Tokyo: Springer-Verlag, 1991, pp 13–26.

Gerber MA, Thung SN. Histology of the liver. *Am J Surg Pathol* 1987; **11**: 709–722.

Kitani K. Aging and the liver. In Popper H, Schaffner F (eds): Progress in Liver Diseases, Vol. IX. Philadelphia: W.B. Saunders, 1990, pp 603–623.

MacSween RNM, Scothorne RJ. Developmental anatomy and normal structure. In MacSween RNM, Anthony PP, Scheuer PJ, Portmann B, Burt AD (eds): Pathology of the Liver, 3rd edn. Edinburgh: Churchill Livingstone, 1994.

4

EXAMINATION OF THE ABNORMAL BIOPSY

MACROSCOPIC APPEARANCES

Naked-eye examination and description of biopsy specimens, while of limited diagnostic value, reduce the possibility of specimen identification error and help in the selection of samples for special investigations such as electron microscopy. Needle-biopsy specimens from cirrhotic liver are often irregular in calibre or obviously nodular, with brown or green nodules separated by grey or white fibrous tissue. The specimen may easily break into smaller pieces on handling or processing. Normal liver, on the other hand, gives rise to cylinders of even colour and thickness which do not fragment easily. Cholestasis imparts a green colour, while fatty liver is pale brown or yellow and may float in the fixative. In cholesterol ester storage disease and Wolman's disease the specimen is bright orange; this should warn the pathologist of the need to keep some tissue for frozen sectioning and electron microscopy. A black or very dark brown colour is characteristic of the Dubin–Johnson syndrome. Metastatic tumour, like fibrous tissue, is often white. Congested liver is deep red in colour. The clinician should record if the specimen was difficult to obtain from the patient and whether the liver felt hard when the needle was inserted, as in many cases of cirrhosis, or very hard as in congenital hepatic fibrosis.

MICROSCOPIC APPEARANCES

Routine microscopy of liver biopsies should include assessment of overall structure, portal tracts and their contents, terminal hepatic venules, hepatocytes and sinusoidal cells. The following notes may help in the evaluation of pathological changes. Most of the information is also to be found in other parts of the book, under individual diseases.

Structural Changes, Collapse and Fibrosis

Minor structural changes are difficult to assess in sections stained with haematoxylin and eosin, and may indeed be missed altogether. Examination of a connective tissue preparation is therefore often important. For detection of the most minor abnormalities an uncounterstained silver impregnation for reticulin is generally best, although pericellular fibrosis is most easily detected in sections stained for collagen.

Using these methods, an impression may be gained that structural relationships are undisturbed, with regular spacing of portal tracts and terminal hepatic venules, but that the portal tracts themselves are enlarged and perhaps even linked by fibrous septa. This is consistent with mild chronic viral hepatitis or with one of the conditions in which portal changes typically predominate; these include biliary tract disease (p. 38), haemochromatosis (p. 222), congenital hepatic fibrosis (p. 201) and schistosomiasis (p. 244). If on the other hand the reticulin framework of the parenchyma is distorted, lesions characterized by intra-acinar damage should be considered. These include acute or chronic hepatitis and forms of biliary disease in which there is also hepatocellular damage, notably primary biliary cirrhosis (p. 51). Venous congestion (p. 188) leads to regular condensation of perivenular reticulin.

Recent collapse and fibrosis are sometimes difficult to distinguish, even with the help of good collagen stains. A stain for elastic tissue can help to resolve this problem because the presence of elastic fibres outside the portal tracts is an indication of disease of long standing (p. 70). In livers with extensive collapse or fibrosis, collagen stains enable vein walls to be identified. Collagen staining is important for the detection of pericellular fibrosis, as already indicated, and should therefore be used whenever there is substantial fatty change or a suspicion of steatohepatitis (pp. 81 and 86). It is also useful for the recognition of blocked veins in alcoholic liver disease, venous outflow obstruction (p. 188) and epithelioid haemangioendothelioma (p. 166).

The histological diagnosis of cirrhosis is fully discussed in Chapter 10. Once cirrhosis has developed, the pattern of fibrosis is one of the features that may help to determine its cause. In primary or secondary biliary cirrhosis, for example, fibrosis expanding and linking the portal tracts is a more important early factor in pathogenesis than hepatocellular regeneration; this is reflected in the morphological picture of broad perilobular septa surrounding irregularly shaped islands of parenchyma (Fig. 5.11, p. 46). In genetic haemochromatosis and chronic venous outflow obstruction the impression is also of fibrosis rather than regeneration as the principal pathogenetic factor. In these diseases with a long pre-cirrhotic phase of fibrosis, transected parenchymal peninsulas may be mistaken for true regenerative nodules. This is particularly common just deep to the liver capsule. Isolated subcapsular nodules in an otherwise not nodular biopsy should therefore be interpreted with caution.

LIVER-CELL NECROSIS AND INFLAMMATION

Death of individual hepatocytes or small groups of these cells is called **focal** necrosis. It is associated with accumulation of inflammatory cells of various types, including macrophages (Fig. 15.26, p. 254). **Spotty** necrosis is used for the same lesion in the context of acute hepatitis. Focal necrosis is a common finding which does not in itself indicate primary disease of the liver, because it is often part of a non-specific reaction to disease elsewhere in the body. While degenerating hepatocytes or cell fragments are sometimes seen within the focal inflammatory infiltrate, the inflammatory reaction is usually more obvious than the necrosis, and the latter is assumed to have taken place because of a gap in a liver-cell plate (liver-cell "drop-out"). Some authors distinguish between cell necrosis and apoptosis, the latter representing a specific form of cell death.[1] In practice, the term focal necrosis is used to cover both processes.

Confluent necrosis (Fig. 8.3, p. 106) refers to substantial areas of liver-cell death. The commonest cause of this type of necrosis in biopsy material is hepatitis, either viral (p. 62) or drug-related (p. 105), in which case the necrosis is accompanied by an inflammatory reaction. Confluent necrosis with little or no inflammation is seen in hypoperfusion of the

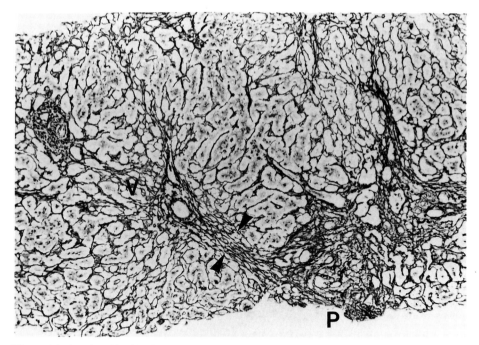

Figure 4.1. *Acute hepatitis with bridging necrosis.* Collapsed reticulin here gives a false impression of chronic liver disease. A bridge or passive septum (arrowheads) links an expanded portal tract (P) with a terminal hepatic venule (V). Needle biopsy, reticulin.

hepatic parenchyma, as in shock or left ventricular failure (Chapter 12). Some liver poisons including paracetamol (acetaminophen) produce a similar lesion (p. 105). In all the above examples the necrosis is typically perivenular but, if severe and extensive, forms bridges linking vascular structures (see below). Haphazardly distributed areas of necrosis are found in disseminated herpes virus infections (e.g. herpes simplex, varicella) in patients with altered immune reactivity and in mycobacterial infections. Tumour necrosis may be so extensive that no recognizable tumour tissue is present in the section; in such cases the reticulin pattern may help to establish a diagnosis.

   Bridging necrosis describes the location rather than the type of necrosis. It usually results from extensive necrosis of confluent type. The term has been used for necrosis linking any of the vascular structures, but it is now more often restricted to the linking of terminal hepatic venules (centrilobular veins) to portal tracts (Fig. 4.1). A possible explanation of this type of bridging is that it represents necrosis of acinar zones 3, which touch both the veins and the larger portal tracts (Fig. 3.1, p. 17). Linking of portal tracts to each other is common in conditions in which portal tracts are widened, for example by chronic hepatitis or biliary tract disease; this is partly because the chance of obtaining a longitudinal section of a widened portal tract is greater than for one of normal width. Linking of perivenular areas to each other may represent necrosis of the periphery of complex acini, and is found in some examples of parenchymal hypoperfusion and venous outflow obstruction.

   Bridging of terminal hepatic venules to portal tracts is a fairly common feature of acute hepatitis of viral type, when the bridges contain few or no elastic fibres (p. 70). It is also seen in exacerbations of chronic hepatitis. Old bridges contain elastic fibres as well as collagen fibres. Such bridging fibrosis is an important component both of the more severe examples of chronic viral hepatitis and of alcoholic hepatitis. Contraction of collagen-rich bridges may produce rapid and severe distortion of the normal hepatic microstructure, with correspondingly rapid progression to cirrhosis.

Panacinar and **multiacinar** necrosis are terms used to describe confluent necrosis involving entire single acini or several adjacent acini, respectively. They are further discussed in the chapter on acute viral hepatitis (p. 62).

Piecemeal necrosis, or **interface hepatitis** (Fig. 9.4, p. 121), is a process of erosion of the hepatic parenchyma at its junction with portal tracts or fibrous septa. It is common in chronic viral hepatitis but is also found in other conditions (Table 9.1, p. 118). It is characterized by an inflammatory infiltrate composed mainly of lymphocytes, with or without recognizable plasma cells, and is accompanied by fibrosis of the affected areas with new formation of collagens and other extracellular matrix components.[2] The process is sometimes referred to as classical or lymphocytic piecemeal necrosis in order to distinguish it from biliary, ductular and fibrotic piecemeal necrosis, processes found in chronic biliary tract disease[3] and described in the section on primary biliary cirrhosis in the next chapter.

CHOLESTASIS

In morphological terms, cholestasis is the presence of visible bile in tissue sections. It is therefore also known as bilirubinostasis. Bile is rarely seen in normal liver and then only in minute amounts, and cholestasis should therefore be regarded as pathological. The location of the bile varies. The commonest is in dilated bile canaliculi between hepatocytes. This canalicular form of cholestasis may be accompanied by bile accumulation in the cytoplasm of hepatocytes and in Kupffer cells. Canalicular cholestasis is typically perivenular and is sometimes called acute cholestasis. In contrast, in patients with chronic biliary tract disease, bile may accumulate in periportal hepatocytes. This is sometimes known as cholate stasis, because abnormal bile salts are thought to contribute to its pathogenesis.[4] Bile within canals of Hering, bile ductules and bile ducts is, paradoxically, not usually seen in large bile-duct obstruction (p. 38) even though the biliary tree may be dilated. The commonest cause of ductular cholestasis is sepsis (p. 241). Dense bile is also visible in ducts in different forms of ductal plate malformation (p. 200).

Canalicular cholestasis takes the form of bile plugs (bile thrombi) in dilated canaliculi (Fig. 5.1, p. 39). There is often brown or yellow pigment in nearby hepatocytes and Kupffer cells, but the distinction of this pigment from others such as lipofuscin and ceroid is not a serious practical problem; this is because the presence of bile in the canaliculi makes the diagnosis of cholestasis obvious. In general cholestasis should only be diagnosed with great caution in the absence of bile plugs in canaliculi but hepatocellular bilirubinostasis without canalicular bile is quite common after liver transplantation. The perivenular location of canalicular cholestasis is partly an artefact of paraffin embedding but also reflects real functional differences between the various parts of the acinus.

The colour of bile under the microscope varies according to pigment concentration and the degree of oxidation. It may be dark brown, green or yellow, and is occasionally so pale as to make detection difficult at first glance. The van Gieson stain, which stains bilirubin green, may then be helpful (Fig. 4.2). Pale counterstaining, as commonly used in Perls' method for iron, also makes bile easier to see. Specific histochemical methods for bilirubin are rarely necessary in ordinary diagnostic work.

When acute cholestasis is prolonged, the relationship of hepatocytes to each other may undergo focal change. Instead of the normal arrangement of two or three hepatocytes around a small bile canaliculus, the number of cells is increased and the lumen of the canaliculus considerably enlarged. The new structures are called cholestatic rosettes (Fig. 4.3). The lumens of the rosettes are part of the biliary tree but the bile may be lost during processing. Other hepatocellular changes in cholestasis are described in the next chapter,

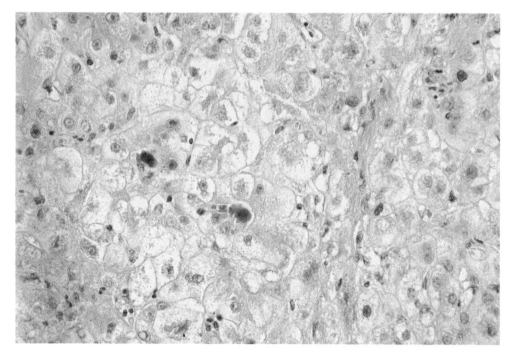

Figure 4.2. *Cholestasis*. Bile thrombi in dilated canaliculi are stained bright green. The red material is collagen. Needle biopsy, haematoxylin & van Gieson.

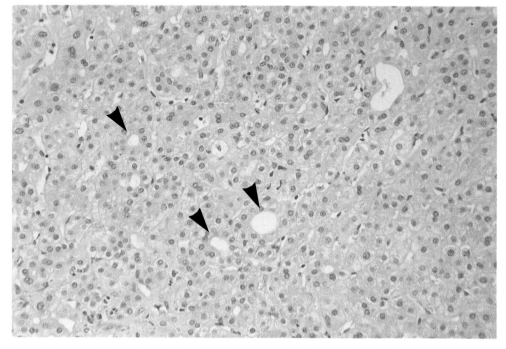

Figure 4.3. *Cholestasis*. Several liver-cell rosettes, glandular formations around prominent lumens, are marked by arrowheads. Wedge biopsy, H & E.

Table 4.1. Common Causes of Canalicular Cholestasis

Obstruction to major bile ducts (p. 38)
Acute hepatitis (p. 62)
Cholestatic drug jaundice (p. 110)
Sepsis
Cholestatic syndromes (Table 4.2)

Table 4.2. Main Causes of Bland Intrahepatic Cholestasis

Drugs (e.g. contraceptive steroids) (p. 110)
Benign recurrent cholestasis (p. 212)
Cholestasis of pregnancy (p. 257)
Lymphomas (p. 170)

in the section on large bile-duct obstruction. Very occasionally prolonged canalicular cholestasis is associated with the accumulation of copper and copper-associated protein, but this is much more characteristic of the chronic periportal form of cholestasis, discussed below.

Canalicular cholestasis in perivenular areas is mainly seen in the conditions listed in Tables 4.1 and 4.2. Cholestasis of less regular distribution is common in chronic liver diseases with severe hepatocellular dysfunction or with associated sepsis.

Chronic cholestasis (Fig. 5.10, p. 45) is seen in chronic liver diseases, especially those involving the biliary tree, and is the result of interference with bile flow at the level of the portal tracts. Bile (i.e. bilirubinostasis) may or may not be obvious, and the lesion is more easily recognized by hepatocellular swelling and pallor, and by the accumulation of copper and copper-associated protein in the affected cells. Mallory bodies may also be present. In some instances these are associated with an infiltrate of neutrophils, in which case the distinction from steatohepatitis (p. 86) must be made on the overall appearances and clinical context. The connective tissue adjacent to an area of chronic cholestasis is often oedematous. It may contain proliferated ductule-like structures which are probably derived from hepatocytes but have the cytokeratin profile of bile ducts;[5,6] they express cytokeratins 7 and 19 which are not normally demonstrable in hepatocytes. They also express neuroendocrine markers including chromogranin.[7] Because the proliferation of ductules is often associated with disruption of the limiting plates of hepatocytes around the portal tracts, it has given rise to the concept of ductular piecemeal necrosis.[3] Chronic cholestasis, unlike acute canalicular cholestasis, is not necessarily associated with clinical jaundice or a high level of serum bilirubin, but the serum alkaline phosphatase level is characteristically raised.

Differentiation of Causes of Acute Cholestatic Jaundice

Modern imaging methods have greatly reduced the need for liver biopsy in acutely jaundiced patients. Nevertheless, biopsy is still helpful in some instances, when the cause of a presumed intrahepatic jaundice is in doubt, when there is a need to distinguish between acute and chronic liver disease and when other investigations give equivocal results. Liver transplantation has given rise to a striking increase in liver biopsies for evaluation of the cause of jaundice. The pathologist may also need to assess operative biopsy specimens from jaundiced patients. Accurate histological diagnosis is important

Table 4.3. Decisions in the Acutely Jaundiced Patient

1. Are the patient's major bile ducts obstructed?
2. Has the patient got an acute viral or drug-related hepatitis?
3. Is there evidence for a diagnosis of sepsis?
4. Does the patient have one of the intrahepatic conditions listed in Table 4.2?
5. Does the patient have steatohepatitis?
6. Does the patient have chronic disease with an acute exacerbation rather than acute disease?

because correct treatment may depend upon it, and a wrong answer can lead to dangerous mismanagement. It has to be admitted, however, that the pathologist cannot always give a clear answer to the questions posed by the clinician.

In essence, the pathologist faced with a liver biopsy from an acutely jaundiced patient is asked to decide between the options in Table 4.3. The last two items are discussed in detail in the relevant chapters, and it is only necessary here to note that it is sometimes difficult at first to distinguish between chronic hepatitis and severe acute hepatitis with bridging necrosis. This clinically important distinction is made more easily with the help of a stain for elastic fibres (p. 13). The main problem lies in the differentiation of the first four possibilities, bile-duct obstruction, acute hepatitis and various other forms of intrahepatic cholestasis, including that due to sepsis. These can usually be distinguished by careful and methodical examination of abnormalities in the acini and in the portal tracts.

Acinar Changes

Obstruction to large bile ducts within or outside the liver leads to morphological cholestasis in perivenular areas. Bile canaliculi are dilated and contain bile thrombi (canalicular cholestasis). There is a variable degree of liver-cell swelling, inflammatory cell infiltration and Kupffer-cell hypertrophy in the cholestatic areas, but elsewhere the parenchyma appears substantially normal. The inflammatory infiltration is usually modest or even absent, and liver-cell plates remain for the most part intact. A few apoptotic bodies and liver-cell mitoses may be seen, reflecting increased liver-cell turnover. Bile infarcts (p. 38) sometimes develop. It should be noted that in the elderly, in whom duct obstruction is a very important cause of acute jaundice, there is sometimes more liver-cell damage than in the young.

By contrast, in acute hepatitis there is usually disruption of cell plates and widespread swelling, shrinking and loss of hepatocytes, usually most striking in perivenular areas but often widely distributed. In some forms of viral hepatitis, especially hepatitis A,[8] there is substantial necrosis and lymphocytic infiltration of the periportal parenchyma. Cholestasis may be seen in acute hepatitis, again commonly in hepatitis A, but canalicular dilatation is slight and hepatocellular changes are not confined to areas of cholestasis. In patients on immunosuppressive therapy, for example, after liver transplantation, the inflammatory infiltrate of an acute viral hepatitis may be relatively inconspicuous.[9,10]

In other forms of intrahepatic cholestasis such as drug-induced cholestasis, benign recurrent cholestasis and cholestasis of pregnancy, the changes within the acini are much the same as in bile-duct obstruction except that bile infarcts are unusual and, if present, small. Canaliculi are less dilated than in bile-duct obstruction, except in liver-cell rosettes which often form in intrahepatic cholestases, and which are described and illustrated above. There may be striking liver-cell swelling and multinucleation. Inflammatory infiltration is variable; in most forms of intrahepatic cholestasis, inflammation and liver-cell damage are absent or slight,[11] but in a minority of cases of idiosyncratic drug cholestasis they are sufficient to justify a label of cholestatic hepatitis.

Portal Changes

Examination of portal tracts provides further discrimination, particularly between bile-duct obstruction and the other conditions. In bile-duct obstruction the portal tracts are typically expanded and oedematous, with a pale watery appearance to the connective tissue. There is an increased number of bile-duct profiles at the margins of the tracts, most of these ducts lying roughly parallel to the portal-parenchymal interface. An associated inflammatory infiltrate includes neutrophils. Not all portal tracts are equally affected. Bile extravasates (p. 44) may be seen. The margins of the portal tracts are usually irregular, leading to possible confusion with piecemeal necrosis. The latter is accompanied by a lymphocytic infiltrate rather than neutrophils, and the cholestasis, portal oedema and duct proliferation of duct obstruction are absent.

The apparent proliferation of marginal bile ducts described above is thought to represent elongation and tortuosity of pre-existing interlobular ducts and ductules rather than formation of new structures (Fig. 5.7, p. 42). The process, loosely called bile-duct proliferation, is different from the ductular proliferation of chronic liver disease, especially biliary tract disease (Fig. 5.21, p. 55). In the latter new duct-like structures (neocholangioles) appear to form from hepatocytes, and acquire the cytokeratin profile of ducts.[5,12] The newly formed structures mostly lie at right angles to the portal-parenchymal interface, rather than parallel as in bile-duct obstruction. Irregularly orientated tangles of new ductular structures are also found in chronic biliary disease in areas of bile-duct loss. Finally it must be said, however, that the duct "proliferation" of large bile-duct obstruction is not always easy to distinguish from ductular proliferation and other criteria must also be taken into account when making a diagnosis.

Paradoxically, the portal bile ducts are not always strikingly dilated when major ducts are obstructed, although the main duct system is seen to be dilated on cholangiography. When small ducts or canals of Hering are dilated, filled with bile and infiltrated or surrounded by neutrophils, sepsis rather than bile-duct obstruction should be suspected as the cause of the patient's jaundice (Fig. 15.11, p. 241).

In acute hepatitis the portal infiltrate is mainly composed of lymphocytes, although a few other cells are commonly seen. Bile-duct proliferation is not conspicuous but ducts may be damaged.[13,14] In the rare examples of acute hepatitis in which the portal reaction mimics that of duct obstruction, the parenchymal changes of hepatitis make the diagnosis clear.

In other forms of acute intrahepatic cholestasis the portal tract changes are less severe. There is usually some degree of portal inflammation in idiosyncratic drug jaundice. Eosinophils may be present and, if numerous, support the diagnosis; on the other hand they are neither necessary for the diagnosis nor specific for drug jaundice, being found in many examples of viral hepatitis. Interlobular bile ducts may show irregularity of the epithelium with or without inflammatory infiltration (Fig. 8.10, p. 111). In some of the intrahepatic cholestatic syndromes, portal tracts are normal or at most lightly infiltrated, but bile-duct loss has been postulated as the basis of the intrahepatic cholestasis which occasionally complicates Hodgkin's disease,[15] and should always be looked for.

The differential diagnosis of bland cholestasis, that is canalicular cholestasis not accompanied by portal inflammation, includes not only intrahepatic cholestatic syndromes such as benign recurrent cholestasis but also large bile-duct obstruction in which the typical portal changes have failed to develop or have regressed. Drug-induced cholestasis must be considered.

Summary

In the patient with normal immunological responses perivenular cholestasis with little or no portal inflammation suggests drug cholestasis or other forms of intrahepatic cholestasis, but large bile-duct obstruction should be considered. Widespread liver-cell damage and inflammation favour hepatitis, irrespective of the nature of the portal changes. Conversely, substantial portal inflammation with parenchymal cholestasis but a poorly developed hepatitic reaction may result from infection with the hepatitis A virus. If canals of Hering and bile ductules at the portal-tract margins contain bile, sepsis should be considered as the cause of the patient's jaundice. Finally, acute portal inflammation with oedema and duct proliferation, but without widespread liver-cell damage and acinar inflammation, make it likely that the patient's biliary tree is obstructed.

REFERENCES

1. Wyllie AH. Apoptosis: cell death in tissue regulation. *J Pathol* 1987; **153**: 313–316.
2. Takahara T, Nakayama Y, Itoh H et al. Extracellular matrix formation in piecemeal necrosis: immunoelectron microscopic study. *Liver* 1992; **12**: 368–380.
3. Portmann B, Popper H, Neuberger J, Williams R. Sequential and diagnostic features in primary biliary cirrhosis based on serial histologic study in 209 patients. *Gastroenterology* 1985; **88**: 1777–1790.
4. Popper H. Cholestasis: the future of a past and present riddle. *Hepatology* 1981; **1**: 187–191.
5. van Eyken P, Sciot R, Desmet VJ. A cytokeratin immunohistochemical study of cholestatic liver disease: evidence that hepatocytes can express "bile duct-type" cytokeratins. *Histopathology* 1989; **15**: 125–135.
6. van Eyken P, Desmet VJ. Cytokeratins and the liver. *Liver* 1993; **13**: 113–122.
7. Roskams T, van den Oord JJ, De Vos R, Desmet VJ. Neuroendocrine features of reactive bile ductules in cholestatic liver disease. *Am J Pathol* 1990; **137**: 1019–1025.
8. Teixeira MR Jr, Weller IVD, Murray AM et al. The pathology of hepatitis A in man. *Liver* 1982; **2**: 53–60.
9. Demetris AJ, Todo S, Van Thiel DH et al. Evolution of hepatitis B virus liver disease after hepatic replacement. Practical and theoretical considerations. *Am J Pathol* 1990; **137**: 667–676.
10. Davies SE, Portmann BC, O'Grady JG et al. Hepatic histological findings after transplantation for chronic hepatitis B virus infection, including a unique pattern of fibrosing cholestatic hepatitis. *Hepatology* 1991; **13**: 150–157.
11. Brenard R, Geubel AP, Benhamou JP. Benign recurrent intrahepatic cholestasis. A report of 26 cases. *J Clin Gastroenterol* 1989; **11**: 546–551.
12. Thung SN. The development of proliferating ductular structures in liver disease. An immunohistochemical study. *Arch Pathol Lab Med* 1990; **114**: 407–411.
13. Schmid M, Pirovino M, Altorfer J, Gudat F, Bianchi L. Acute hepatitis non-A, non-B; are there any specific light microscopic features? *Liver* 1982; **2**: 61–67.
14. Bach N, Thung SN, Schaffner F. The histological features of chronic hepatitis C and autoimmune chronic hepatitis: a comparative analysis. *Hepatology* 1992; **15**: 572–577.
15. Hubscher SG, Lumley MA, Elias E. Vanishing bile duct syndrome: a possible mechanism for intrahepatic cholestasis in Hodgkin's lymphoma. *Hepatology* 1993; **17**: 70–77.

GENERAL READING

Ludwig J. Practical Liver Biopsy Interpretation: Diagnostic Algorithms. Chicago: ASCP Press, 1992.

5

BILIARY DISEASE

The biliary tree may be damaged or obstructed at any level from its smallest intrahepatic branches to the duodenum. Diseases of the larger ducts must be distinguished from diffuse intrahepatic diseases because of different clinical management, and liver biopsy is often helpful in this respect. However, diseases of large bile ducts outside and within the liver share pathological features and may be amenable to similar forms of treatment; for this reason the term "extrahepatic biliary obstruction" is not used in this chapter. Carcinoma of the main hepatic ducts, for example, may be situated wholly within the liver, yet lead to the changes of large-duct obstruction described below.

Intrahepatic cholestasis is not by itself an acceptable final diagnosis because it covers many acute and chronic cholestatic diseases, some of which can be distinguished by their pathological features. Of these intrahepatic diseases, primary biliary cirrhosis and primary sclerosing cholangitis are described in the present chapter. Others, such as viral hepatitis, drug-induced cholestasis and the cholestasis of sepsis, are discussed elsewhere.

LARGE BILE-DUCT OBSTRUCTION

From the first weeks of obstruction there is cholestasis in perivenular areas; that is to say, bile is visible under the microscope in the form of bile thrombi (bile plugs) in canaliculi and as yellow–brown pigment in hepatocytes and Kupffer cells (Fig. 5.1). The presence of canalicular bile thrombi distinguishes cholestasis from other pigmentations (Table 3.1, p. 22). Kupffer cells in cholestatic areas are enlarged and pigmented, containing both bile and diastase-resistant PAS-positive material. In recovering obstruction the Kupffer-cell changes persist while bile thrombi become smaller and less numerous. Finally, as in residual acute hepatitis, a few diastase-PAS-positive Kupffer cells may provide the only histological evidence of a recent episode of jaundice.

At first the hepatocytes in areas of cholestasis show little change, but with time they often become swollen. Their nuclei increase in size and number, and a few apoptotic bodies and mitoses may be seen, indicating increased cell turnover. Individual hepatocytes or small groups of cells undergo **feathery degeneration**, characterized by rarefied and reticular cytoplasm (Fig. 5.2). The lesion is focal and the affected cells are typically surrounded by more or less normal hepatocytes. Feathery degeneration may be difficult to distinguish from the ballooning degeneration of hepatitis (Fig. 6.1, p. 63) or following liver transplantation, but in ballooning the cytoplasm is often granular rather than feathery and the lesion is more widespread in the acinus.

In a minority of patients with obstructed ducts **bile infarcts** form (Fig. 5.3). These

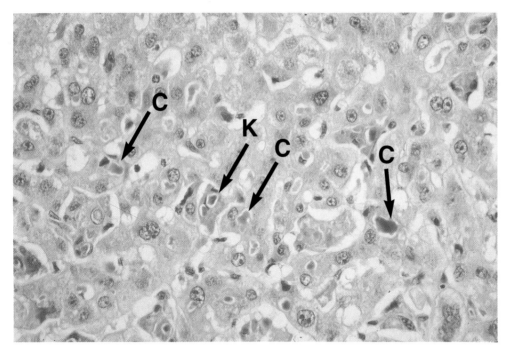

Figure 5.1. *Cholestasis.* Bile is seen in the form of bile thrombi (bile plugs) in dilated canaliculi (C), as well as in Kupffer cells (K). Needle biopsy, H & E.

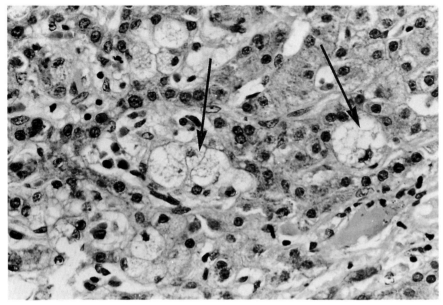

Figure 5.2. *Cholestasis.* Small groups of swollen hepatocytes (arrows) have undergone feathery degeneration. Adjacent hepatocytes appear normal. Wedge biopsy, H & E.

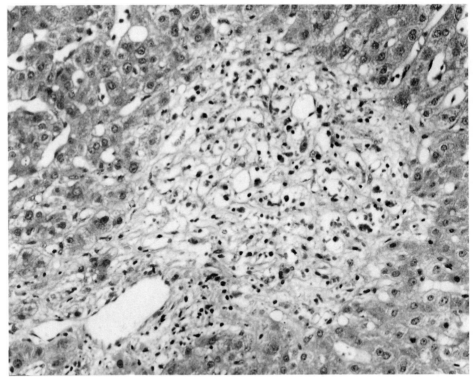

Figure 5.3. *Large bile-duct obstruction.* A bile infarct at the edge of a portal tract contains pyknotic nuclei. Wedge biopsy, H & E.

are substantial areas of hepatocellular degeneration or death containing pale or bile-stained hepatocytes or discrete rounded cells difficult to distinguish from macrophages. There are variable amounts of bile and fibrin, the latter often abundant (Fig. 5.4). Reticulin fibres become progressively more difficult to demonstrate. Bile eventually leaches out of the infarct to leave a barely pigmented and scarcely stained lesion containing the ghosts of hepatocytes. Small bile infarcts may be found in severe cholestasis from any cause; larger infarcts such as the one shown in Fig. 5.4, especially if adjacent to a portal tract, are highly suggestive of bile-duct obstruction. However, because such infarcts are only seen in a minority of patients with obstructed ducts, the diagnosis must usually be established by other criteria.

As a result of these various forms of hepatocellular damage in biliary obstruction and indeed in cholestasis generally, a certain amount of inflammatory infiltration of the parenchyma is commonly seen after a period of some weeks. This infiltration is usually mild and restricted to the cholestatic areas, unlike the inflammation of an acute hepatitis. When cholestasis resulting from duct obstruction is prolonged, especially in older patients, inflammation and liver-cell damage are occasionally severe enough to raise the alternative possibility of an acute hepatitis (Fig. 5.5). It is then helpful to note that in bile-duct obstruction the liver-cell plates remain for the most part intact, whereas in hepatitis they become irregular as a result of cell loss, swelling and regeneration. Zone 3 (central-portal) bridging necrosis is not a feature of biliary obstruction.

Within a few days or weeks of the onset of duct obstruction an acute inflammatory reaction develops in the portal tracts. The enlarged tracts become oedematous (Fig. 5.6) and show increased numbers of bile-duct profiles at their margins (Fig. 5.7). This marginal bile-duct proliferation, thought to represent increased tortuosity of pre-existing ducts, is the most consistent single finding in the portal tracts and is rarely absent.[1] The proliferated ducts may be dilated or of normal calibre, and there may be variation in the

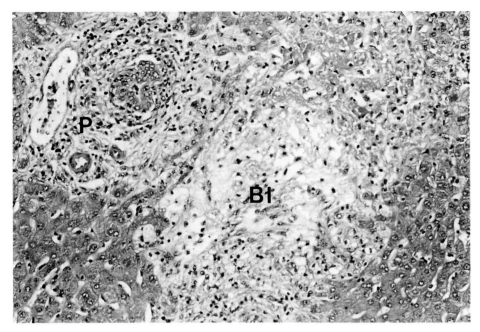

Figure 5.4. *Large bile-duct obstruction.* A bile infarct (BI) is seen near a portal tract (P). The infarct is rich in fibrin (top right). Wedge biopsy, H & E.

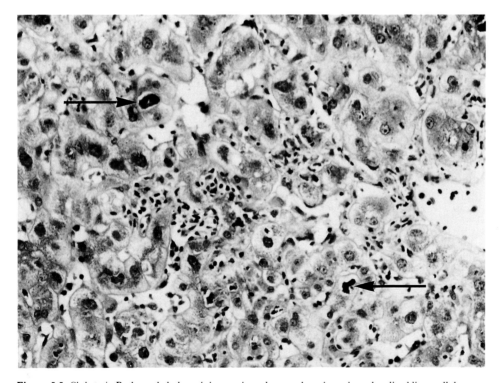

Figure 5.5. *Cholestasis.* Prolonged cholestasis in a perivenular area has given rise to localized liver-cell damage and inflammation. Canaliculi contain bile thrombi (arrows). Needle biopsy, H & E.

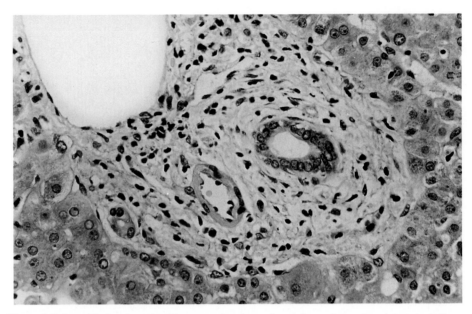

Figure 5.6. *Large bile-duct obstruction.* The connective tissue of a small portal tract is oedematous. Inflammatory infiltration is mild in this example. Wedge biopsy, H & E.

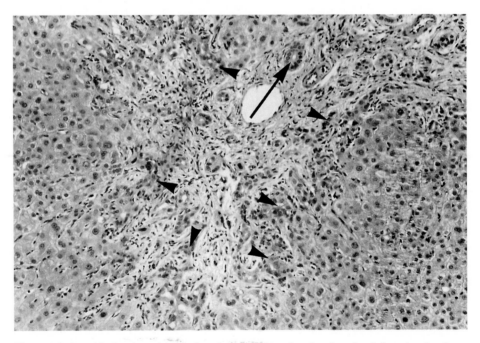

Figure 5.7. *Large bile-duct obstruction.* Bile ducts have proliferated at the edge of an inflamed and oedematous portal tract (arrowheads). The original interlobular duct is marked by an arrow. Needle biopsy, H & E.

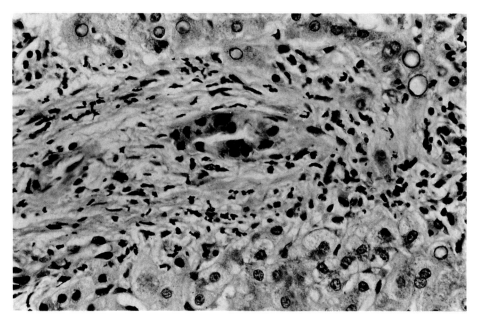

Figure 5.8. *Large bile-duct obstruction.* Inflammation is mild and bile ducts have not proliferated in this portal tract from a biopsy taken 2 weeks after onset of jaundice. The duct epithelium (centre) is irregular and nuclei are hyperchromatic. Needle biopsy, H & E.

location, size and staining of their nuclei (Fig. 5.8). Surprisingly, bile is not usually seen within dilated ducts or ductules in uncomplicated obstruction; when it is present, sepsis should be suspected (p. 241). The differentiation of the proliferated bile ducts of biliary obstruction from the ductular proliferation of chronic liver disease has already been discussed in the previous chapter, on p. 36. Fibrosis around damaged interlobular ducts is occasionally seen in patients with no evidence of primary sclerosing cholangitis.[2]

Within the oedematous, swollen portal tracts, especially around proliferated bile ducts, there is an inflammatory infiltrate. Neutrophils are prominent but there may be other cells including lymphocytes and eosinophils. The presence of a few eosinophils is therefore not in itself sufficient evidence for a diagnosis of drug jaundice. As a result of the proliferative and inflammatory changes of bile-duct obstruction, the outlines of the portal tracts become irregular and the limiting plates of hepatocytes are disrupted to a variable extent. This disruption should be distinguished from piecemeal necrosis (p. 32) in which the infiltrate is predominantly composed of lymphocytes and plasma cells and in which the acute inflammatory changes of bile-duct obstruction are not seen.

In a few patients with bile-duct obstruction the portal changes are inconspicuous (Fig. 5.8) or even absent. Biliary obstruction should therefore be considered in the differential diagnosis of canalicular cholestasis without portal reaction (so-called pure or bland cholestasis). Conversely, portal changes resembling those of duct obstruction are occasionally found in severe acute hepatitis, when the parenchymal alterations make the diagnosis clear. Sometimes similar portal changes are seen without cholestasis near space-occupying lesions such as metastases,[3] usually together with sinusoidal dilatation. Portal inflammation without cholestasis is also found in patients with disease affecting one or other part of the biliary tree but without current obstruction of the segment biopsied. It is seen in chronic pancreatitis[2] and in patients with acute cholecystitis or chole-docholithiasis.[4]

In a few instances of biliary obstruction, bile escapes from a duct into the connective tissue of a portal tract, giving rise to a **bile extravasate**. This leads to a phagocytic reaction, with or without foreign-body giant cells (Fig. 5.9). Bile extravasates, like large

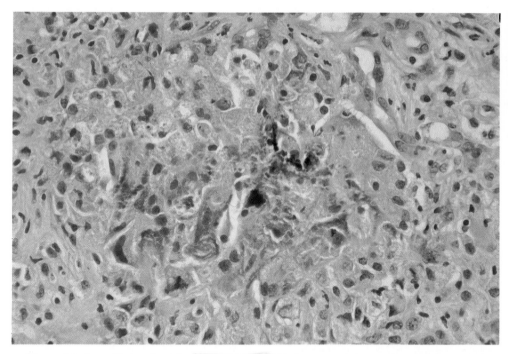

Figure 5.9. *Large bile-duct obstruction.* Bile extravasate. Bile has escaped from a duct and has evoked a phagocytic reaction. Needle biopsy, H & E.

bile infarcts, are almost diagnostic of obstruction but are only seen in a minority of patients. If the extravasate extends beyond the confines of a portal tract into the adjacent parenchyma, the appearances at the periphery of the lesion are very like those of a bile infarct.

Chronic Bile-duct Obstruction and Biliary Cirrhosis

When bile duct obstruction persists, the acute inflammatory reaction in the portal tracts is followed by increasing fibrosis. Eventually the tracts are linked by broad fibrous septa. There is a variable degree of acute and chronic inflammatory infiltration, the chronic element less striking than in primary biliary cirrhosis. In some patients the lesion appears to progress more by cholangitis than by obstruction, and cholestasis is therefore not always prominent or even present.

Interference with normal secretion of bile leads to several changes in hepatocytes adjacent to portal tracts and fibrous septa. The cells become swollen and separated by fibrous tissue, inflammatory cells and proliferated ductules (neocholangioles) derived from the hepatocytes themselves. Their cytoplasm is rarefied and may contain visible bile pigment, Mallory bodies, copper and copper-associated protein (Fig. 5.10). The latter is seen in the form of fine brown granules staining variably with diastase-PAS and strongly with orcein or Victoria blue. The combination of all these changes is known as **chronic cholestasis**, or cholate stasis on the basis that some of the alterations probably result from the accumulation of toxic bile salts. Canalicular cholestasis is sometimes seen between the affected hepatocytes. The hepatocellular changes, ductular proliferation and associated fibrosis respectively constitute the biliary, ductular and fibrotic forms of piecemeal necrosis described by Portmann et al.[5]

The fibrous septa which eventually form in chronic biliary tract disease surround and

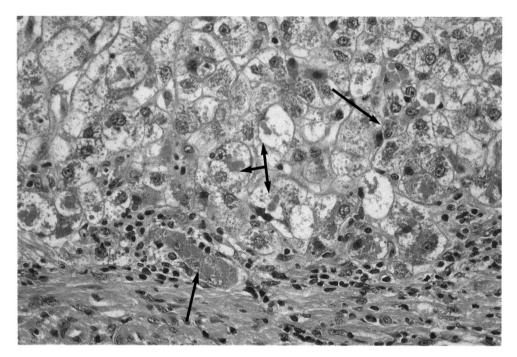

Figure 5.10. *Chronic cholestasis.* Hepatocytes near a portal tract (below) are swollen and pale-staining. Many contain Mallory bodies (lower arrow and triple arrow). Bile thrombi are also seen (top arrow). Wedge biopsy, H & E.

outline groups of classical hepatic lobules, leaving the normal vascular relationships essentially intact. Islands of parenchyma with characteristic protruding studs resemble the pieces of a jigsaw puzzle or land masses on a map (Fig. 5.11). Spherical nodules are sparse at first, in spite of evidence of liver-cell hyperplasia in the form of thickened liver-cell plates, seen particularly in patients with associated portal hypertension.[6] An occasional rounded parenchymal island may merely represent a tangential section of a complex parenchymal mass such as the one shown in Fig. 5.11, rather than a true regeneration nodule of cirrhosis. This is especially common just deep to the liver capsule. A histological diagnosis of cirrhosis should therefore be made with caution, because at a fibrotic, pre-cirrhotic stage considerable resolution can occasionally result if an obstruction is relieved.[7] Eventually, true **secondary biliary cirrhosis** develops, its biliary origin still evident from nodule shape and the regular, broad fibrous septa composed of loose collagen bundles with parallel arrangement (Fig. 5.12). A zone of oedema containing proliferated ductules is often diagnostically helpful and may be striking even at low magnification (Fig. 5.11). Thus many different structural characteristics make it possible to diagnose chronic biliary tract disease even in the absence of cholestasis. Finally, however, an end-stage cirrhosis forms, no longer recognizable as biliary in origin.

CHOLANGITIS: INFECTION OF THE BILIARY TREE

In biliary obstruction the inflammatory infiltrate around bile ducts in small portal tracts typically includes neutrophils. There is therefore cholangitis in a strictly histological sense, but this does not imply that there must be bacterial infection of the biliary tree or clinical ascending cholangitis. In the latter, neutrophils are more numerous and are found not only around ducts but also in their walls and lumens (Fig. 5.13). Paradoxically,

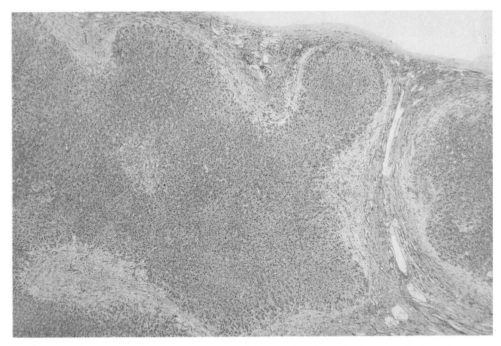

Figure 5.11. *Secondary biliary cirrhosis*. Irregular nodules resemble pieces of a jigsaw puzzle. Note the narrow zone of oedema and ductular proliferation at the nodule margin. Wedge biopsy, H & E.

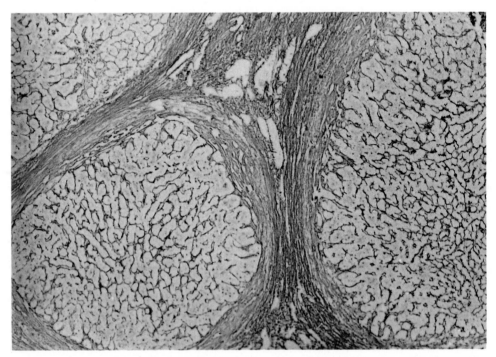

Figure 5.12. *Secondary biliary cirrhosis*. Nodules are surrounded by loose bundles of parallel collagen fibres showing little compression. Wedge biopsy, reticulin.

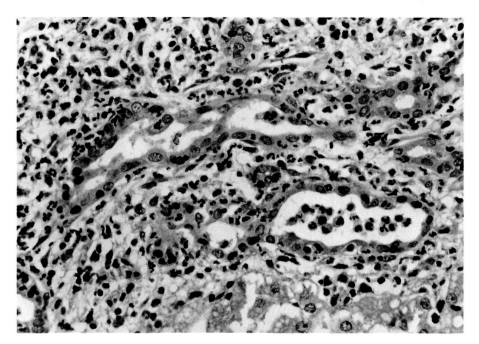

Figure 5.13. *Acute cholangitis.* Many neutrophil leucocytes are seen in the walls and dilated lumens of the bile ducts, and in the surrounding connective tissue. Wedge biopsy, H & E.

interlobular bile ducts are most affected, and larger ducts may appear histologically normal. The wall of a small duct may rupture, leading to abscess formation in the portal tract. Neutrophils are seen in the sinusoids and abscesses may form in the acini. Associated lesions include fibrin thrombi in portal vein branches, pylephlebitis and various degrees of parenchymal necrosis,[8] the latter probably related to hypoperfusion of the parenchyma. Cholestasis is more often absent than present. Causes of ascending cholangitis include cholecystitis and choledocholithiasis, strictures including those due to primary sclerosing cholangitis, pancreatitis, neoplasia of the biliary tree and Caroli's disease (p. 202). In patients with AIDS, cholangitis is frequently associated with infection by *Cryptosporidium*, CMV or by species of microsporidia.[9,10] If cholangitis persists or recurs over a period of years, secondary biliary cirrhosis may develop. The histological features are then as described above in the section on bile-duct obstruction.

Septicaemia and other forms of sepsis (p. 241) are associated with a particular form of histological cholangitis principally affecting the canals of Hering.[11] Affected ductules are dilated and filled with inspissated bile. Neutrophils accumulate around and sometimes within them (Fig. 15.11, p. 241). Larger ducts may be affected, as may the periportal parenchyma in which bile is seen in dilated bile canaliculi. These changes are easily confused with those of large bile-duct obstruction, but in obstruction the inspissated bile in the canals of Hering is not a feature unless there is concomitant sepsis. Sepsis can also give rise to widespread canalicular cholestasis, with or without the ductular lesions. In the toxic shock syndrome the appearances of the small bile ducts can closely mimic ascending bacterial cholangitis.[12]

PRIMARY SCLEROSING CHOLANGITIS

This condition is characterized by inflammation, strictures and saccular dilatations in the biliary tree. Typically found in adults with ulcerative colitis, it is also seen in neonates

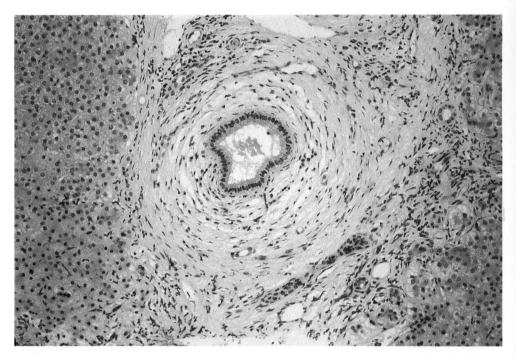

Figure 5.14. *Primary sclerosing cholangitis.* A bile duct is surrounded by a cuff of oedematous, inflamed fibrous tissue with an onion-skin appearance. Needle biopsy, H & E.

and children[13] and in the absence of inflammatory bowel disease. In a few cases the latter is Crohn's disease rather than ulcerative colitis.[14] Any part of the biliary tree may be affected, and involvement of the gallbladder[15] and pancreas[16] has been reported. Patients do not necessarily have symptoms referable to the liver or abnormal liver function tests.[17] Lesions similar to those of primary sclerosing cholangitis have been found in patients given arterial infusion of the anti-cancer drug fluorodeoxyuridine (FUDR) and other chemotherapeutic agents.[18,19] Obliteration or narrowing of hepatic arteries and portal vein branches suggests that in drug-related cases at least, the bile-duct damage may have an ischaemic origin.[20]

Final diagnosis of primary sclerosing cholangitis normally rests on cholangiographic demonstration of the characteristic beading of bile ducts, but similar histological features, as described below, may be found in patients with normal cholangiograms. This can be explained on the basis of involvement of the smallest ducts, too small to be seen radiographically.[21] This small-duct primary sclerosing cholangitis corresponds approximately to the now obsolete label of "pericholangitis", when applied to patients without cholangiographic abnormalities. Large- and small-duct forms of the disease frequently co-exist.

The features seen on liver biopsy depend in part on the location of strictures in relation to the biopsy site. If the biopsy is taken from a part of the liver unaffected by the primary disease proximal to a stricture, then the changes, if any, will simply be those of bile-duct obstruction or cholangitis. If on the other hand the biopsy site is affected by the primary disease, there may be one or more features suggesting the diagnosis. These include periduct oedema and concentric fibrosis (Fig. 5.14), ductular proliferation, portal inflammation and atrophy or disappearance of the small ducts (Fig. 5.15). Loss of ducts is the commonest finding in the smallest portal tracts, while periduct fibrosis is typical of medium-sized tracts.[22] Major bile ducts, as seen, for example, in explanted livers at transplantation, may be inflamed, ulcerated or dilated.

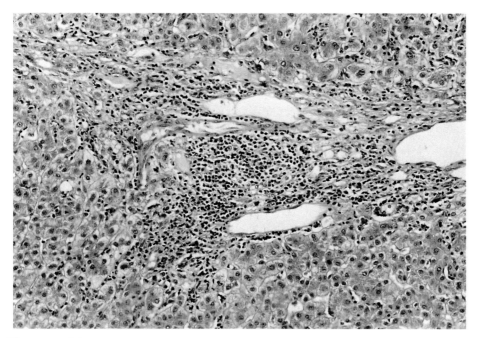

Figure 5.15. *Primary sclerosing cholangitis.* The inflamed portal tract lacks a bile duct. Inflammation extends into the adjacent parenchyma and there is piecemeal necrosis. Wedge biopsy, H & E.

Loss of interlobular bile ducts from the smallest portal tracts can be assessed only in biopsy samples of adequate size, that is to say containing several portal tracts. While interlobular ducts are not necessarily seen in all tracts because of the plane of section, arteries provide a useful guide; 70–80% of arteries are normally accompanied by a duct lying near the centre of a portal tract.[23] If there is doubt, for instance because ducts are difficult to identify in an inflammatory infiltrate, immunostaining of duct-associated cytokeratins is helpful.[24] Suitable antibodies include AE-1 (Signet) and other antibodies against cytokeratins 7 and 19. In the presence of ductular proliferation, identification and counting of interlobular bile ducts is sometimes difficult.

The concentric fibrosis around medium-sized ducts is not entirely diagnostic, since it is occasionally found in other forms of biliary disease such as hepatolithiasis.[25] It is, however, a very helpful finding. The lamellar pattern of the fibrosis gives an "onion-skin" appearance. The cuff of connective tissue around the duct may be oedematous and pale-staining or sclerotic, depending on the stage of the process. Inflammatory cells are seen in small numbers lying between the layers of collagen. The duct epithelium may show various degrees of atrophy, and sometimes disappears entirely, leaving a characteristic rounded scar[26,27] (Fig. 5.16). Staining with diastase-PAS often reveals irregular or regular thickening of the basement membrane material around both scarred and unscarred ducts.[28] In long-standing or severe cases, portal fibrosis gradually increases, fibrous septa form and secondary biliary cirrhosis may develop. In some patients, on the other hand, the lesions remain mild and clinically insignificant for many years.[14,17]

Parenchymal changes in primary sclerosing cholangitis are usually less striking than the portal ones. Cholestasis may be seen as a result of large-duct obstruction or small-duct loss. In the later stages, the cholestasis is typically of the chronic type, with accumulation of copper and copper-associated protein. Piecemeal necrosis of the classical, lymphoplasmacytic type is common but not as a rule severe (Fig. 5.15). However, more severe piecemeal necrosis may be seen in patients with an unfavourable clinical course.[14] Liver cells may undergo hyperplasia, indicated by thickening of cell plates.

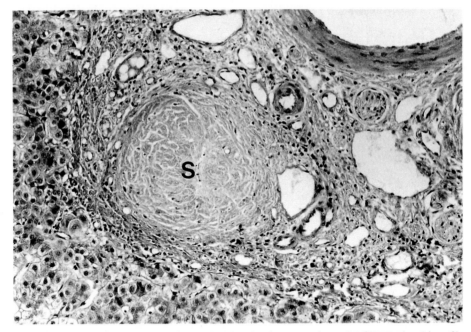

Figure 5.16. *Primary sclerosing cholangitis.* The bile duct in a large portal tract has been replaced by a fibrous scar (*S*). Wedge biopsy, H & E.

Histological assessment of liver biopsies in patients with an established diagnosis of primary sclerosing cholangitis is important for prognosis. Ludwig[21,29,30] has proposed a histological staging system based on essential and non-essential features. The stages correspond approximately to those of primary biliary cirrhosis (p. 51): they are, respectively, designated portal, periportal, septal and cirrhotic.

There is an increased risk of carcinoma of the biliary tree in patients with sclerosing cholangitis.[31-33] Severe dysplasia has been reported throughout the mucosa of the gallbladder, cystic duct and common bile duct, in association with carcinoma of the common hepatic duct.[34]

The main **differential diagnosis** is from chronic hepatitis, primary biliary cirrhosis and other forms of chronic biliary tract disease. In **chronic hepatitis** bile duct numbers are normal, periduct fibrosis is not seen and cholestasis is very uncommon. Stains for copper and copper-associated protein are negative or near-negative unless cirrhosis has developed.[35] **Primary biliary cirrhosis** closely resembles primary sclerosing cholangitis in its later stages, and firm diagnosis usually requires cholangiography and/or testing for antimitochondrial antibodies. However, the typical granulomatous cholangitis of primary biliary cirrhosis is not a feature of sclerosing cholangitis, although granulomas are very occasionally found in the liver. Substantial chronic inflammation of portal tracts with or without lymphoid follicles favours primary biliary cirrhosis. Conversely, fibrous obliteration of ducts is much more characteristic of sclerosing cholangitis, and there is often dense portal fibrosis with relatively little inflammation. The main difference from **other chronic biliary diseases** is the loss of ducts and piecemeal necrosis. There is occasionally confusion between the focal duct dilatations of **Caroli's disease** and the cholangiectases which are typically seen in the large and medium-sized bile ducts in primary sclerosing cholangitis.[36]

PRIMARY BILIARY CIRRHOSIS

Primary biliary cirrhosis, generally regarded as an autoimmune disease, is characterized by a chronic non-suppurative destructive cholangitis which can eventually lead to cirrhosis.[37] For much of its course the term cirrhosis is not strictly applicable but the name survives despite this inconsistency. It typically presents in middle life, but may also be found in the elderly or in younger adults. Women are about ten times as commonly affected as men. In symptomatic patients the onset is insidious, with itching as the commonest presenting symptom. Jaundice and histological cholestasis are usually absent in the early years of the disease. Characteristic findings on investigation of both symptomatic and asymptomatic patients include a raised serum alkaline phosphatase and the presence of antimitochondrial antibodies. Several of these antibodies have been found. An antibody against the M2 antigen, part of the pyruvate dehydrogenase complex of mitochondria,[38] is the most specific and can be detected in more than 90% of patients. The antigen has been demonstrated on the surface of cultured human biliary epithelial cells, suggesting a link between the antimitochondrial antibodies and bile-duct damage.[39]

Primary biliary cirrhosis is associated with a wide range of other conditions, many of them regarded as autoimmune in origin. The commonest association is with the sicca complex of dry eyes and mouth.[40] Others include scleroderma, thyroiditis, rheumatoid arthritis, membranous glomerulonephritis and coeliac disease.

Liver biopsy plays an important part in diagnosis throughout the often long course of the disease. Four histological stages have been described[29,37,41] (Table 5.1). These are not always easy to determine in needle biopsies, partly because the lesions of primary biliary cirrhosis are unevenly distributed within the liver and partly because the stages overlap. For example, stage 1 bile duct lesions and granulomas are sometimes seen in an

Table 5.1. Stages of Primary Biliary Cirrhosis

1. The florid duct lesion; portal hepatitis
2. Ductular proliferation and periportal hepatitis
3. Scarring; bridging necrosis, septal fibrosis
4. Cirrhosis

established cirrhosis. From a practical point of view, however, the pathologist is usually able to decide whether the disease appears to be still in stage 1, with lesions more or less restricted to enlarged portal tracts, or whether it has extended to a significant degree into the adjacent parenchyma, with consequent alteration of acinar structure (the progressive lesion; stages 2, 3 or 4). This is of some clinical importance, because stage 1 often lasts for many years and the prognosis is therefore relatively favourable, especially in patients without symptoms referable to the liver. Having established in other patients that the disease has progressed beyond stage 1, the pathologist may also be able to determine with reasonable confidence that cirrhosis has developed. The patient is then at increased risk for hepatocellular carcinoma,[42] sometimes preceded by macroregenerative nodule formation.[43] Because different sets of differential diagnoses should be considered for the portal and the progressive lesion, these are considered separately in the following section.

The Portal Lesion of Primary Biliary Cirrhosis

The bile-duct damage characteristic of early primary biliary cirrhosis mainly affects the septal and larger interlobular ducts, while the smaller interlobular ducts remain intact

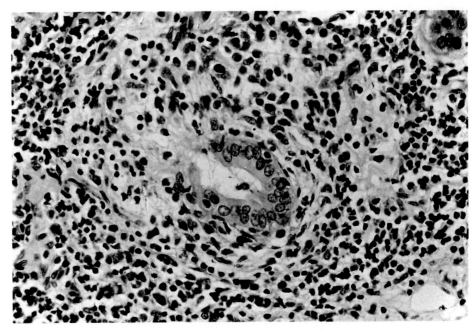

Figure 5.17. *Primary biliary cirrhosis.* A damaged large interlobular bile duct has ruptured, and is surrounded by lymphocytes and plasma cells. Wedge biopsy, H & E.

until later. The epithelium of the affected ducts becomes irregular and is infiltrated with lymphocytes. The basement membrane becomes disrupted and the duct may rupture (Fig. 5.17). An inflammatory infiltrate is seen around or to one side of the duct. The denser parts of this infiltrate are mainly composed of lymphocytes, which may form aggregates or follicles with germinal centres (Fig. 5.18). Elsewhere there is a mixture of plasma cells, often abundant, eosinophils and neutrophils. In a minority of patients some portal tracts are infiltrated by large numbers of eosinophils, containing immunochemically-demonstrable eosinophilic cationic protein.[44] Granulomas are present in many patients, although they are not necessarily seen in small biopsies; their absence does not therefore exclude the diagnosis. They take a variety of forms,[45] ranging from well-defined granulomas like those of sarcoidosis or tuberculosis (Fig. 5.19) to small focal collections of histiocytoid cells (Fig. 5.18). Alternatively there may be a substantial component of histiocytes or epithelioid cells within the inflammatory infiltrate, without formation of identifiable localized granulomas (Fig. 5.20). A relationship between presence of granulomas and a good prognosis has been found in some series[46] but not in others.[47]

Not all liver biopsies from patients in this stage of the disease show the typical bile-duct lesions, so that a firm histological diagnosis cannot always be made. Small portal tracts may merely show "non-specific" portal inflammation, in which case step sections may make the true diagnosis clear by revealing bile-duct lesions or granulomas.

Although in the first stage of primary biliary cirrhosis the lesions are by definition mainly portal, slight disruption of the limiting plate is common. Sinusoids may be infiltrated by lymphocytes, Kupffer cells are prominent and there may be focal necrosis[48] and thickening of liver-cell plates. Nodular regenerative hyperplasia (p. 155), best recognized in reticulin preparations, is common even at this stage[49,50] and together with portal-vein narrowing[51] helps to explain the portal hypertension which frequently precedes the development of significant fibrosis or cirrhosis. Foci of small hepatocytes with basophilic cytoplasm and hyperchromatic nuclei (small-cell dysplasia) or hepatocytes with enlarged pleomorphic nuclei (large-cell dysplasia) are occasionally found.[52]

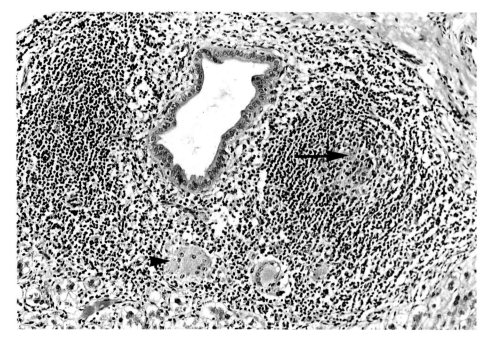

Figure 5.18. *Primary biliary cirrhosis.* Lymphoid follicles, one with a germinal centre (arrow), are seen near a duct of irregular outline. The arrowhead marks a group of large histiocyte-like cells. Wedge biopsy, H & E.

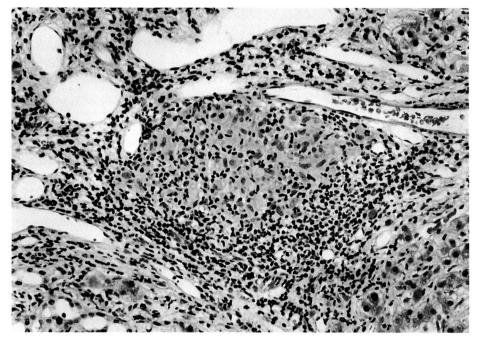

Figure 5.19. *Primary biliary cirrhosis.* A well-formed epithelioid-cell granuloma is infiltrated and surrounded by lymphocytes. Wedge biopsy, H & E.

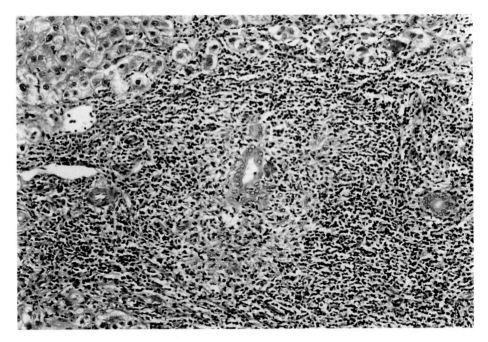

Figure 5.20. *Primary biliary cirrhosis.* An ill-defined collection of pale-staining histiocytes is seen around a damaged bile duct (centre). Beyond the histiocytes the infiltrate is mainly lymphocytic. Wedge biopsy, H & E.

Canalicular cholestasis is unusual in early primary biliary cirrhosis unless there is a complicating factor such as steroid-induced jaundice. Cholestasis of the chronic type (cholate stasis) does not develop until later, although small amounts of copper-associated protein are occasionally seen in periportal hepatocytes.

The **differential diagnosis of early primary biliary cirrhosis** includes other causes of portal inflammation and of bile-duct damage. The differentiation from **primary sclerosing cholangitis** is discussed on p. 50. In this disease, duct atrophy and fibrosis predominate and granulomas are unusual. **Drug injury** (p. 110) occasionally leads to bile-duct damage but the ducts affected are smaller than in early primary biliary cirrhosis, and the lesion is seen in the clinical context of an acutely jaundiced patient. Bile ducts are often abnormal in acute and chronic **viral hepatitis**, especially hepatitis C.[53] In hepatitis the epithelium of the affected ducts may be abnormal in only part of its circumference (Fig. 6.7, p. 67), and is typically stratified and vacuolated.[54] The surrounding infiltrate is almost entirely composed of lymphocytes, with few plasma cells or segmented leucocytes and no granulomas. Large numbers of eosinophils, sometimes seen in primary biliary cirrhosis, are rare.[44] In doubtful cases the clinical context and laboratory investigations usually make the diagnosis clear. Because in viral hepatitis the duct damage is focal and does not lead to extensive duct loss, the clinical and biochemical picture is not necessarily cholestatic. Other causes of bile duct damage include **bile-duct obstruction with suppuration**, **graft-versus-host disease and rejection of a grafted liver**. The latter two situations are discussed in Chapter 16. Two rare causes of bile-duct damage associated with granulomas are **fascioliasis** and **sarcoidosis**, but in general this association strongly supports a diagnosis of primary biliary cirrhosis.

The Progressive Lesion of Primary Biliary Cirrhosis

The disease now extends beyond the confines of the portal tracts and there is increasing fibrosis and alteration of acinar architecture. Bile-duct damage is less dramatic and

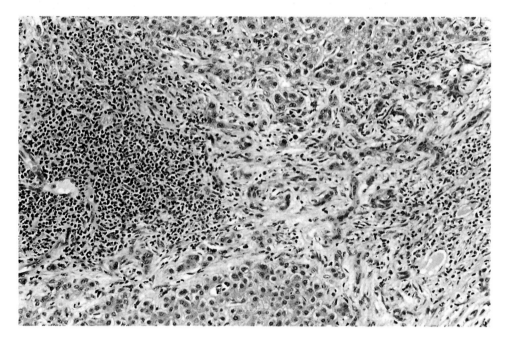

Figure 5.21. *Primary biliary cirrhosis.* A widened portal tract contains proliferated ductules and a lymphoid aggregate (left). The margins of the tract are blurred by piecemeal necrosis of fibrotic type. Wedge biopsy, H & E.

granulomas are fewer but there is a progressive fall in duct numbers. Duct numbers are best assessed in relation to arteries,[23] as already discussed in relation to primary sclerosing cholangitis (p. 49). The sites of former ducts are marked by aggregates of lymphocytes (Figs 5.21 and 5.22). These sometimes show compression artefact, with rupture of lymphocyte nuclei.

The portal tracts expand progressively as the inflammatory process begins to extend from them into the adjacent parenchyma. At this time two apparently separate processes affect the future course of the disease. The first comprises a combination of biliary and cholestatic features probably related to bile duct loss, while the second closely resembles the piecemeal necrosis of chronic hepatitis.[5,55] The earliest and often most obvious biliary feature is ductular proliferation (Fig. 5.21). As discussed previously, this partly represents transformation of hepatocytes into duct-like structures. For a time it allows bile to drain from the parenchyma into the main ducts in spite of destruction of the medium-sized ducts.[56] It is almost always associated with an infiltrate of neutrophils, so that it needs to be distinguished from the duct tortuosity and inflammation of mechanical bile-duct obstruction (p. 40). The ductular proliferation of primary biliary cirrhosis, and indeed of primary sclerosing cholangitis, is often focal, representing a system of bypass channels in relation to a local interruption of bile flow through the duct system.

Loss of bile ducts also leads to the chronic form of cholestasis (p. 34), marked by swelling of hepatocytes, bile staining, Mallory body formation and accumulation of copper (Fig. 5.23) and copper-associated protein (Fig. 5.24). Bile plugs are sometimes seen in canaliculi in the affected areas around portal tracts and septa, but more widespread canalicular cholestasis often reflects hepatocellular failure or associated sepsis. There may be many lipid-laden macrophages, forming diffuse or localized xanthomas.

In addition to the cholestatic features described above, piecemeal necrosis of the classical, lymphocytic type is common in the progressive stage of primary biliary cirrhosis.[5] It is accompanied by an infiltrate rich in activated T cells.[55] Lymphocytes also form bridge-like extensions into the acini and may be the forerunners of fibrous septa.[57]

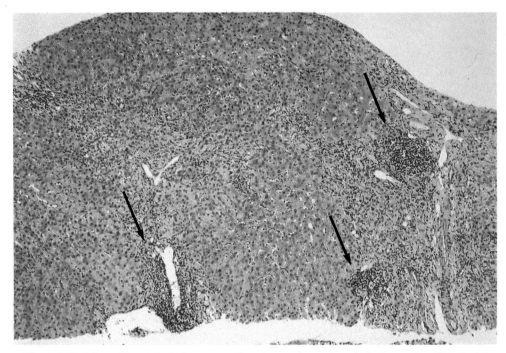

Figure 5.22. *Primary biliary cirrhosis.* Aggregates of lymphocytes (arrows) mark the former sites of bile ducts in this inflamed, fibrotic liver. The picture is very typical of the progressive phase of the disease. Needle biopsy, H & E.

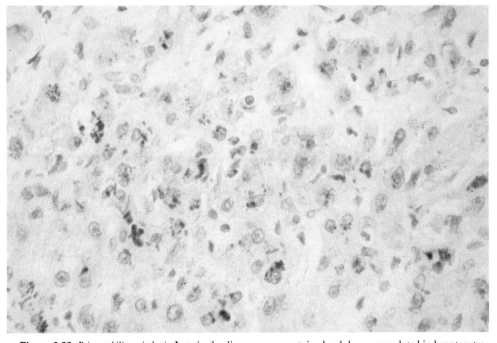

Figure 5.23. *Primary biliary cirrhosis.* Late in the disease, copper, stained red, has accumulated in hepatocytes. Bile thrombi are green. Needle biopsy, rhodanine.

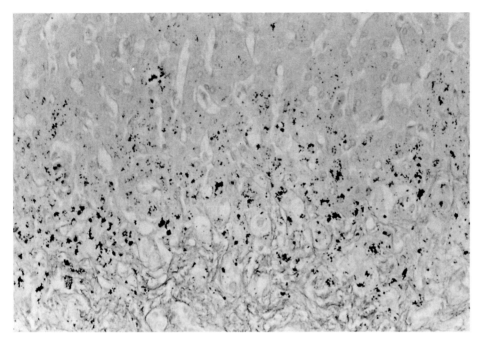

Figure 5.24. *Primary biliary cirrhosis.* Granular deposits of copper-associated protein have accumulated in hepatocytes near a fibrous septum (below) at a late stage of the disease. Needle biopsy, orcein.

Necrosis of perivenular hepatocytes has been noted.[48] There is therefore a histological resemblance to hepatitis. Hepatocellular dysplasia of small- or large-cell type may be present.[52]

The combination of cholestatic and hepatitic processes leads to increasing fibrosis. Portal inflammation diminishes, but lymphoid aggregates continue to mark the former sites of bile ducts (Fig. 5.25). Septa extend from the portal tracts and eventually come to link portal tracts to each other and to terminal hepatic venules.[57] In patients in whom the biliary and cholestatic features predominate, the cirrhosis which ultimately develops is generally of the biliary type. When hepatitic features predominate, the cirrhosis tends to be of a post-hepatitis type. All combinations of the two patterns may be seen. Nodules often develop unevenly throughout the liver, so that nodular areas with the appearance of cirrhosis co-exist with areas in which the acinar architecture remains preserved.

The **differential diagnosis of the progressive lesion** includes **primary sclerosing cholangitis** and **other forms of chronic biliary disease** on the one hand, and **chronic hepatitis** on the other.[58] The differentiation from primary sclerosing cholangitis is discussed on p. 50; in the later stages of the two diseases it is often impossible to make the distinction histologically. With respect to other forms of chronic biliary obstruction and chronic hepatitis, the most important observation is that bile duct numbers remain normal in both whereas they are characteristically reduced in primary biliary cirrhosis and in primary sclerosing cholangitis (Table 5.2). Granulomas favour primary biliary cirrhosis over chronic hepatitis, as does chronic cholestasis particularly when it is seen in the absence of cirrhosis.[35] Difficulties remain even after these factors are taken into account, especially if the biopsy specimen is small or fragmented. They can usually be resolved by consideration of the clinical context and laboratory investigations; a middle-aged woman with itching, high serum alkaline phosphatase and antimitochondrial antibodies is unlikely to be suffering from chronic viral hepatitis. There do, however, appear to be rare overlap syndromes, discussed briefly below.

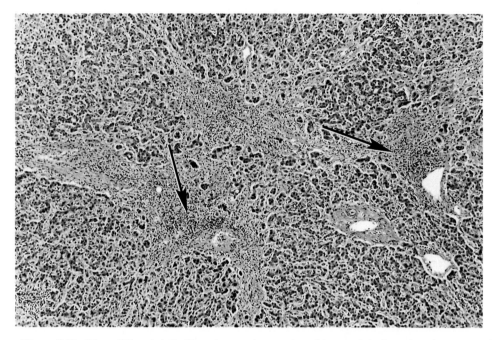

Figure 5.25. *Primary biliary cirrhosis.* There is extensive scarring without nodule formation. Aggregates of lymphocytes (arrows) mark the former sites of bile ducts, as in Fig. 5.22. Post-mortem liver, H & E.

Table 5.2. Causes of Bile-duct Damage and Loss

Loss of Ducts	Little or No Loss
Primary sclerosing cholangitis	Bile-duct obstruction
Primary biliary cirrhosis	Viral hepatitis
Idiopathic ductopenia (p. 197)	Drug jaundice
Graft-versus-host disease (p. 276)	Parasitic duct disease
Rejection of liver grafts (p. 267)	
Sarcoidosis	

Overlap Syndromes

A few patients have been reported in whom features of primary biliary cirrhosis co-exist with an unusually severe degree of piecemeal necrosis. In spite of the presence of antimitochondrial antibodies, these are sometimes regarded as examples of chronic hepatitis with cholestatic features and may respond to treatment with corticosteroids. Other patients have the histological features of primary biliary cirrhosis or primary sclerosing cholangitis but the serum antibody profile of autoimmune hepatitis.[59-63]

REFERENCES

1. Christoffersen P, Poulsen H. Histological changes in human liver biopsies following extrahepatic biliary obstruction. *Acta Pathol Microbiol Scand Suppl* 1970; **212**: 150–157.
2. Wilson C, Auld CD, Schlinkert R et al. Hepatobiliary complications in chronic pancreatitis. *Gut* 1989; **30**: 520–527.

3. Gerber MA, Thung SN, Bodenheimer HC Jr, Kapelman B, Schaffner F. Characteristic histologic triad in liver adjacent to metastatic neoplasm. *Liver* 1986; **6**: 85–88.

4. Flinn WR, Olson DF, Oyasu R, Beal JM. Biliary bacteria and hepatic histopathologic changes in gallstone disease. *Ann Surg* 1977; **185**: 593–597.

5. Portmann B, Popper H, Neuberger J, Williams R. Sequential and diagnostic features in primary biliary cirrhosis based on serial histologic study in 209 patients. *Gastroenterology* 1985; **88**: 1777–1790.

6. Weinbren K, Hadjis NS, Blumgart LH. Structural aspects of the liver in patients with biliary disease and portal hypertension. *J Clin Pathol* 1985; **38**: 1013–1020.

7. Yeong ML, Nicholson GI, Lee SP. Regression of biliary cirrhosis following choledochal cyst drainage. *Gastroenterology* 1982; **82**: 332–335.

8. Shimada H, Nihmoto S, Matsuba A, Nakagawara G. Acute cholangitis: a histopathologic study. *J Clin Gastroenterol* 1988; **10**: 197–200.

9. Bouche H, Housset C, Dumont J-L et al. AIDS-related cholangitis. Diagnostic features and course in 15 patients. *J Hepatol* 1993; **17**: 34–39.

10. Pol S, Romana CA, Richard S et al. Microsporidia infection in patients with the human immunodeficiency virus and unexplained cholangitis. *N Engl J Med* 1993; **328**: 95–99.

11. Lefkowitch JH. Bile ductular cholestasis: an ominous histopathologic sign related to sepsis and "cholangitis lenta". *Hum Pathol* 1982; **13**: 19–24.

12. Ishak KG, Rogers WA. Cryptogenic acute cholangitis – association with toxic shock syndrome. *Am J Clin Pathol* 1981; **76**: 619–626.

13. Amedee-Manesme O, Bernard O, Brunelle F et al. Sclerosing cholangitis with neonatal onset. *J Pediatr* 1987; **111**: 225–229.

14. Aadland E, Schrumpf E, Fausa O et al. Primary sclerosing cholangitis: a long-term follow-up study. *Scand J Gastroenterol* 1987; **22**: 655–664.

15. Jeffrey GP, Reed DW, Carrello S, Shilkin KB. Histological and immunohistochemical study of the gall bladder lesion in primary sclerosing cholangitis. *Gut* 1991; **32**: 424–429.

16. Kawaguchi K, Koike M, Tsuruta K, Okamoto A, Tabata I, Fujita N. Lymphoplasmacytic sclerosing pancreatitis with cholangitis: a variant of primary sclerosing cholangitis extensively involving pancreas. *Hum Pathol* 1991; **22**: 387–395.

17. Broome U, Glaumann H, Hultcrantz R. Liver histology and follow up of 68 patients with ulcerative colitis and normal liver function tests. *Gut* 1990; **31**: 468–472.

18. Kemeny MM, Battifora H, Blayney DW et al. Sclerosing cholangitis after continuous hepatic artery infusion of FUDR. *Ann Surg* 1985; **202**: 176–181.

19. Herrmann G, Lorenz M, Kirkowa-Reimann M, Hottenrott C, Hubner K. Morphological changes after intra-arterial chemotherapy of the liver. *Hepatogastroenterology* 1987; **34**: 5–9.

20. Ludwig J, Kim CH, Wiesner RH, Krom RA. Floxuridine-induced sclerosing cholangitis: an ischemic cholangiopathy? *Hepatology* 1989; **9**: 215–218.

21. Ludwig J. Small-duct primary sclerosing cholangitis. *Semin Liver Dis* 1991; **11**: 11–17.

22. Harrison RF, Hubscher SG. The spectrum of bile duct lesions in end-stage primary sclerosing cholangitis. *Histopathology* 1991; **19**: 321–327.

23. Nakanuma Y, Ohta G. Histometric and serial section observations of the intrahepatic bile ducts in primary biliary cirrhosis. *Gastroenterology* 1979; **76**: 1326–1332.

24. van Eyken P, Sciot R, Desmet VJ. A cytokeratin immunohistochemical study of cholestatic liver disease: evidence that hepatocytes can express "bile duct-type" cytokeratins. *Histopathology* 1989; **15**: 125–135.

25. Nakanuma Y, Yamaguchi K, Ohta G, Terada T. The Japanese Hepatolithiasis Study Group. Pathological features of hepatolithiasis in Japan. *Hum Pathol* 1988; **19**: 1181–1186.

26. Bhathal PS, Powell LW. Primary intrahepatic obliterating cholangitis: a possible variant of "sclerosing cholangitis". *Gut* 1969; **10**: 886–893.

27. MacSween RN, Burt AD, Haboubi NY. Unusual variant of primary sclerosing cholangitis. *J Clin Pathol* 1987; **40**: 541–545.

28. Fleming KA. Interlobular bile duct basement membrane thickening – a specific marker for primary sclerosing cholangitis (PSC)? *J Pathol* 1993; **169** Suppl. (Abstract).

29. Ludwig J, Dickson ER, McDonald GS. Staging of chronic nonsuppurative destructive cholangitis (syndrome of primary biliary cirrhosis). *Virchows Arch Pathol Anat* 1978; **379**: 103–112.

30. Ludwig J, LaRusso NF, Wiesner RH. The syndrome of primary sclerosing cholangitis. In Popper H, Schaffner F (eds): Progress in Liver Diseases, Vol. IX. Philadelphia: WB Saunders, 1990, pp 555–566.

31. Wee A, Ludwig J, Coffey RJJ, LaRusso NF, Wiesner RH. Hepatobiliary carcinoma associated with primary sclerosing cholangitis and chronic ulcerative colitis. *Hum Pathol* 1985; **16**: 719–726.

32. Mir-Madjlessi SH, Farmer RG, Sivak MVJ. Bile duct carcinoma in patients with ulcerative colitis. Relationship to sclerosing cholangitis: report of six cases and review of the literature. *Dig Dis Sci* 1987; **32**: 145–154.

33. Miros M, Kerlin P, Walker N, Harper J, Lynch S, Strong R. Predicting cholangiocarcinoma in patients with primary sclerosing cholangitis before transplantation. *Gut* 1991; **32**: 1369–1373.

34. Haworth AC, Manley PN, Groll A, Pace R. Bile duct carcinoma and biliary tract dysplasia in chronic ulcerative colitis. *Arch Pathol Lab Med* 1989; **113**: 434–436.

35. Guarascio P, Yentis F, Cevikbas U, Portmann B, Williams R. Value of copper-associated protein in diagnostic assessment of liver biopsy. *J Clin Pathol* 1983; **36**: 18–23.

36. Ludwig J. Surgical pathology of the syndrome of primary sclerosing cholangitis. *Am J Surg Pathol* 1989; **13** (Suppl. 1): 43–49.

37. Rubin E, Schaffner F, Popper H. Primary biliary cirrhosis. Chronic non-suppurative destructive cholangitis. *Am J Pathol* 1965; **46**: 387–407.
38. Fussey SP, West SM, Lindsay JG et al. Clarification of the identity of the major M2 autoantigen in primary biliary cirrhosis. *Clin Sci* 1991; **80**: 451–455.
39. Joplin R, Lindsay JG, Johnson GD, Strain A, Neuberger J. Membrane dihydrolipoamide acetyltransferase (E2) on human biliary epithelial cells in primary biliary cirrhosis. *Lancet* 1992; **339**: 93–94.
40. Culp KS, Fleming CR, Duffy J, Baldus WP, Dickson ER. Autoimmune associations in primary biliary cirrhosis. *Mayo Clin Proc* 1982; **57**: 365–370.
41. Scheuer P. Primary biliary cirrhosis. *Proc R Soc Med* 1967; **60**: 1257–1260.
42. Nakanuma Y, Terada T, Doishita K, Miwa A. Hepatocellular carcinoma in primary biliary cirrhosis: an autopsy study. *Hepatology* 1990; **11**: 1010–1016.
43. Terada T, Kurumaya H, Nakanuma Y, Hayakawa Y, Matsuda H. Macroregenerative nodules of the liver in primary biliary cirrhosis: report of two autopsy cases. *Am J Gastroenterol* 1989; **84**: 418–421.
44. Terasaki S, Nakanuma Y, Yamazaki M, Unoura M. Eosinophilic infiltration of the liver in primary biliary cirrhosis: a morphological study. *Hepatology* 1993; **17**: 206–212.
45. Nakanuma Y, Ohta G. Quantitation of hepatic granulomas and epithelioid cells in primary biliary cirrhosis. *Hepatology* 1983; **3**: 423–427.
46. Lee RG, Epstein O, Jauregui H, Sherlock S, Scheuer PJ. Granulomas in primary biliary cirrhosis: a prognostic feature. *Gastroenterology* 1981; **81**: 983–986.
47. Roll J, Boyer JL, Barry D, Klatskin G. The prognostic importance of clinical and histologic features in asymptomatic and symptomatic primary biliary cirrhosis. *N Engl J Med* 1983; **308**: 1–7.
48. Nakanuma Y. Necroinflammatory changes in hepatic lobules in primary biliary cirrhosis with less well-defined cholestatic changes. *Hum Pathol* 1993; **24**: 378–383.
49. McMahon RF, Babbs C, Warnes TW. Nodular regenerative hyperplasia of the liver, CREST syndrome and primary biliary cirrhosis: an overlap syndrome? *Gut* 1989; **30**: 1430–1433.
50. Colina F, Pinedo F, Solis JA, Moreno D, Nevado M. Nodular regenerative hyperplasia of the liver in early histological stages of primary biliary cirrhosis. *Gastroenterology* 1992; **102**: 1319–1324.
51. Nakanuma Y, Ohta G, Kobayashi K, Kato Y. Histological and histometric examination of the intrahepatic portal vein branches in primary biliary cirrhosis without regenerative nodules. *Am J Gastroenterol* 1982; **77**: 405–413.
52. Nakanuma Y, Hirata K. Unusual hepatocellular lesions in primary biliary cirrhosis resembling but unrelated to hepatocellular neoplasms. *Virchows Arch (A)* 1993; **422**: 17–23.
53. Bach N, Thung SN, Schaffner F. The histological features of chronic hepatitis C and autoimmune chronic hepatitis: a comparative analysis. *Hepatology* 1992; **15**: 572–577.
54. Christoffersen P, Poulsen H, Scheuer PJ. Abnormal bile duct epithelium in chronic aggressive hepatitis and primary biliary cirrhosis. *Hum Pathol* 1972; **3**: 227–235.
55. Nakanuma Y, Saito K, Unoura M. Semiquantitative assessment of cholestasis and lymphocytic piecemeal necrosis in primary biliary cirrhosis: a histologic and immunohistochemical study. *J Clin Gastroenterol* 1990; **12**: 357–362.
56. Yamada S, Howe S, Scheuer PJ. Three-dimensional reconstruction of biliary pathways in primary biliary cirrhosis: a computer-assisted study. *J Pathol* 1987; **152**: 317–323.
57. Nakanuma Y. Pathology of septum formation in primary biliary cirrhosis: a histological study in the non-cirrhotic stage. *Virchows Arch (A)* 1991; **419**: 381–387.
58. Williamson JM, Chalmers DM, Clayden AD, Dixon MF, Ruddell WS, Losowsky MS. Primary biliary cirrhosis and chronic active hepatitis: an examination of clinical, biochemical, and histopathological features in differential diagnosis. *J Clin Pathol* 1985; **38**: 1007–1012.
59. Brunner G, Klinge O. Ein der chronisch-destruierenden nicht-eitrigen Cholangitis ähnliches Krankheitsbild mit antinukleären Antikörpern (Immuncholangitis). *Dtsch Med Wochenschr* 1987; **112**: 1454–1458.
60. Carrougher JG, Shaffer RT, Canales LI, Goodman ZD. A 33-year-old woman with an autoimmune syndrome. *Semin Liver Dis* 1991; **11**: 256–262.
61. Rabinovitz M, Demetris AJ, Bou-Abboud CF, Van Thiel DH. Simultaneous occurrence of primary sclerosing cholangitis and autoimmune chronic active hepatitis in a patient with ulcerative colitis. *Dig Dis Sci* 1992; **37**: 1606–1611.
62. Ben-Ari Z, Dhillon AP, Sherlock S. Autoimmune cholangiopathy: part of the spectrum of autoimmune chronic active hepatitis. *Hepatology* 1993; **18**: 10–15.
63. Michieletti P, Wanless IR, Katz A et al. Are patients with antimitochondrial antibody negative primary biliary cirrhosis a distinct syndrome of autoimmune cholangitis? *Gut* 1994; **35**: 260–265.

GENERAL READING

Chapman RW. Aetiology and natural history of primary sclerosing cholangitis – a decade of progress? *Gut* 1991; **32**: 1433–1435.

Desmet VJ. Cholestasis: extrahepatic obstruction and secondary biliary cirrhosis. In

MacSween RNM, Anthony PP, Scheuer PJ, Portmann B, Burt AD (eds): Pathology of the Liver, 3rd edn. Edinburgh: Churchill Livingstone, 1994.

Farrant JM, Hayllar KM, Wilkinson ML et al. Natural history and prognostic variables in primary sclerosing cholangitis. *Gastroenterology* 1991; **100**: 1710–1717.

Ludwig J, LaRusso NF, Wiesner RH. The syndrome of primary sclerosing cholangitis. In Popper H, Schaffner F (eds): Progress in Liver Diseases, Vol. IX. Philadelphia: WB Saunders, 1990, pp 555–566.

MacSween RNM, Burt AD. Pathology of the intrahepatic bile ducts. In Anthony PP, MacSween RNM (eds): Recent Advances in Histopathology 14. Edinburgh: Churchill Livingstone, 1989, pp 161–183.

Portmann B, MacSween RNM. Diseases of the intrahepatic bile ducts. In MacSween RNM, Anthony PP, Scheuer PJ, Portmann B, Burt AD (eds): Pathology of the Liver, 3rd edn. Edinburgh: Churchill Livingstone, 1994.

Wiesner RH, Grambsch PM, Dickson ER et al. Primary sclerosing cholangitis: natural history, prognostic factors and survival analysis. *Hepatology* 1989; **10**: 430–436.

6

ACUTE VIRAL HEPATITIS

The last few years have seen an explosion of knowledge in the field of viral hepatitis. Hepatitis C and E have been added to the hepatitic alphabet, and F and G postulated[1-5] (Table 6.1). Testing of serum for antibodies to hepatitis A, B, C and D has become routine, and in the case of the hepatitis C virus is supplemented by the polymerase chain reaction for viral nucleic acid. Liver biopsy continues to be used to establish or confirm a diagnosis of acute viral hepatitis, and to assess severity and evolution to chronic disease.

Table 6.1. The Hepatitis Viruses

Virus	Type	Spread and Disease
Hepatitis A (HAV)	RNA hepatovirus	Faecal–oral; acute
Hepatitis B (HBV)	DNA hepadnavirus	Parenteral; acute or chronic
Hepatitis C (HCV)	RNA, flavi- and pestivirus-like	Parenteral or sporadic; acute, often chronic
Hepatitis D (HDV)	Defective RNA virus	Pathogenic when combined with HBV infection
Hepatitis E (HEV)	RNA virus	Faecal–oral; epidemic or sporadic acute disease

Note: Other possible human hepatitis viruses include a togavirus-like agent causing fulminant disease,[4] sometimes referred to as hepatitis F virus, and a paramyxovirus implicated in some examples of giant-cell hepatitis.[5] The term hepatitis G for this disease remains tentative.

The pathological features of viral hepatitis were discussed briefly in Chapter 4 in the context of acute jaundice. The present chapter deals with them in more detail, and outlines the variations in pattern and sequelae which may be seen in liver biopsies. The characteristics of hepatitis caused by different viruses are described but for more information on the viruses themselves larger texts should be consulted.

Four main histological patterns of acute hepatitis can be distinguished (Table 6.2). Because they are relevant to diagnosis and in some cases to prognosis, each pattern will be discussed separately.

CLASSICAL ACUTE HEPATITIS (ACUTE HEPATITIS WITH SPOTTY NECROSIS)

In contrast to classical acute inflammation, the dominant changes in acute viral hepatitis are damage to the hepatic parenchymal cells and infiltration by cells of the

Table 6.2. Histological Patterns of Acute Hepatitis

Classical acute hepatitis
   (acute hepatitis with focal or spotty necrosis)
Acute hepatitis with bridging necrosis
Acute hepatitis with panacinar necrosis
Acute hepatitis with periportal necrosis

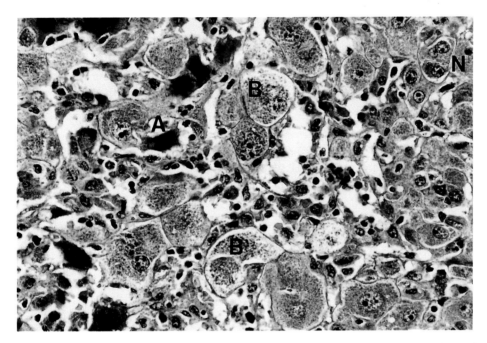

Figure 6.1. *Acute viral hepatitis.* Many hepatocytes in this perivenular area have undergone ballooning degeneration (B) and are much larger than normal hepatocytes (N). Other hepatocytes show acidophilic change (A). The inflammatory infiltrate is mainly composed of lymphocytes, plasma cells and macrophages. Wedge .biopsy, H & E.

lymphocyte and macrophage series. The parenchymal damage takes two main forms. **Ballooned** liver cells (Fig. 6.1) are swollen and have granular pale-staining cytoplasm, unlike the reticular cytoplasm of cells undergoing feathery degeneration in cholestasis (Fig. 5.2, p. 39). Other hepatocytes undergo **acidophilic degeneration**, becoming densely stained and irregular in shape, their borders often concave. These cells are probably the precursors of **apoptotic bodies**,[6,7] also known as acidophil or Councilman bodies, which are shrunken cells or cell fragments separated from the liver-cell plates (Fig. 6.2). Apoptotic bodies are usually rounded in shape and sometimes bulge beyond the plane of the section. They may or may not contain pyknotic nuclear material. While very characteristic and often abundant in acute hepatitis they are by no means diagnostic, being found in many other forms of liver injury and even rarely in normal liver. Fatty change is found in a minority of patients with acute hepatitis from any cause and is almost always mild.

Prominence of syncytial giant hepatocytes, typical of neonatal hepatitis, is also sometimes a feature of acute hepatitis in adults. Some cases have been attributed to paramyxovirus infection.[5] Others are associated with a variety of infective agents including hepatitis viruses while some have the features of autoimmune hepatitis.[8,9]

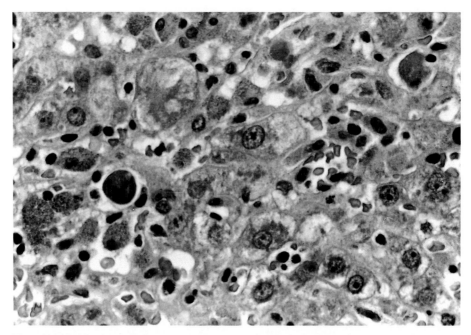

Figure 6.2. *Acute viral hepatitis.* Two rounded and deeply-stained acidophil bodies are seen (left and top right). Kupffer cells (left) contain granular ceroid pigment. Needle biopsy, H & E.

The combination of hepatocellular swelling, shrinkage, apoptosis and cell dropout, together with regenerative hyperplasia of surviving hepatocytes, leads to a diagnostically helpful loss of the normal regular liver-cell plate pattern[10] (Fig. 6.1). This disarray of cell plates helps to distinguish hepatitis from liver-cell damage secondary to cholestasis.

The above changes may be present throughout the acini but are usually most severe in zones 3, near terminal hepatic venules (Fig. 6.3). Damage predominantly in zone 1 is less common but is sometimes a feature of type A hepatitis[11] (p. 73). Within zone 3 the severity of the hepatocellular damage varies, some cells being more severely affected than others; this is expressed in the term spotty necrosis, synonymous with focal necrosis. In the more severe forms of acute hepatitis confluent necrosis may also develop. The sinusoidal collapse which results is thought to be a factor in the portal hypertension found in some patients with acute hepatitis.[12]

Some degree of morphological cholestasis is very common in acute hepatitis. It results from damage to the bile secretory and contractile functions of hepatocytes and sometimes also from interference with bile flow at the level of the portal tracts.[13] Bile canaliculi contain bile thrombi but are not as widely dilated as in bile-duct obstruction. The term "cholestatic hepatitis" is best confined to patients with a prolonged cholestatic course clinically; in such patients histological cholestasis may dominate the picture or persist after resolution of the other changes.

In addition to these various forms of liver-cell damage, there is infiltration of the acini by inflammatory cells. These are predominantly activated memory T cells.[14] The accumulation of lymphocytes is probably mediated by increased expression of adhesion molecules on sinusoidal endothelium.[15] Plasma cells may also be found from the earliest stages,[16] and a few segmented leucocytes are sometimes seen. Kupffer cells are enlarged and form clumps which are most easily seen in diastase-PAS preparations, especially in zones 3 (Fig. 6.4). Their cytoplasm contains brown, lipid-rich ceroid pigment and is sometimes iron-positive (Fig. 6.5). In the absence of ceroid pigment and iron, PAS-

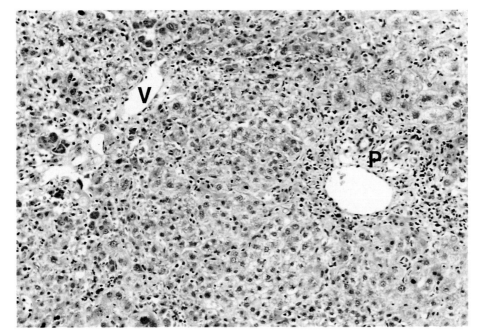

Figure 6.3. *Acute viral hepatitis.* Hepatocellular swelling and inflammatory infiltration are most severe near a terminal venule (V). The portal tract (P) also contains inflammatory cells. Needle biopsy, H & E.

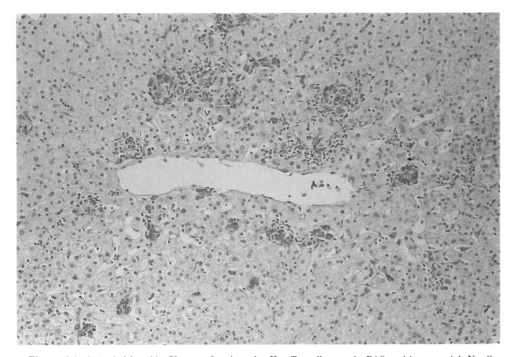

Figure 6.4. *Acute viral hepatitis.* Clumps of perivenular Kupffer cells contain PAS-positive material. Needle biopsy, diastase-PAS.

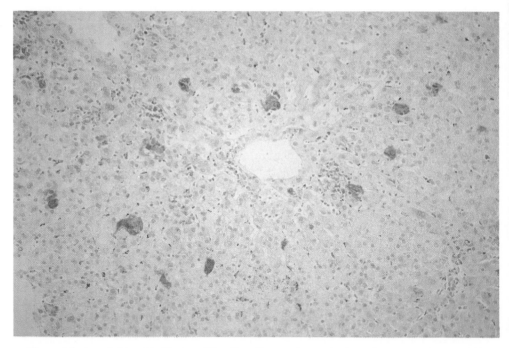

Figure 6.5. *Acute viral hepatitis.* Clumps of Kupffer cells around a terminal venule are strongly iron-positive. Needle biopsy, Perls' stain.

positive macrophages are less specific, being found also during and after episodes of cholestasis.

While the parenchymal lesions are the most characteristic part of the histological picture of an acute hepatitis, most portal tracts are also involved. They are infiltrated with inflammatory cells, and as in the acini these are mainly lymphocytes and plasma cells[14,16] (Fig. 6.6). Neutrophils, eosinophils and pigment-laden macrophages are also commonly present. The infiltrate often spills out into the adjacent parenchyma, blurring the outlines of the portal tracts and giving rise to possible confusion with the piecemeal necrosis of chronic hepatitis. Emperipolesis, periportal apoptosis and trapping of hepatocytes deep within the infiltrate suggest chronicity, but the distinction is not always easy to make; both acinar changes and clinical information need to be taken into account.

Proliferation of bile ducts or ductules is not usually a prominent feature in acute hepatitis unless there is sepsis or very severe liver-cell necrosis. In the latter case the portal changes can mimic those of bile-duct obstruction but the correct diagnosis is easily made by assessment of the whole histological picture.[17] Damage to the epithelium of interlobular bile ducts is quite common in acute hepatitis,[18] particularly in hepatitis C.[19,20] The damaged ducts usually lie within or adjacent to lymphoid follicles (Fig. 6.7). Biliary epithelial cells are focally stratified, irregular in shape and vacuolated. The clinical context helps to prevent diagnostic confusion with primary biliary cirrhosis. Granuloma formation is not a feature of the bile-duct lesion of hepatitis.

Evolution of the Lesion of Acute Hepatitis

Acute viral hepatitis evolves through an early stage, rarely seen in biopsies, to the above fully developed lesion. This gradually subsides, leaving late and residual changes which may persist for some months. Ultimately the liver returns to normal in many patients. The

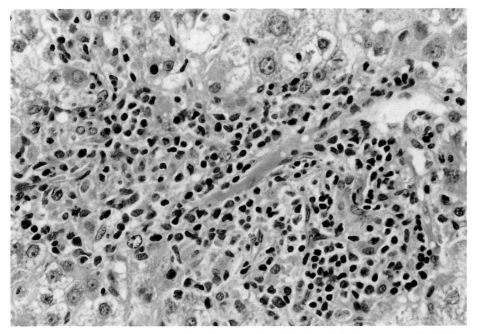

Figure 6.6. *Acute viral hepatitis*. A small portal tract is heavily infiltrated by lymphocytes. Needle biopsy, H & E.

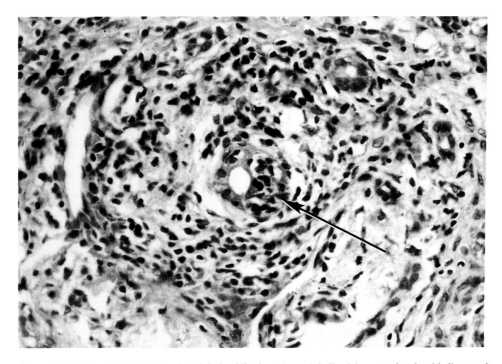

Figure 6.7. *Acute viral hepatitis*. An interlobular bile duct (arrow) is lined by vacuolated epithelium and infiltrated by lymphocytes. Wedge biopsy, H & E.

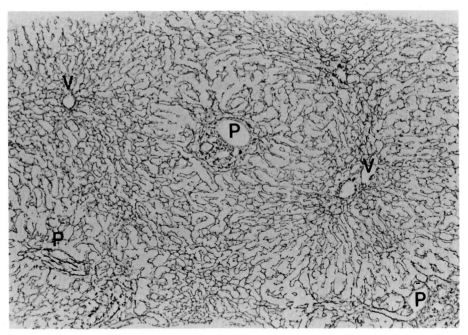

Figure 6.8. *Acute viral hepatitis.* Reticulin framework is condensed near terminal venules (V) but not near portal tracts (P). Needle biopsy, reticulin.

rate of this evolution varies from patient to patient and no accurate assessment can therefore be made by the pathologist in terms of weeks or even months. However, the fully developed stage commonly lasts for at least several weeks, so that a near-normal biopsy 2 or 3 weeks after an episode of jaundice provides some evidence against a diagnosis of acute viral hepatitis. The rate of evolution of idiosyncratic drug hepatitis (p. 105) depends partly on how quickly the offending drug is withdrawn.

In the later stages of an acute self-limited hepatitis the degenerative liver-cell changes diminish, leaving some inflammation and prominent macrophages in acini and portal tracts. Condensation of the reticulin framework provides further evidence of recent liver-cell loss (Fig. 6.8). Occasionally canalicular cholestasis is slow to resolve. Finally, the histological pattern becomes less specific and more difficult to identify. Residual changes, which may persist for many months, include mild portal inflammation, focal necrosis and inflammation in the acini, prominence of pigmented macrophages and increased variation in liver-cell and nuclear size for the patient's age (Fig. 6.9). Accentuation of residual changes in acinar zones 3 helps to suggest the correct diagnosis. Slender fibrous septa may extend from portal tracts (Fig. 6.10).

ACUTE HEPATITIS WITH BRIDGING NECROSIS

In some patients with acute hepatitis death of hepatocytes is so extensive that necrotic bridges come to link portal tracts to terminal hepatic venules (Fig. 6.11). One explanation for the distribution of this lesion is that it represents confluent necrosis of entire acinar zones 3.[21] These bridges, also called central–portal bridges, are fundamentally different from portal–portal bridges which result principally from periportal necrosis and portal-tract widening. The term "bridging hepatic necrosis" (BHN) will therefore be restricted here to central–portal lesions. Any of the hepatitis viruses may be responsible. BHN is an

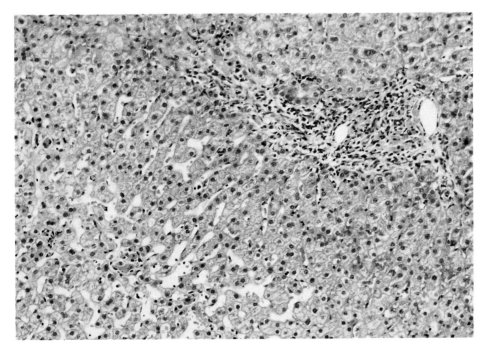

Figure 6.9. *Acute viral hepatitis, residual stage.* In acinar zone 3 (below left) liver-cell plates are irregular and there is slight lymphocytic infiltration. The portal tract (top right) is inflamed. Needle biopsy, H & E.

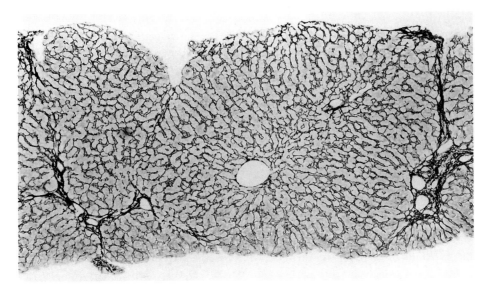

Figure 6.10. *Acute viral hepatitis, residual stage.* Slender septa link portal tracts (left and right), but the perivenular area (centre) is unaffected and architectural relationships are preserved. Needle biopsy, reticulin.

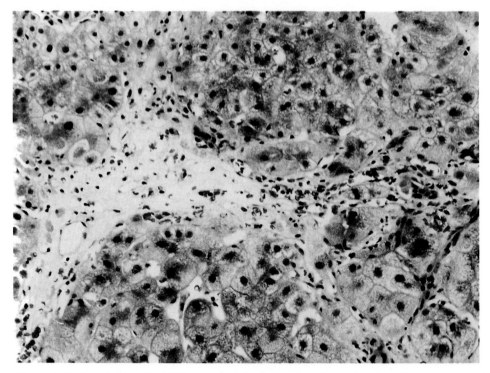

Figure 6.11. *Acute viral hepatitis: bridging necrosis.* A bridge has been formed by the collapse of an area of confluent necrosis, and links a portal tract (right) with a terminal venule (left). See also Figure 4.1. Needle biopsy, H & E.

indication of a severe hepatitis, and patients with it are more prone to die within weeks or months of onset or to develop chronic liver disease than those with spotty necrosis alone.[22] Nevertheless, BHN is compatible with full recovery provided that regeneration is adequate.

The necrotic bridges are composed of collapsed connective tissue framework in which there are ceroid-rich macrophages, other inflammatory cells and blood vessels. The bridges are often curved, probably reflecting the shape of acinar zones 3. They may be mistaken for the fibrous septa of chronic liver disease; this error can usually be avoided by means of stains for elastic fibres, since recently formed bridges are devoid of these fibres whereas older septa are positive[23] (Figs 6.12 and 6.13). Substantial amounts of elastic tissue take many months to develop but small amounts can be detected by sensitive methods such as Victoria blue as early as 1 or 2 months after onset of hepatitis.[24]

ACUTE HEPATITIS WITH PANACINAR OR MULTIACINAR NECROSIS

In a minority of patients confluent necrosis extends throughout entire acini (panacinar necrosis) or several adjacent acini (multiacinar necrosis). This pattern is typical of clinically fulminant, coma-producing hepatitis. It is also found in some less severely affected patients, especially immediately deep to the liver capsule. A similar lesion is sometimes seen in subcapsular areas in chronic rather than acute hepatitis. Under the microscope the hepatic parenchyma in panacinar necrosis is seen to be replaced by collapsed stroma, inflammatory cells and ceroid-rich macrophages (Fig. 6.14). In and

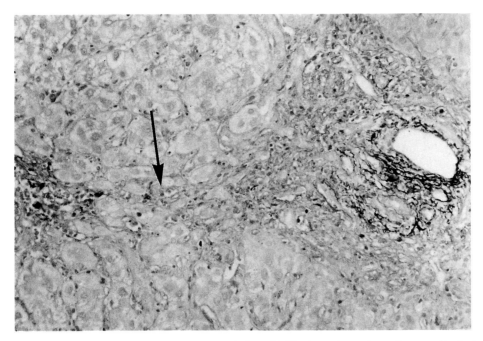

Figure 6.12. *Viral hepatitis: bridging necrosis.* A recently formed bridge (arrow) contains no demonstrable elastic fibres. Orcein has stained elastic fibres in the portal tract (right) and ceroid-containing macrophages in the perivenular area (left). Needle biopsy, orcein.

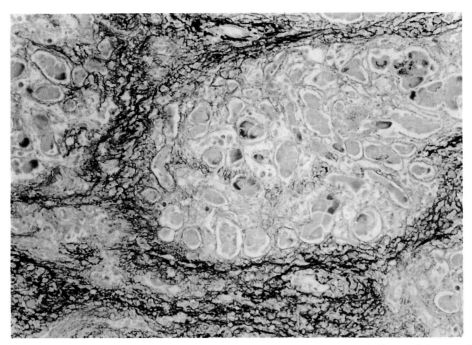

Figure 6.13. *Cirrhosis.* Old fibrous septa in a cirrhotic liver contain abundant elastic fibres, staining strongly with orcein. Hepatitis B surface antigen and scanty copper-associated protein granules are also orcein-positive. Contrast with the recently formed, orcein-negative septum in Figure 6.12. Wedge biopsy, orcein.

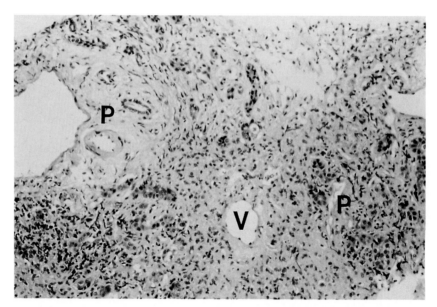

Figure 6.14. *Acute viral hepatitis: panacinar necrosis.* Hepatocytes between two approximated portal tracts (P) have been destroyed. Duct-like structures have proliferated in periportal areas. V = terminal venule. Needle biopsy, H & E.

around the portal tracts there are proliferated duct-like structures. Some of the cells which make up these structures have neuroendocrine features and may represent a population of stem cells capable of differentiating into hepatocytes.[25] They are thought to provide a special mechanism of regeneration which comes into play when hepatocellular regeneration is inadequate. Occasionally the portal changes in panacinar necrosis mimic those of bile-duct obstruction.[17]

ACUTE HEPATITIS WITH PERIPORTAL NECROSIS

While in most examples of acute hepatitis the necrosis and inflammation are most severe in acinar zones 3, a predominantly portal and periportal lesion may also be found in some patients (Fig. 6.15). Substantial portal infiltration and periportal liver-cell damage may also co-exist with one or more of the other patterns already described. The periportal lesion closely resembles the piecemeal necrosis of chronic hepatitis so that there is a risk of misdiagnosis. However, full recovery from acute hepatitis with periportal necrosis is possible. The periportal pattern is indeed common in type A hepatitis, which does not lead to chronic disease. This emphasizes the need for clinical and serological information when assessing liver biopsies from patients with hepatitis.

INDIVIDUAL CAUSES OF VIRAL HEPATITIS

There are more similarities than differences between hepatitis A, B, C, D and E (Table 6.1, page 62), and the cause of an acute hepatitis cannot be diagnosed with certainty on histological grounds alone. There are, however, common trends and patterns which will be described in this section. The histological picture may be confused by the presence of more than one virus or by additional liver damage due to alcohol abuse. This applies to both acute and chronic hepatitis.

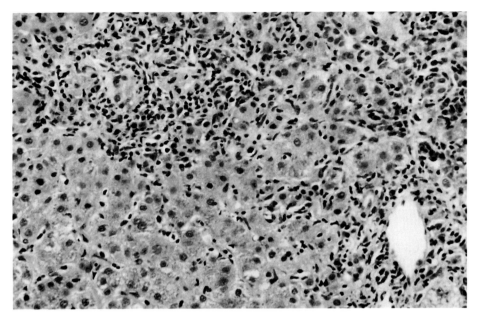

Figure 6.15. *Acute viral hepatitis: periportal necrosis.* In this example of hepatitis A, inflammation and necrosis are most severe in a periportal area, above and to the right. The appearances are very like those of chronic hepatitis. Needle biopsy, H & E.

Type A Hepatitis

Two main patterns are described, occurring separately or together.[11,26,27] One is a histological picture of perivenular cholestasis with little liver-cell damage or inflammation, easily mistaken for other causes of cholestasis. The second is a hepatitis with periportal necrosis and a dense portal infiltrate which includes abundant, often aggregated plasma cells (Fig. 6.15). These two patterns may indeed be related, the cholestasis resulting from interruption of bile flow by the periportal necrosis.[13] Other patterns of hepatitis as described above are also found but fulminant hepatitis with multiacinar necrosis is rare. Extensive microvesicular change of hepatocytes, previously described in hepatitis D infection,[28,29] has also been seen in severe acute hepatitis A (Fig. 6.16). Fibrin-ring granulomas have been reported.[30,31] Viral RNA can be demonstrated in tissue sections by *in situ* hybridization.[32]

Type B Hepatitis

The histological appearances are broadly similar to those of other forms of viral hepatitis.[26,27,33,34] Differences reported in the literature may well reflect patient selection rather than features specific for HBV infection. However, lymphocytes and macrophages sometimes lie in close contact with hepatocytes (peripolesis) or even invaginate them deeply (emperipolesis), which probably reflects the immunological nature of the cell damage.[35] Liver-cells and their nuclei may show a moderate degree of pleomorphism. Hepatitis B core and surface antigens (HBcAg and HBsAg) are only demonstrable, if at all, in very small amounts early in the acute attack,[36] and positive staining of any substantial degree therefore indicates chronic disease. Recurrence of HBV infection after liver transplantation is an exception, both antigens being found in large amounts.[37] Ground-glass hepatocytes are not seen in acute hepatitis. In any parenterally-transmitted hepatitis, including types B and C, birefringent spicules of talc may be found in portal tracts as a result of intravenous drug abuse.[38,39]

Type C Hepatitis

Usually the histological features are those of any acute hepatitis (Fig. 6.17), but two distinguishing features have been noted in acute hepatitis C or in parenterally transmitted non-A, non-B hepatitis, most of which have proved to be due to hepatitis C virus (HCV) infection. First, there may be prominent infiltration of sinusoids by lymphocytes in the absence of severe liver-cell damage,[40] giving rise to a picture reminiscent of infectious mononucleosis (Fig. 6.18). Secondly, features usually associated with chronic hepatitis, notably lymphoid follicles and bile-duct damage, may also be seen within a few weeks or months of onset. There may be cholestasis and fatty change is relatively common.[33] Fulminant hepatitis with multiacinar necrosis is only very rarely due to HCV infection, at least in the Western world. Demonstration of HCV antigens in tissue sections by immunohistochemistry has been achieved[41-43] but is not, at the time of writing, available as a routine procedure. The histological characteristics of chronic type C hepatitis are discussed in Chapter 9.

Type D Hepatitis (Delta Virus Infection)

Coinfection or superinfection with the hepatitis D virus (HDV) alters the course of type B hepatitis, encouraging chronicity and enhancing severity.[44-47] The antigen, HDAg, can easily be demonstrated immunohistochemically in paraffin sections and is mainly found in hepatocyte nuclei[36] (Fig. 6.19). These may have finely granular eosinophilic centres (so-

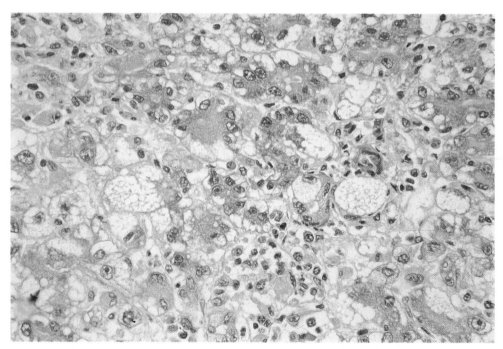

Figure 6.16. *Hepatitis A*. In this patient with fulminant hepatitis, hepatocytes are swollen and microvesicular. There is cholestasis, and a lymphoplasmacytic infiltrate is present. Needle biopsy, H & E.

called "sanded" nuclei[48]). Cytoplasmic and membrane-associated staining is also some-times seen. Viral RNA can be demonstrated in routine sections by *in situ* hybridization.[49-51]

Severe acute hepatitis in a patient with markers of HBV infection may in fact be due to superinfection by HDV of a chronic HBV carrier.[52] In an outbreak of HDV infection among Venezuelan Indians, notable features included early small-droplet fatty change, sparse lymphocytes and abundant macrophages in the parenchyma, and substantial portal infiltration.[53] Later in the attack there was extensive necrosis and collapse. Microvesicular fatty change and acidophilic necrosis of hepatocytes have been reported from Colombia[28] and North America.[29] In non-immunosuppressed patients with current HDV infection, liver biopsy is likely to show substantial necrosis and inflammation.[46,54,55] Following liver transplantation, on the other hand, HDV without HBV is sometimes demonstrable in the absence of hepatitic changes, indicating that HDV can survive in the absence of HBV. It does not then appear, however, to be capable of causing liver damage.[56]

Type E Hepatitis

This is the result of infection by the enteric route with an RNA virus.[57-59] The disease causes epidemics in Asia, and has also been found in Africa and North America. In the Western world it is most often seen in travellers. Infection does not appear to lead to chronic disease. There is so far little detailed information on pathological changes in man. In a small group of patients studied, the appearances were like those of hepatitis A with prominent cholestasis and a predominantly portal and periportal inflammatory infil-trate.[60] The liver of a pregnant woman with fatal hepatitis E showed little portal

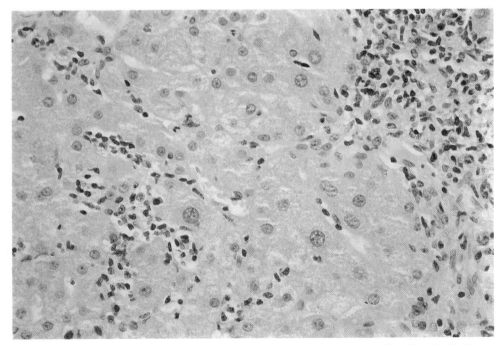

Figure 6.17. *Acute hepatitis C.* There is patchy liver-cell drop-out and lymphocytic infiltration. Needle biopsy, H & E.

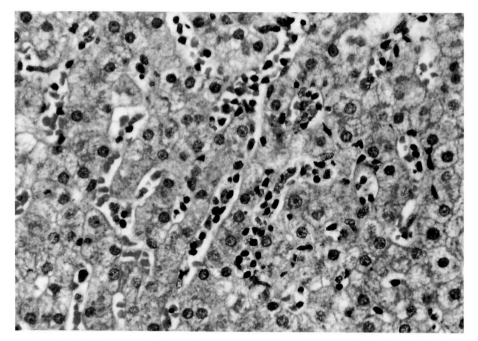

Figure 6.18. *Acute hepatitis C.* Liver-cell damage is mild but sinusoids are infiltrated by lymphocytes. Needle biopsy, H & E.

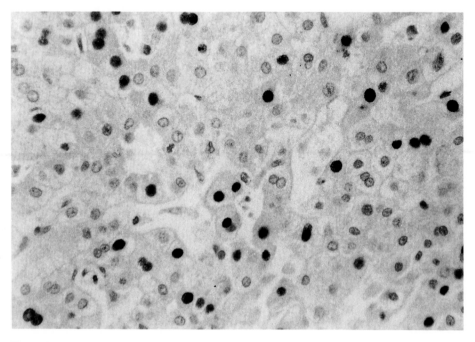

Figure 6.19. *Delta (HDV) hepatitis.* Many hepatocyte nuclei contain the delta antigen. Needle biopsy, specific immunoperoxidase.

inflammation, much cholestasis and prominent phlebitis.[61] Virus particles were seen by electron microscopy in proliferated bile ductules.

Other Types of Acute Hepatitis

A togavirus-like agent has been reported as a possible cause of acute fulminant hepatitis with panacinar necrosis.[4] Livers removed surgically at transplantation showed extensive necrosis and collapse, and map-like areas of surviving parenchyma with much cholestasis.

Intracytoplasmic paramyxovirus-like structures have been reported in hepatocytes of adult patients with giant-cell hepatitis.[5] In other patients with this pattern the cause may be one of the hepatitis viruses listed above, or an autoimmune form of liver disease[8,9] (p. 130).

In some patients with acute hepatitis no viral or other agent can be identified. It is therefore possible that other agents will be added to the list of hepatitis viruses in the future.

DIFFERENTIAL DIAGNOSIS OF ACUTE VIRAL HEPATITIS

The distinction of acute hepatitis from **bile-duct obstruction** rests mainly on the finding of typical hepatitic changes in the acini. **Drug-related hepatitis** may be indistinguishable from viral hepatitis and should always be suspected if the cause of the hepatitis is in doubt. Features commoner in drug-induced than in viral hepatitis include sharply defined perivenular necrosis, granulomas, abundant neutrophils or eosinophils, damaged small bile ducts in the absence of lymphoid follicles and a poorly developed portal inflammatory reaction. Absence of these features does not exclude drug hepatitis. **Autoimmune hepatitis** may have an acute onset, histologically indistinguishable from viral hepatitis. In **alcoholic hepatitis** there is usually conspicuous fatty change. Mallory bodies may be present in ballooned hepatocytes and the infiltrate typically includes neutrophils. The key to the diagnosis is the presence of pericellular fibrosis in affected areas. The differentiation of acute from **chronic hepatitis** is briefly discussed in the section on bridging necrosis above. Generally the parenchymal changes predominate in acute hepatitis, especially in acinar zones 3, while the portal and periportal changes predominate in chronic disease. The distinction is, however, sometimes very difficult.

FATE AND MORPHOLOGICAL SEQUELAE OF ACUTE VIRAL HEPATITIS (Table 6.3)

Resolution. This is the commonest outcome overall but in parenterally transmitted type C hepatitis a chronic course is probably commoner than resolution. Residual changes may persist for many months after clinical recovery from an acute hepatitis.

Table 6.3. Fate and Sequelae of Acute Viral Hepatitis

Resolution; return to normal liver
Death in the acute phase
Post-hepatitic scarring
Chronic virus carrier state without significant disease
Chronic hepatitis
Cirrhosis
Hepatocellular carcinoma

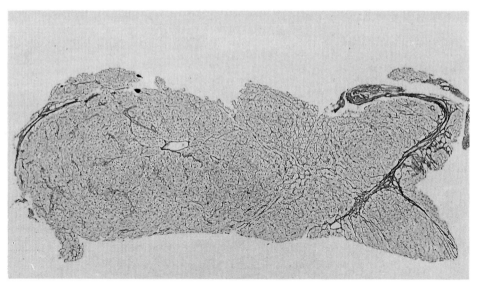

Figure 6.20. *Post-hepatitic scarring.* There is irregular scarring and evidence of regeneration, as indicated by the nodular area to the left. The patient had no clinical or other evidence of cirrhosis. Contrast with residual viral hepatitis in Figure 6.10. Needle biopsy, reticulin.

Fatal outcome. There is usually severe necrosis, and regenerative hyperplasia may be seen.

Post-hepatitic scarring. Localized collapse, scarring and regeneration following severe hepatitis with bridging or panacinar necrosis sometimes produce a histological picture very like that of cirrhosis (Fig. 6.20). Distinction requires full clinical and serological information.

Chronic hepatitis and virus carrier states. These are discussed in Chapter 9.

Cirrhosis. Post-hepatitis cirrhosis almost always follows a period of chronic hepatitis, with repeated or continuous hepatocellular necrosis and regeneration. Occasionally it may follow directly after a single episode of severe acute hepatitis, in much the same way as post-hepatitic scarring but diffusely throughout the liver.

Hepatocellular carcinoma. This may develop on the basis of cirrhosis in patients infected with HBV or HCV. Occasionally, however, hepatocellular carcinoma is found in HBV-infected patients in the absence of cirrhosis.

REFERENCES

1. Anon. The A to F of viral hepatitis. *Lancet* 1990; **336**: 1158–1160.
2. Lau JYN, Alexander GJM, Alberti A. Viral hepatitis. *Gut Suppl* 1991; S47–S62.
3. Anon. Hepatitis G? *Lancet* 1991; **337**: 1070.
4. Fagan EA, Ellis DS, Tovey GM et al. Toga virus-like particles in acute liver failure attributed to sporadic non-A, non-B hepatitis and recurrence after liver transplantation. *J Med Virol* 1992; **38**: 71–77.
5. Phillips MJ, Blendis LM, Poucell S et al. Syncytial giant-cell hepatitis. Sporadic hepatitis with distinctive pathological features, a severe clinical course, and paramyxoviral features. *N Engl J Med* 1991; **324**: 455–460.
6. Powell LW. The nature of cell death in piecemeal necrosis: is order emerging from chaos? *Hepatology* 1987; **7**: 794–796.
7. Wyllie AH. Apoptosis: cell death in tissue regulation. *J Pathol* 1987; **153**: 313–316.
8. Devaney K, Goodman ZD, Ishak KG. Postinfantile giant-cell transformation in hepatitis. *Hepatology* 1992; **16**: 327–333.
9. Lau JYN, Koukoulis G, Mieli-Vergani G, Portmann BC, Williams R. Syncytial giant-cell hepatitis – a specific disease entity? *J Hepatol* 1992; **15**: 216–219.

10. Peters RL. Viral hepatitis: a pathologic spectrum. *Am J Med Sci* 1975; **270**: 17–31.
11. Teixeira MR Jr, Weller IVD, Murray AM et al. The pathology of hepatitis A in man. *Liver* 1982; **2**: 53–60.
12. Valla D, Flejou J-F, Lebrec D et al. Portal hypertension and ascites in acute hepatitis: clinical, hemodynamic and histological correlations. *Hepatology* 1989; **10**: 482–487.
13. Sciot R, Van Damme B, Desmet VJ. Cholestatic features in hepatitis A. *J Hepatol* 1986; **3**: 172–181.
14. Volpes R, van den Oord JJ, Desmet VJ. Memory T cells represent the predominant lymphocyte subset in acute and chronic liver inflammation. *Hepatology* 1991; **13**: 826–829.
15. Volpes R, van den Oord JJ, Desmet VJ. Vascular adhesion molecules in acute and chronic liver inflammation. *Hepatology* 1992; **15**: 269–275.
16. Mietkiewski JM, Scheuer PJ. Immunoglobulin-containing plasma cells in acute hepatitis. *Liver* 1985; **5**: 84–88.
17. Schmid M, Cueni B. Portal lesions in viral hepatitis with submassive hepatic necrosis. *Hum Pathol* 1972; **3**: 209–216.
18. Poulsen H, Christoffersen P. Abnormal bile duct epithelium in liver biopsies with histological signs of viral hepatitis. *Acta Pathol Microbiol Scand* 1969; **76**: 383–390.
19. Schmid M, Pirovino M, Altorfer J, Gudat F, Bianchi L. Acute hepatitis non-A, non-B; are there any specific light microscopic features? *Liver* 1982; **2**: 61–67.
20. Bach N, Thung SN, Schaffner F. The histological features of chronic hepatitis C and autoimmune chronic hepatitis: a comparative analysis. *Hepatology* 1992; **15**: 572–577.
21. Rappaport AM. The microcirculatory acinar concept of normal and pathological hepatic structure. *Beitr Pathol* 1976; **157**: 215–243.
22. Boyer JL, Klatskin G. Pattern of necrosis in acute viral hepatitis. Prognostic value of bridging (subacute hepatic necrosis). *N Engl J Med* 1970; **283**: 1063–1071.
23. Scheuer PJ, Maggi G. Hepatic fibrosis and collapse: histological distinction by orcein staining. *Histopathology* 1980; **4**: 487–490.
24. Thung SN, Gerber MA. The formation of elastic fibers in livers with massive hepatic necrosis. *Arch Pathol Lab Med* 1982; **106**: 468–469.
25. Roskams T, De Vos R, van den Oord JJ, Desmet V. Cells with neuroendocrine features in regenerating human liver. *APMIS* 1991; Suppl. 23: 32–39.
26. Abe H, Beninger PR, Ikejiri N, Setoyama H, Sata M, Tanikawa K. Light microscopic findings of liver biopsy specimens from patients with hepatitis type A and comparison with type B. *Gastroenterology* 1982; **82**: 938–947.
27. Okuno T, Sano A, Deguchi T et al. Pathology of acute hepatitis A in humans. Comparison with acute hepatitis B. *Am J Clin Pathol* 1984; **81**: 162–169.
28. Buitrago B, Popper H, Hadler SC et al. Specific histologic features of Santa Marta hepatitis: a severe form of hepatitis delta-virus infection in northern South America. *Hepatology* 1986; **6**: 1285–1291.
29. Lefkowitch JH, Goldstein H, Yatto R, Gerber MA. Cytopathic liver injury in acute delta virus hepatitis. *Gastroenterology* 1987; **92**: 1262–1266.
30. Ponz E, Garcia-Pagan JC, Bruguera M, Bruix J, Rodes J. Hepatic fibrin-ring granulomas in a patient with hepatitis A. *Gastroenterology* 1991; **100**: 268–270.
31. Ruel M, Sevestre H, Henry-Biabaud E, Courouce AM, Capron JP, Erlinger S. Fibrin ring granulomas in hepatitis A. *Dig Dis Sci* 1992; **37**: 1915–1917.
32. Taylor M, Goldin RD, Ladva S, Scheuer PJ, Thomas HC. In situ hybridization studies of hepatitis A viral RNA in patients with acute hepatitis A. *J Hepatol* 1994; **20**: 380–387.
33. Kryger P, Christoffersen P. Liver histopathology of the hepatitis A virus infection: a comparison with hepatitis type B and non-A, non-B. *J Clin Pathol* 1983; **36**: 650–654.
34. Rugge M, Vanstapel M-J, Ninfo V et al. Comparative histology of acute hepatitis B and non-A, non-B in Leuven and Padova. *Virchows Arch (A)* 1983; **401**: 275–288.
35. Dienes HP, Popper H, Arnold W, Lobeck H. Histologic observations in human hepatitis non-A, non-B. *Hepatology* 1982; **2**: 562–571.
36. Bianchi L, Gudat F. Chronic hepatitis. In MacSween RNM, Anthony PP, Scheuer PJ, Portmann B, Burt AD (eds): Pathology of the Liver, 3rd edn. Edinburgh: Churchill Livingstone, 1994.
37. Davies SE, Portmann BC, O'Grady JG et al. Hepatic histological findings after transplantation for chronic hepatitis B virus infection, including a unique pattern of fibrosing cholestatic hepatitis. *Hepatology* 1991; **13**: 150–157.
38. Min KW, Gyorkey F, Cain GD. Talc granulomata in liver disease in narcotic addicts. *Arch Pathol* 1974; **98**: 331–335.
39. Molos MA, Litton N, Schubert TT. Talc liver. *J Clin Gastroenterol* 1987; **9**: 198–203.
40. Bamber M, Murray A, Arborgh BA et al. Short incubation non-A, non-B hepatitis transmitted by factor VIII concentrates in patients with congenital coagulation disorders. *Gut* 1981; **22**: 854–859.
41. Hiramatsu N, Hayashi N, Haruna Y et al. Immunohistochemical detection of hepatitis C virus-infected hepatocytes in chronic liver disease with monoclonal antibodies to core, envelope and NS3 regions of the hepatitis C virus genome. *Hepatology* 1992; **16**: 306–311.
42. Krawczynski K, Beach MJ, Bradley DW et al. Hepatitis C virus antigen in hepatocytes: immunomorphologic detection and identification. *Gastroenterology* 1992; **103**: 622–629.
43. Yamada G, Nishimoto H, Endou H et al. Localization of hepatitis C viral RNA and capsid protein in human liver. *Dig Dis Sci* 1993; **38**: 882–887.
44. Craig JR, Govindarajan S, DeCock KM. Delta viral hepatitis. Histopathology and course. *Pathol Annu* 1986; **21**(2): 1–21.

45. Govindarajan S, De-Cock KM, Redeker AG. Natural course of delta superinfection in chronic hepatitis B virus-infected patients: histopathologic study with multiple liver biopsies. *Hepatology* 1986; **6**: 640–644.
46. Verme G, Amoroso P, Lettieri G et al. A histological study of hepatitis delta virus liver disease. *Hepatology* 1986; **6**: 1303–1307.
47. Lin H-H, Liaw Y-F, Chen T-J, Chu C-M, Huang M-J. Natural course of patients with chronic type B hepatitis following acute hepatitis delta virus superinfection. *Liver* 1989; **9**: 129–134.
48. Moreno A, Ramón y Cahal S, Marazuela M et al. Sanded nuclei in delta patients. *Liver* 1989; **9**: 367–371.
49. Negro F, Bonino F, Di Bisceglie A, Hoofnagle JH, Gerin JL. Intrahepatic markers of hepatitis delta virus infection: a study by *in situ* hybridization. *Hepatology* 1989; **10**: 916–920.
50. Pacchioni D, Negro F, Chiaberge E, Rizzetto M, Bonino F, Bussolati G. Detection of hepatitis delta virus RNA by a nonradioactive in situ hybridization procedure. *Hum Pathol* 1992; **23**: 557–561.
51. Lopez-Talavera JC, Buti M, Casacuberta J et al. Detection of hepatitis delta virus RNA in human liver tissue by non-radioactive in situ hybridization. *J Hepatol* 1993; **17**: 199–203.
52. Smedile A, Farci P, Verme G et al. Influence of delta infection on severity of hepatitis B. *Lancet* 1982; **ii**: 945–947.
53. Popper H, Thung SN, Gerber MA et al. Histologic studies of severe delta agent infection in Venezuelan Indians. *Hepatology* 1983; **3**: 906–912.
54. Sagnelli E, Felaco FM, Filippini P et al. Influence of HDV infection on clinical, biochemical and histological presentation of HBsAg positive chronic hepatitis. *Liver* 1989; **9**: 229–234.
55. Lau JYN, Hansen LJ, Bain VG et al. Expression of intrahepatic hepatitis D viral antigen in chronic hepatitis D virus infection. *J Clin Pathol* 1991; **44**: 549–553.
56. Davies SE, Lau JYN, O'Grady JG, Portmann BC, Alexander GJM, Williams R. Evidence that hepatitis D virus needs hepatitis B virus to cause hepatocellular damage. *Am J Clin Pathol* 1992; **98**: 554–558.
57. Zuckerman AJ. Hepatitis E virus. The main cause of enterically transmitted non-A, non-B hepatitis. *Br Med J* 1990; **300**: 1475–1476.
58. Khuroo MS, Dar MY, Zargar SA, Khan BA, Boda MI, Yattoo GN. Hepatitis C virus antibodies in acute and chronic liver disease in India. *J Hepatol* 1993; **17**: 175–179.
59. Jameel S, Durgapal H, Habibullah CM, Khuroo MS, Panda SK. Enteric non-A, non-B hepatitis: epidemics, animal transmission, and hepatitis E virus detection by the polymerase chain reaction. *J Med Virol* 1992; **37**: 263–270.
60. Dienes HP, Hütteroth T, Bianchi L, Grün M, Thoenes W. Hepatitis A-like non-A, non-B hepatitis: light and electron microscopic observations of three cases. *Virchows Arch (A)* 1986; **409**: 657–667.
61. Asher LVS, Innis BL, Shrestha MP, Ticehurst J, Baze WB. Virus-like particles in the liver of a patient with fulminant hepatitis and antibody to hepatitis E virus. *J Med Virol* 1990; **31**: 229–233.

GENERAL READING

Bonino F, Brunetto MR, Negro F, Smedile A, Ponzetto A. Hepatitis delta virus, a model of liver cell pathology. *J Hepatol* 1991; **13**: 260–266.

Jameel S, Durgapal H, Habibullah CM, Khuroo MS, Panda SK. Enteric non-A, non-B hepatitis: epidemics, animal transmission, and hepatitis E virus detection by the polymerase chain reaction. *J Med Virol* 1992; **37**: 263–270.

Lau JYN, Alexander GJM, Alberti A. Viral hepatitis. *Gut Suppl* 1991; S47–S62.

7

FATTY LIVER AND LESIONS IN THE ALCOHOLIC

Fatty liver (fatty change, steatosis) results from the accumulation of triglycerides in hepatocytes and is a frequent finding in biopsy and autopsy specimens. Its clinical presentation includes hepatomegaly as well as elevated activity of serum aminotransferases, alkaline phosphatase, and/or gamma glutamyl transpeptidase. Among the many aetiologies of fatty liver,[1] alcohol use, obesity, diabetes and malnutrition are the most common. In inflammatory and debilitating diseases such as tuberculosis, acquired immune deficiency syndrome and leukaemias the liver is also often fatty. The pathogenetic factors contributing to fatty liver include abnormalities in lipoprotein metabolism[2] and actions of cytokine mediators such as tumour necrosis factor.[3]

The pathologist's evaluation of the **type** of fat, **acinar distribution**, and possible **complications** (e.g. steatohepatitis, cirrhosis) provides important information concerning aetiology, the stage of architectural damage and prognosis. The complete pathological assessment of the fatty liver should take these elements into account (Table 7.1).

FATTY LIVER

Type of Fat and Acinar Distribution

Fatty change ranges from vacuolation of a few liver cells, usually in acinar zones 2 or 3, to severe involvement of all zones. While hepatocytes may contain fat droplets of various sizes, **macrovesicular steatosis** (large droplet fat) is the most common form (Fig. 7.1). Here, large single fat vacuoles displace the nuclei to one side. This is in contrast to **microvesicular steatosis** (small droplet fat) in which finely divided fat droplets occupy the hepatocyte cytoplasm, with the nucleus maintained in a more or less central position (Fig. 7.2). Specific fat stains such as Oil Red O on frozen sections may be necessary to identify microvesicular fat which is small in amount or extremely finely divided.

Histology alone is usually not sufficient to distinguish between the many respective causes of either large droplet or small droplet fat (Table 7.2). However, notation of the acinar zone involved may be helpful. Fat seen in alcoholism, obesity, diabetes and corticosteroid therapy is found predominantly in zone 3 (pericentral region). **Periportal** (zone 1) fat deposition (Fig. 7.3) is favoured in kwashiorkor,[4] the acquired immune deficiency syndrome[5] and total parenteral nutrition.[6] Fatty change is typically well distributed throughout the liver but occasionally **focal fat**[7] is encountered, which is often

Table 7.1. Pathological Evaluation of the Fatty Liver

Type
    Macrovesicular (large droplet)
    Microvesicular (small droplet)
    Mixed
    Focal fat
    Lipogranulomas (fat granulomas)
Acinar zone(s) involved
Complications
    Steatohepatitis (fatty liver hepatitis)
      Alcoholic hepatitis
      Non-alcoholic steatohepatitis (NASH)
    Steatohepatitis with cirrhosis
    Portal fibrosis

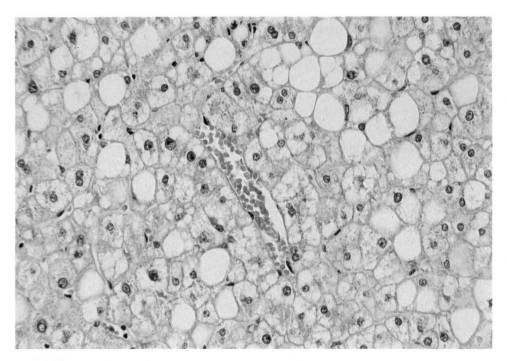

Figure 7.1. *Macrovesicular steatosis.* Large vacuoles of lipid are present in perivenular hepatocytes. The hepatocyte nuclei are compressed to the edge of the cytoplasm. Needle biopsy, H & E.

subcapsular. In an otherwise normal or minimally fatty liver, these mass-like lesions of macrovesicular fat may be confused with tumours on ultrasound or other imaging studies;[8] magnetic resonance imaging (MRI) is discriminating.[9]

Rupture of fat-laden hepatocytes evokes an inflammatory response which may take the form of focal accumulations of macrophages and leucocytes, or of **lipogranulomas** (fat granulomas) (Fig. 7.4). The latter can resemble granulomas of other aetiology, but serial sectioning sometimes reveals a fatty core.[10] Lipogranulomas lead to focal fibrosis, and this must be distinguished from the pericellular fibrosis of alcoholic hepatitis by the associated hepatocellular changes and more diffuse distribution of the latter. Focal fibrosis due to lipogranulomas seems to play no significant part in the development of serious chronic liver disease in the alcoholic. Clusters of vacuoles may also be seen in portal tracts, usually within macrophages[11] (Fig. 7.5).

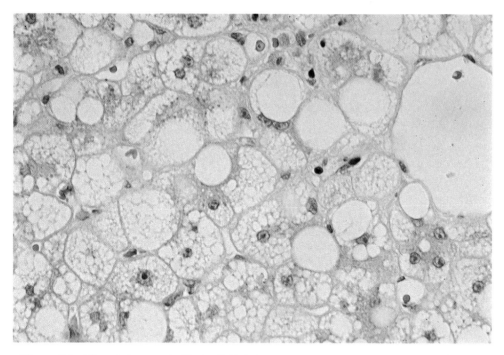

Figure 7.2. *Microvesicular steatosis.* Finely divided fat vacuoles are present in hepatocytes with nuclei maintained in a central position. Some large vacuoles are also seen. The terminal hepatic venule is at right. Needle biopsy, H & E.

Table 7.2. Causes of Large and Small Droplet Fatty Liver

Macrovesicular fat	Microvesicular fat
Alcohol	Fatty liver of pregnancy
Obesity	Reye's syndrome
Diabetes mellitus	Tetracycline toxicity
Corticosteroids	Valproate toxicity
Malnutrition	Alcoholic foamy degeneration
Chronic hepatitis C	Jamaican vomiting sickness
	Total parenteral nutrition
	Wolman's disease
	Cholesterol ester storage disease

In some series, no relationship was found between lipogranulomas and parenchymal fatty change. The fairly common isolated lipogranuloma that is attached to or near the wall of terminal hepatic venules (Fig. 7.6), as well as portal lipogranulomas, in non-fatty livers are probably reactions to ingested mineral oils rather than to neutral lipid of hepatocellular origin.[12-14]

Complications

Studies of alcoholics and other individuals with fatty liver have shown that under certain circumstances steatosis is associated with other pathological complications which are prognostically more serious. These complications include **steatohepatitis** (fatty liver hepatitis), an inflammatory and fibrosing condition associated with liver-cell injury, **portal fibrosis** and **cirrhosis**.

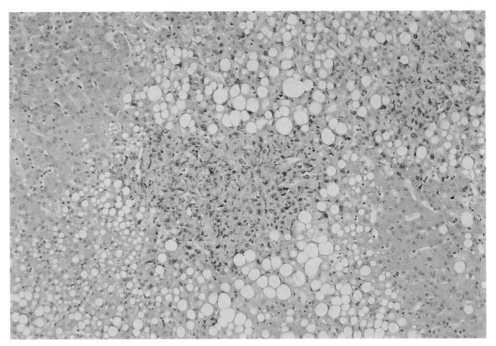

Figure 7.3. *Periportal steatosis.* Liver biopsy from a patient with AIDS and portal tract infiltration by large cell lymphoma. Periportal hepatocytes contain large fat vacuoles. Needle biopsy, H & E.

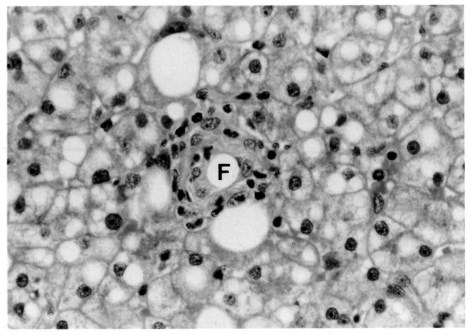

Figure 7.4. *Fat granuloma (lipogranuloma).* Macrophages and lymphocytes have accumulated around a fat vacuole (F). Needle biopsy, H & E.

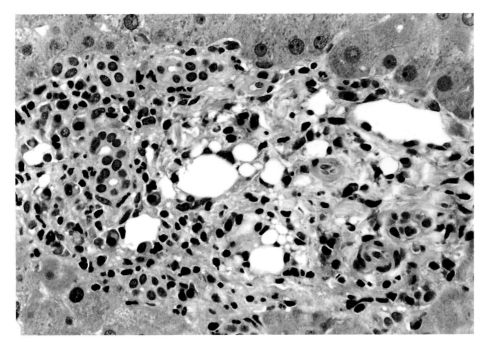

Figure 7.5. *Mineral oil granuloma.* Multiple vacuoles are seen in this portal tract of a patient who was not an alcohol abuser and whose hepatic parenchyma showed only very mild fatty change. The mineral oil nature of the vacuoles is presumed but not proved. Needle biopsy, H & E.

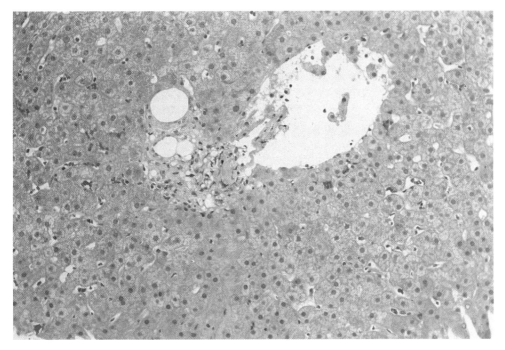

Figure 7.6. *Perivenular lipogranuloma.* A cluster of Kupffer cells and lymphocytes surrounding large vacuoles (lipogranuloma) is present to the left of the terminal hepatic venule. Needle biopsy, H & E.

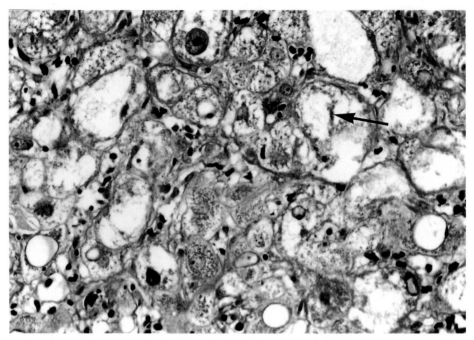

Figure 7.7. *Diabetes mellitus.* Steatohepatitis characterized by ballooned hepatocytes containing scanty Mallory material (arrow), inflammatory infiltration and pericellular fibrosis. Enlarged, vacuolated nuclei are seen in the lower part of the field. Needle biopsy, chromotrope-aniline blue (CAB).

Table 7.3. Causes of Steatohepatitis

Alcohol		
	Non-alcoholic steatohepatitis	
Obesity		Therapeutic drugs
Diabetes mellitus		Amiodarone
Jejunoileal bypass		Perhexilene maleate
Gastroplasty		Corticosteroids
Small bowel resection		Synthetic oestrogens
Weber–Christian disease		

The early stage of **steatohepatitis** is localized to acinar zone 3 and consists of a constellation of changes, including liver-cell ballooning, intracytoplasmic Mallory bodies, inflammatory infiltrates (predominantly neutrophils), and both perivenular and pericellular ("chicken-wire") fibrosis (Fig. 7.7). All these components need not be present in the individual case. Steatohepatitis has been best characterized in alcoholics, where the term **alcoholic hepatitis** is used. In individuals with fatty liver and steatohepatitis due to causes other than alcohol, such as obesity or diabetes[4,15,16] (Table 7.3), the term **non-alcoholic steatohepatitis** (NASH) is applied.[17–20] NASH has been well documented in obese and diabetic patients, though in the minority. Rapid weight loss in obese individuals and poor diabetic control may precipitate steatohepatitis.[21] Most patients with NASH show little, if any, progression of the condition. In some cases, however, inactive cirrhosis may develop, with disappearance of fat and hepatitis.[21]

While the features of non-alcoholic steatohepatitis are virtually identical to alcoholic hepatitis, non-alcoholics may have more marked fatty change. In the alcoholic, Mallory bodies are more plentiful and better formed, and neutrophils are in greater abundance.[17,18]

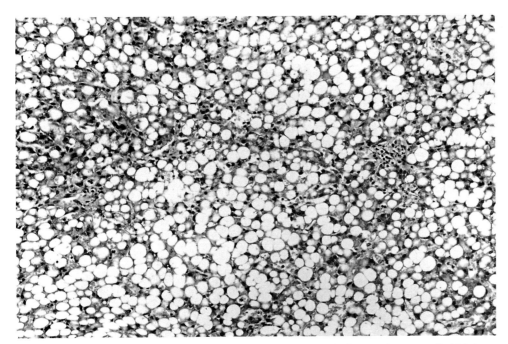

Figure 7.8. *Fatty liver in kwashiorkor.* Most of the hepatocytes contain fat vacuoles, some of which have coalesced. Needle biopsy, H & E.

In alcoholic and non-alcoholic fatty liver, there may be fibrosis without the other features of hepatitis, either within acini or resulting in **portal fibrosis**[4,16,22,23] and cirrhosis can develop.[16,24]

Small areas of fatty liver hepatitis or scarring are easily missed in haematoxylin and eosin-stained sections of fatty liver. Their presence has a marked effect on prognosis. Perivenular areas should therefore be carefully examined. In particular, a stain for collagen should be examined for pericellular and perivenular fibrosis.

Differential Diagnosis of Fatty Liver

In patients with fatty liver, a complete history should exclude alcohol and other chemicals or drugs. Other causes are shown in Table 7.2. Protein malnutrition, as seen in **kwashiorkor**, is characterized by severe macrovesicular fatty change (Fig. 7.8). There are fat vacuoles of regular size in periportal areas or throughout the acini.[25] Portal inflammation is at most mild, and while stellate fibrosis is sometimes seen there is no clear evidence that protein malnutrition alone leads to cirrhosis in man.[26] Electron microscopy shows lipid droplets within hepatocytes, depletion of peroxisomes and mitochondrial swelling. Canalicular cholestasis with loss of microvilli may be seen.[27]

Fatty change is also a regular finding in **obesity**, whether mild or severe[23,24,28–30] and may be accompanied by non-alcoholic steatohepatitis.[18,19] Fatty liver and fibrosis have been reported in obese children as well as adults.[31] Weight loss can lead to resolution of the fatty change.[32]

Steatohepatitis has been seen in severe form following **intestinal bypass operations** for obesity,[33] after **gastric partitioning**[34] and following **intestinal resection**.[35]

The commonest abnormality in the livers of patients with **diabetes mellitus** is fatty change. This is often accompanied by glycogen vacuolation of hepatocyte nuclei.

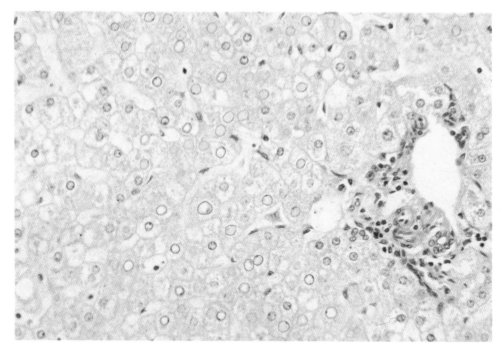

Figure 7.9. *Diabetes mellitus.* Numerous glycogenated nuclei are present in periportal hepatocytes. Needle biopsy, H & E.

Affected nuclei are moderately enlarged and appear empty (Fig. 7.9). Glycogen may no longer be demonstrable after fixation and processing, apart from a few clumps which remain next to the clearly defined nuclear membrane. It should be noted that glycogen vacuolation of nuclei is not confined to diabetics; it is found in normal subjects, especially children, and in Wilson's disease. Sometimes vacuolation is due not to glycogen but to the accumulation of lipid,[36] or to invagination of cytoplasm into the nucleus.

Steatohepatitis (Fig. 7.7) has been reported in patients with maturity onset diabetes,[17,37] and may precede the appearance of glucose intolerance.[38] It is probably responsible for the increased incidence of cirrhosis among diabetic patients. Conversely, patients with severe chronic active hepatitis and cirrhosis often have abnormalities of carbohydrate metabolism such as fasting hyperglycaemia or glucose intolerance.[39] Correction of hyperglycaemia in diabetics may result in regression of fatty change and steatohepatitis.[40] Even in the absence of steatohepatitis, insulin-dependent and non-insulin-dependent diabetics may show increased collagen, basement membrane material, laminin and fibronectin in the space of Disse.[41] A statistical association between diabetes mellitus and hepatocellular carcinoma has been reported.[42]

Patients with **chronic hepatitis C** (pp. 127–129) often have fatty change, predominantly large droplet.[43-45] Severe steatosis is seen in some cases but the majority show mild to moderate fat. Mallory body-like material is also occasionally present in hepatocytes.[45]

Reye's syndrome and **fatty liver of pregnancy**, both associated with small droplet fatty liver, are discussed in Chapter 15.

LESIONS IN THE ALCOHOLIC

Ethanol is a liver toxin, the effects of which depend largely on the duration and level of excess intake. However, the response of individuals to a given level of intake varies

Table 7.4. Liver Disease in the Alcoholic: Main Conditions and Related Lesions

Fatty liver
    Fat granulomas
    Alcoholic foamy degeneration
Alcoholic hepatitis and fibrosis
    Perivenular fibrosis
    Venous occlusion
Cirrhosis
Other syndromes and lesions
    Chronic hepatitis
    Fetal alcohol syndrome
    Pancreatitis
    Siderosis
    Hepatocellular carcinoma

greatly. In some subjects who habitually drink fairly heavily, the liver is histologically normal or only mildly fatty as judged by light microscopy. In others a variety of lesions is found[46] (Table 7.4).

Alcoholic fatty change typically consists of large fat vacuoles within hepatocytes in acinar zone 3 (Fig. 7.1), progressing further outward from perivenular regions with increasing severity of steatosis. Some alcoholics develop an acute fatty liver with finely vacuolated hepatocytes in perivenular areas (**alcoholic foamy degeneration**), usually in addition to the more common large fat droplets elsewhere. The condition may be transient but can also be fatal.[47,48] Other features include canalicular cholestasis, focal liver-cell necrosis and the formation of delicate collagen fibres in affected areas. Scanty Mallory bodies have been described, but inflammatory infiltration is minimal or absent and foamy degeneration thus appears to be distinct from alcoholic hepatitis.

Megamitochondria are seen by light microscopy as round or sometimes spindle-shaped cytoplasmic inclusions between 2 and 10 μm across; they are present in hepatocytes in many patients with different forms of alcoholic liver disease, and were found to be particularly abundant in the vacuolated perivenular hepatocytes of alcoholic foamy degeneration by Uchida et al.[49] Their presence does not prove that the patient has alcoholic liver disease, however, as they are sometimes seen in non-alcoholic patients. Bruguera et al,[50] in a study of alcoholics, found the megamitochondria to be a good indicator of recent heavy drinking, whereas Chedid et al[51] saw them more often in mild than in severe alcoholic hepatitis. Junge et al[52] found them much more often in livers with alcohol-related than in those with non-alcoholic fibrosis. They are well seen in trichrome stains such as chromotrope-aniline blue (CAB) in which they appear red (Fig. 7.10) but are also easily visible with haematoxylin and eosin. They must be distinguished from Mallory bodies, which have a less distinct outline and usually stain blue with CAB.

Alcoholic Hepatitis and Fibrosis

The term "alcoholic hepatitis" , originally used for a clinical syndrome, is now usually defined by a combination of histological features. "Alcoholic steatonecrosis",[53] "fatty liver hepatitis", and "steatohepatitis" are alternative terms; although they imply the presence of fatty change, it is sometimes scanty. In the following discussion the term "alcoholic hepatitis" will be used.

The lesion is distinctive in its distribution and character. In its early stages it is maximal near terminal hepatic venules. Most or all acini are affected but a few may escape injury, a fact to be kept in mind when a small biopsy specimen is assessed. Later, in more severe examples, as necrotic bridges and fibrous septa come to link terminal hepatic venules to

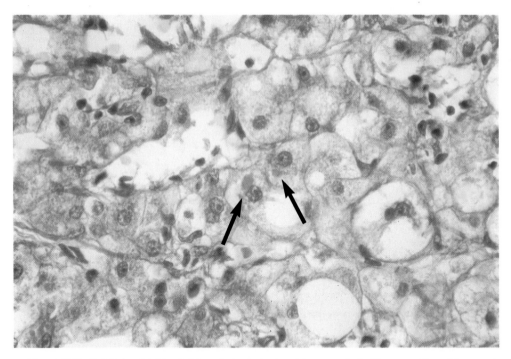

Figure 7.10. *Alcoholic hepatitis.* Two bright-red giant mitochondria are marked with arrows. There is increased collagen, stained blue, around ballooned hepatocytes. Needle biopsy, CAB.

portal tracts, periportal areas are also affected.[54] It may then prove difficult to be sure of the acinar location of the changes but connective tissue staining usually resolves the difficulty.

The essential components of alcoholic hepatitis are liver-cell damage, inflammation and fibrosis.[46] Fatty change is usual but is not invariably present. Liver-cell damage takes the form of ballooning, with loss of the normal polygonal cell shape. Affected cells have abundant pale-staining cytoplasm, with or without fat vacuoles (Figs 7.10 and 7.11). They may contain megamitochondria or Mallory bodies, often seen together in the same liver but usually not in the same cell.[51] Mallory bodies (also known as alcoholic hyalin or hyaline) are clumps, strands or perinuclear rings of dense material composed largely of the intermediate filaments of the cytoskeleton[46,55] (Figs 7.11–7.13). Under the electron microscope a number of different patterns are seen, most commonly clusters of randomly orientated filaments and less often bundles of parallel filaments or granular non-filamentous material[56] (Fig. 17.9, p. 290). Mallory bodies are occasionally seen in bile duct epithelium as well as in hepatocytes.[57] Hepatocytic Mallory bodies are neither specific for alcoholic hepatitis (since they are also found in other forms of fatty liver hepatitis and in cholate stasis) nor necessary for its diagnosis. However, when seen together with the other changes of alcoholic hepatitis in a perivenular location, they help to produce a very striking and characteristic picture. Canalicular cholestasis is sometimes seen in severe alcoholic hepatitis. It can also result from pancreatitis (see below).

The inflammatory infiltrate in alcoholic hepatitis is typically rich in neutrophils, but lymphocytes[57a] and macrophages are also found and sometimes predominate. Neutrophils are seen either among (Fig. 7.12) or even within damaged hepatocytes (Fig. 7.13). Inflammation is sometimes slight (Fig. 7.11) or even lacking from the constellation of changes. This probably reflects a stage of evolution of the lesion, but makes the histological diagnosis of a "hepatitis" difficult. Sometimes an isolated hepatocyte is

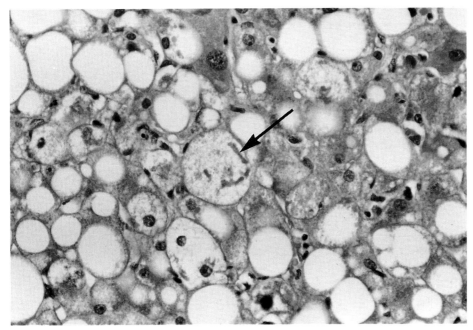

Figure 7.11. *Alcoholic hepatitis*. A ballooned hepatocyte contains Mallory bodies (arrow) and retained protein. Needle biopsy, H & E.

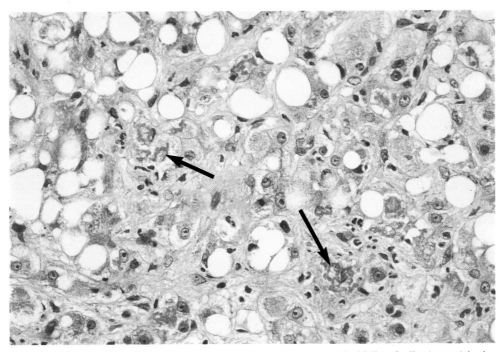

Figure 7.12. *Alcoholic hepatitis*. Hepatocytes are swollen and many contain Mallory bodies (arrows) in the form of strands and clumps of brightly stained cytoplasmic material. There is fatty change. A few neutrophil leucocytes are seen. Needle biopsy, H & E.

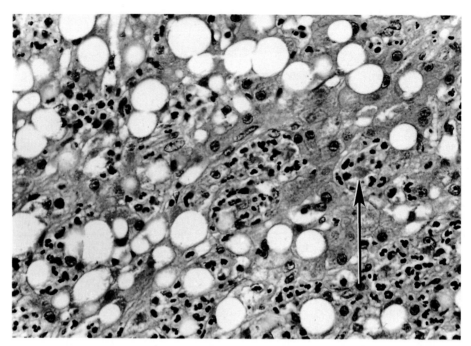

Figure 7.13. *Alcoholic hepatitis.* Clumps of neutrophil leucocytes have accumulated around and within single hepatocytes, some of which contain Mallory bodies (arrow). There is fatty change. Wedge biopsy, H & E.

ballooned and contains scanty Mallory material, in a liver biopsy otherwise showing only fatty change but neither inflammation nor fibrosis.

Fibrosis is a constant feature of alcoholic hepatitis, and is an important factor in its transition to cirrhosis.[58] When it is not clearly seen in a good section appropriately stained for collagen, the diagnosis should at least be questioned. The most characteristic form is pericellular (perisinusoidal) fibrosis, around individual ballooned hepatocytes (Figs 7.10 and 7.14). On three-dimensional reconstruction studies, such apparently isolated hepatocytes form part of parenchymal "pillars" that are surrounded by fibrosis and basement membrane material.[59] This is often visible in reticulin preparations as a meshwork of new fibres in perivenular areas. The fibrosis persists for a variable time after resolution of an alcoholic hepatitis, providing evidence of a previous attack (Fig. 7.15). In some examples of alcoholic hepatitis liver-cell destruction and fibrosis are extensive, leading to large fibrous scars in perivenular areas (Fig. 7.16). Fibrous bridges link these scars to portal tracts. Over time, proliferation of bile ductules at the margins of portal tracts may develop in association with periportal inflammation ("piecemeal necrosis").[60]

Fibrosis also involves the terminal hepatic venules, giving rise to thickening of their walls (Fig. 7.17). It has been suggested that this process of **perivenular fibrosis** is a marker of future cirrhosis in persistent drinkers,[61,62] although others believe that the frequently associated pericellular fibrosis is the more important prognostic feature.[63] Perivenular fibrosis may be seen without histological features of alcoholic hepatitis and, while it could represent residual changes of a previous hepatitis, it has been postulated that it can also develop in its absence, both in laboratory animals and in man.[64] Lipocytes (perisinusoidal or fat-storing cells, Ito cells) are thought to be responsible for the fibrosis; their apparent transformation into fibroblast-like cells has been documented in liver biopsies from patients with alcoholic liver disease.[65]

In some examples of alcoholic hepatitis, fibrosis narrows or occludes the lumens of terminal hepatic venules.[66,67] The occluded veins can easily be seen within fibrous scars by means of collagen stains (Fig. 7.18) but may be missed in sections stained with

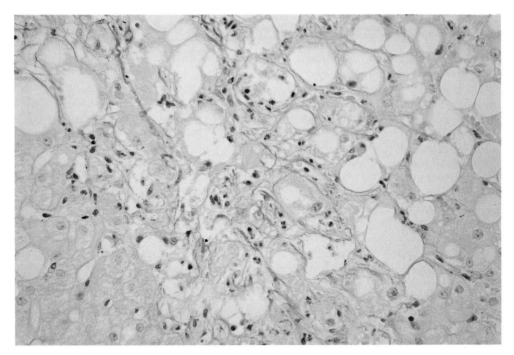

Figure 7.14. *Alcoholic hepatitis.* There is pericellular fibrosis in a perivenular area. Collagen fibres are stained red. Needle biopsy, haematoxylin–van Gieson (HVG).

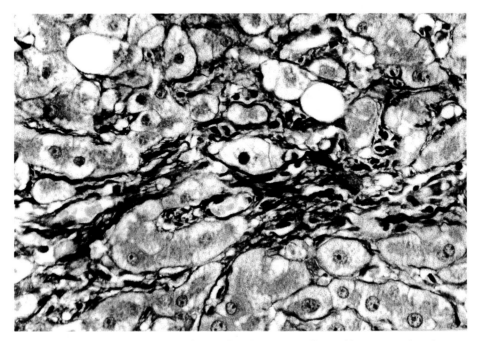

Figure 7.15. *Pericellular fibrosis in an alcoholic.* Deeply stained collagen fibres surround and separate hepatocytes, some of which contain fat. There are no changes of current alcoholic hepatitis, but this patient was known to have had alcoholic hepatitis previously and the fibrosis may therefore represent a residual feature. Needle biopsy, CAB.

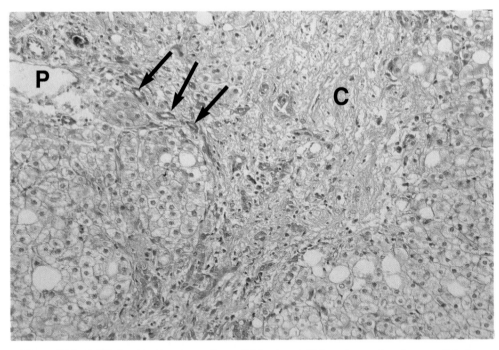

Figure 7.16. *Alcoholic hepatitis.* Abundant collagen (C) has been laid down in a perivenular area, linked to a portal tract (P) by a fibrous bridge containing proliferated bile ducts (arrows). Needle biopsy, Martius Scarlet Blue stain (MSB).

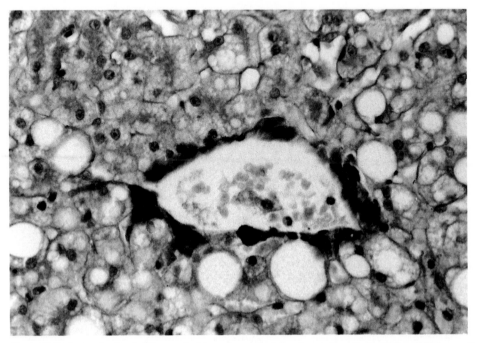

Figure 7.17. *Perivenular fibrosis.* The terminal hepatic venule shown has an irregularly thickened fibrous wall. Surrounding parenchyma is fatty but shows no changes of alcoholic hepatitis. Needle biopsy, HVG.

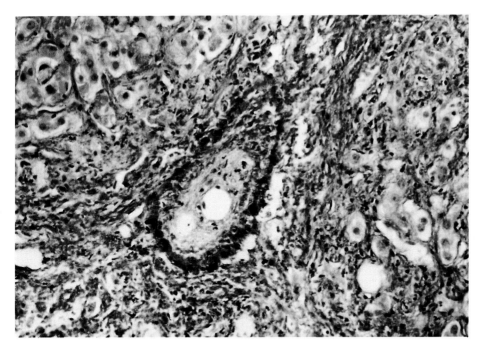

Figure 7.18. *Venous occlusion in alcoholic hepatitis.* An efferent vein in the centre of the field is grossly narrowed by fibrous tissue. Post-mortem liver, HVG.

haematoxylin and eosin. Venous occlusion is sometimes but not always associated with clinical features of venous outflow block.

Differential Diagnosis of Alcoholic Hepatitis

Differentiation from **viral hepatitis** is usually easy; the nature of the liver-cell damage and inflammatory infiltrate is different, and viral hepatitis causes collapse of pre-existing connective tissue rather than formation of new collagen. When inflammation, liver-cell ballooning and Mallory bodies are absent, the perivenular and pericellular fibrosis of alcoholic liver disease may be mistaken for the fibrosis of **chronic venous congestion**. This is seen in patients with **alcoholic cardiomyopathy**, together with other features of chronic congestion.[68]

Hepatocellular ballooning, Mallory bodies, neutrophils and fibrosis may all be found in a number of circumstances and diseases unrelated to alcohol. These include **chronic cholestasis** (p. 44) and **Wilson's disease** (p. 218), in which the risk of confusion is slight because of the anatomical location of the lesions and clinical circumstances. Pericellular fibrosis, sometimes progressing to cirrhosis, may also be seen in **hypervitaminosis A**.[69,70] Fatty change and fibrosis may develop in patients on long-term **methotrexate therapy** but the fibrosis is characteristically periportal rather than perivenular. As discussed earlier, **non-alcoholic steatohepatitis** closely resembling alcoholic hepatitis may be seen in obesity and diabetes,[17,33,37] intestinal bypass operations, treatment with perhexiline maleate,[71,72] amiodarone[73,74] or steroid hormones.[75]

Cirrhosis in the Alcoholic

Cirrhosis in the alcoholic is thought to be the result of alcoholic hepatitis in most instances, although non-hepatitic fibrosis has been postulated as an alternative pathway,

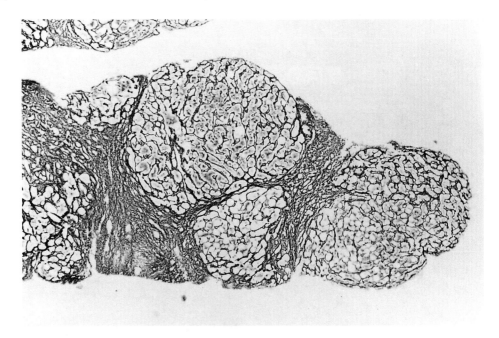

Figure 7.19. *Cirrhosis in an alcoholic.* A micronodular pattern is seen, with nodules of acinar size or smaller. Needle biopsy, reticulin.

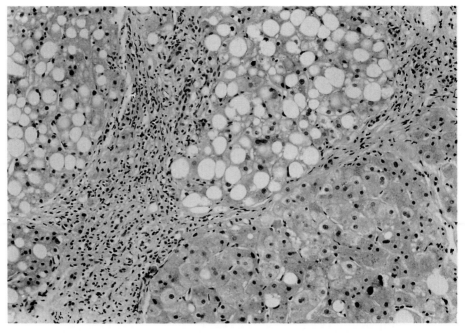

Figure 7.20. *Cirrhosis in an alcoholic.* Some nodules are rich in fat. Needle biopsy, H & E.

as indicated in the previous section. Evolution of alcoholic hepatitis to cirrhosis is accelerated by contraction of fibrous bridges linking perivenular to portal areas.[54] Regeneration of the surviving parenchyma then leads to the formation of small nodules, often showing fatty change (Figs 7.19 and 7.20). Features of alcoholic hepatitis in addition to the cirrhosis make the prognosis worse.[76] In their absence, evidence of an alcoholic aetiology is provided by dense fibrosis blurring the edges of nodules, venous occlusion or fatty change; however, the latter can result from other causes. Regeneration nodules may be seen in some parts of a biopsy while acinar architecture is preserved elsewhere; thus an exact onset of cirrhosis is difficult to determine, and a report of "developing cirrhosis" may be appropriate. Later in the course of the cirrhosis, nodule size increases and the character of the cirrhosis changes. Eventually all histological features of the alcoholic aetiology may be lost.

Lesions other than alcoholic hepatitis and fibrosis may contribute to or cause cirrhosis in the alcoholic. These include **chronic hepatitis**, whether viral or due to alcohol itself[77-79] (see "Other liver lesions in the alcoholic"). Features of chronic active hepatitis, notably piecemeal necrosis and portal or acinar lymphocytic infiltration, may be superimposed on those of alcoholic hepatitis and should prompt serologic studies to exclude hepatitis virus infection, particularly **hepatitis C**.[80] Acute viral hepatitis is a serious complication in patients with established alcoholic cirrhosis.[81]

Other Liver Lesions in the Alcoholic

Portal tract infiltrates of lymphocytes and plasma cells with piecemeal necrosis are unusual in alcoholics unless **chronic hepatitis** is present. While this is possibly due to alcohol itself,[82] in most instances it is due to chronic viral hepatitis, particularly hepatitis C.[80,83] Portal lymphoid follicles or aggregates and lymphocytic inflammation of portal tracts and acini[80] are helpful in recognizing chronic hepatitis C (see Chapter 9) which should be confirmed by serological studies and other techniques such as the polymerase chain reaction for hepatitis C viral RNA.[84,85] Extensive **perivenular necrosis**, on the other hand, may develop in alcoholics taking therapeutic doses of **paracetamol (acetaminophen)**.[86,87]

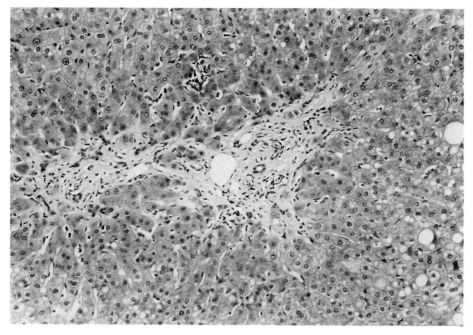

Figure 7.21. *Portal fibrosis in an alcoholic.* Fibrosis extends irregularly from a small portal tract. The parenchyma shows mild fatty change. Needle biopsy, H & E.

In the **fetal alcohol syndrome**, children of mothers abusing alcohol during pregnancy may have fatty livers together with perisinusoidal and portal fibrosis. The fibrosis resembles that seen in alcoholic adults and in laboratory animals.[88]

Chronic alcoholic pancreatitis leads to stricturing of the pancreatic duct system and to bile-duct obstruction.[89,90,90a] The liver changes are those of bile duct obstruction from any cause, with or without cholangitis. Biliary cirrhosis develops in a minority of patients.[91] Fibrosis predominantly or solely portal in distribution (Fig. 7.21) should arouse a suspicion of possible chronic pancreatitis,[92] as should unexplained cholestasis.

Hepatocellular **siderosis** is sometimes seen in alcoholics but is rarely sufficient to cause confusion with genetic haemochromatosis.[93] LeSage et al[94] concluded that severe siderosis was likely to be the result of genetic haemochromatosis, irrespective of alcohol abuse. Difficult cases are best resolved by quantitative tissue iron determination and calculation of the hepatic iron index.[95]

Hepatocellular carcinoma may complicate alcoholic cirrhosis, especially in long-term survivors. Alcohol intake may promote the development of hepatocellular carcinoma in hepatitis B virus carriers[96] and in patients with chronic hepatitis C.[97–99]

REFERENCES

1. Hoyumpa AM, Greene HL, Dunn GD, Schenker SS. Fatty liver: biochemical and clinical considerations. *Dig Dis* 1975; **20**: 1142–1170.
2. Sabesin SM, Ragland JB, Freeman MR. Lipoprotein disturbances in liver disease. In Popper H, Schaffner F (eds): Progress in Liver Diseases, Vol. VI. Orlando: Grune and Stratton, 1979, pp 243–262.
3. Grunfeld C, Kotler DP. Wasting in the acquired immunodeficiency syndrome. *Semin Liver Dis* 1992; **12**: 175–187.
4. Schaffner F, Thaler H. Nonalcoholic fatty liver disease. In Popper H, Schaffner F (eds): Progress in Liver Diseases, Vol. VIII. Orlando: Grune and Stratton, 1986, pp 283–298.
5. Lefkowitch JH. Pathologic aspects of the liver in human immunodeficiency virus (HIV) infection. In McIntyre N, Benhamou J-P, Bircher J, Rizzetto M, Rodés J (eds): Oxford Textbook of Clinical Hepatology. Oxford: Oxford University Press, 1991, pp 630-634.
6. Quigley EMM, Marsh MN, Shaffer JL, Markin RS. Hepatobiliary complications of total parenteral nutrition. *Gastroenterology* 1993; **104**: 286–301.
7. Brawer MK, Austin GE, Lewin KJ. Focal fatty change of the liver, a hitherto poorly recognized entity. *Gastroenterology* 1980; **78**: 247–252.
8. Clain JE, Stephens DH, Charboneau JW. Ultrasonography and computed tomography in focal fatty liver. Report of two cases with special emphasis on changing appearances over time. *Gastroenterology* 1984; **87**: 948–952.
9. Johnson CD. Magnetic resonance imaging of the liver: current clinical applications. *Mayo Clin Proc* 1993; **68**: 147–156.
10. Christoffersen P, Braendstrup O, Juhl E, Poulsen H. Lipogranulomas in human liver biopsies with fatty change. A morphological, biochemical and clinical investigation. *Acta Pathol Microbiol Scand A* 1971; **79**: 150–158.
11. Delladetsima JK, Horn T, Poulsen H. Portal tract lipogranulomas in liver biopsies. *Liver* 1987; **7**: 9–17.
12. Dincsoy HP, Weesner RE, MacGee J. Lipogranulomas in non-fatty human livers. A mineral oil induced environmental disease. *Am J Clin Pathol* 1982; **78**: 35–41.
13. Cruickshank B, Thomas MJ. Mineral oil (follicular) lipidosis: II. Histologic studies of spleen, liver, lymph nodes, and bone marrow. *Hum Pathol* 1984; **15**: 731–737.
14. Wanless IR, Geddie WR. Mineral oil lipogranulomata in liver and spleen. A study of 465 autopsies. *Arch Pathol Lab Med* 1985; **109**: 283–286.
15. Thaler H. Relation of steatosis to cirrhosis. *Clin Gastroenterol* 1975; **4**: 273–280.
16. Adler M, Schaffner F. Fatty liver hepatitis and cirrhosis in obese patients. *Am J Med* 1979; **67**: 811–816.
17. Ludwig J, Viggiano TR, McGill DB, Oh BJ. Nonalcoholic steatohepatitis: Mayo Clinic experiences with a hitherto unnamed disease. *Mayo Clin Proc* 1980; **55**: 434–438.
18. Diehl AM, Goodman Z, Ishak KG. Alcohollike liver disease in nonalcoholics. A clinical and histologic comparison with alcohol-induced liver injury. *Gastroenterology* 1988; **95**: 1056–1062.
19. Lee RG. Nonalcoholic steatohepatitis: a study of 49 patients. *Hum Pathol* 1989; **20**: 594–598.
20. Wanless IR, Lentz JS. Fatty liver hepatitis (steatohepatitis) and obesity: an autopsy study with analysis of risk factors. *Hepatology* 1990; **12**: 1106–1110.
21. Powell EE, Cooksley GE, Hanson R, Searle J, Halliday JW, Powell LW. The natural history of nonalcoholic steatohepatitis: a follow-up study of forty-two patients for up to 21 years. *Hepatology* 1990; **11**: 74–80.

22. Galambos J, Wills CE. Relationship between 505 paired liver tests and biopsies in 242 obese patients. *Gastroenterology* 1978; **74**: 1191–1195.

23. Nasrallah SM, Wills CE Jr, Galambos JT. Hepatic morphology in obesity. *Dig Dis Sci* 1981; **26**: 325–327.

24. Kern WH, Heger AH, Payne JH, DeWind LT. Fatty metamorphosis of the liver in morbid obesity. *Arch Pathol* 1973; **96**: 342–346.

25. Webber BL, Freiman I. The liver in kwashiorkor. A clinical and electron microscopical study. *Arch Pathol* 1974; **98**: 400–408.

26. Nayak NC. Nutritional liver disease. In MacSween RNM, Anthony PP, Scheuer PJ (eds): Pathology of the Liver, 2nd edn. Edinburgh: Churchill Livingstone, 1987, pp 265–280.

27. Brooks SEH, Goldon MHN, Taylor E. Hepatic ultrastructure in children with protein-energy malnutrition. *West Indian Med J* 1992; **42**: 139–145.

28. Massarrat S, Jordan G, Sahrhage G, Korb G, Bode JC, Dolle W. Five-year follow-up study of patients with nonalcoholic and nondiabetic fatty liver. *Acta Hepato-Gastroenterol* 1974; **21**: 176–186.

29. Braillon A, Capron JP, Herve MA, Degott C, Quenum C. Liver in obesity. *Gut* 1985; **26**: 133–139.

30. Clain DJ, Lefkowitch JH. Fatty liver disease in morbid obesity. *Gastroenterol Clin N Amer* 1987; **16**: 239–252.

31. Kinugasa A, Tsunamoto K, Furukawa N, Sawada T, Kusunoki T, Shimada N. Fatty liver and its fibrous changes found in simple obesity of children. *J Ped Gastroenterol Nutr* 1984; **3**: 408–414.

32. Keefe EB, Adesman PW, Stenzel P, Palmer RM. Steatosis and cirrhosis in an obese diabetic. *Dig Dis Sci* 1987; **32**: 441–445.

33. Marubbio AT Jr, Buchwald H, Schwartz MZ, Varco R. Hepatic lesions of central pericellular fibrosis in morbid obesity, and after jejunoileal bypass. *Am J Clin Pathol* 1976; **66**: 684–691.

34. Hamilton DL, Vest TK, Brown BS, Shah AN, Menguy RB, Chey WY. Liver injury with alcoholic-like hyalin after gastroplasty for morbid obesity. *Gastroenterology* 1983; **85**: 722–726.

35. Peura DA, Stromeyer FW, Johnson LF. Liver injury with alcoholic hyaline after intestinal resection. *Gastroenterology* 1980; **79**: 128–130.

36. Haboubi NY, Brown C. 'Vacuolation' and 'glycogenation' not synonymous. *Histopathology* 1985; **9**: 1246–1247.

37. Falchuk KR, Fiske SC, Haggitt RC, Federman M, Trey C. Pericentral hepatic fibrosis and intracellular hyalin in diabetes mellitus. *Gastroenterology* 1980; **78**: 535–541.

38. Batman PA, Scheuer PJ. Diabetic hepatitis preceding the onset of glucose intolerance. *Histopathology* 1985; **9**: 237–243.

39. Kingston ME, Ali MA, Atiyeh M, Donnelly RJ. Diabetes mellitus in chronic active hepatitis and cirrhosis. *Gastroenterology* 1984; **87**: 688–694.

40. Tak PP, ten Kate FJW. Remission of active diabetic hepatitis after correction of hyperglycemia. *Liver* 1993; **13**: 183–187.

41. Latry P, Bioulac-Sage P, Echinard E et al. Perisinusoidal fibrosis and basement membrane-like material in the livers of diabetic patients. *Hum Pathol* 1987; **18**: 775–780.

42. Lawson DH, Gray JM, McKillop C, Clarke J, Lee FD, Patrick RS. Diabetes mellitus and primary hepatocellular carcinoma. *Quart J Med* 1986; **61**: 945–955.

43. Scheuer PJ, Ashrafzadeh P, Sherlock S, Brown D, Dusheiko GM. The pathology of hepatitis C. *Hepatology* 1992; **15**: 567–571.

44. Bach N, Thung SN, Schaffner F. The histological features of chronic hepatitis C and autoimmune chronic hepatitis: a comparative analysis. *Hepatology* 1992; **15**: 572–577.

45. Lefkowitch JH, Schiff ER, Davis GL et al. Pathological diagnosis of chronic hepatitis C: a multicenter comparative study with chronic hepatitis B. *Gastroenterology* 1993; **104**: 595–603.

46. French SW, Nash J, Shitabata P et al. Pathology of alcoholic liver disease. *Semin Liver Dis* 1993; **13**: 154–169.

47. Morgan MY, Sherlock S, Scheuer PJ. Acute cholestasis, hepatic failure, and fatty liver in the alcoholic. *Scand J Gastroenterol* 1978; **13**: 299–303.

48. Uchida T, Kao H, Quispe-Sjogren M, Peters RL. Alcoholic foamy degeneration – a pattern of acute alcoholic injury of the liver. *Gastroenterology* 1983; **84**: 683–692.

49. Uchida T, Kronborg I, Peters RL. Alcoholic hyalin-containing hepatocytes – a characteristic morphologic appearance. *Liver* 1984; **4**: 233–243.

50. Bruguera M, Bertran A, Bombi JA, Rodes J. Giant mitochondria in hepatocytes: a diagnostic hint for alcoholic liver disease. *Gastroenterology* 1977; **73**: 1383–1387.

51. Chedid A, Mendenhall CL, Tosch T et al. Significance of megamitochondria in alcoholic liver disease. *Gastroenterology* 1986; **90**: 1858–1864.

52. Junge J, Horn T, Christoffersen P. Megamitochondria as a diagnostic marker for alcohol induced centrilobular and periportal fibrosis in the liver. *Virchows Arch A Pathol Anat Histopathol* 1987; **410**: 553–558.

53. Birschbach HR, Harinasuta U, Zimmerman HJ. Alcoholic steatonecrosis. II. Prospective study of prevalence of Mallory bodies in biopsy specimens and comparison of severity of hepatic disease in patients with and without this histological feature. *Gastroenterology* 1974; **66**: 1195–1202.

54. Gerber MA, Popper H. Relation between central canals and portal tracts in alcoholic hepatitis. A contribution to the pathogenesis of cirrhosis in alcoholics. *Hum Pathol* 1972; **3**: 199–207.

55. French SW. Present understanding of the development of Mallory's body. *Arch Pathol Lab Med* 1983; **107**: 445–450.

56. Yokoo H, Minick OT, Batti F, Kent G. Morphologic variants of alcoholic hyalin. *Am J Pathol* 1972; **69**: 25–40.

57. Uchida T, Peters RL. The nature and origin of proliferated bile ductules in alcoholic liver disease. *Am J Clin Pathol* 1983; **79**: 326–333.

57a. Chedid A, Mendenhall CL, Moritz TE et al. Cell-mediated hepatic injury in alcoholic liver disease. *Gastroenterology* 1993; **105**: 254–266.

58. Popper H. The pathogenesis of alcoholic cirrhosis. In Fisher MM, Rankin JG (eds): Alcohol and the Liver. New York: Plenum Press, 1977, pp 289–305.

59. Dinges HP, Zatloukal K, Denk H, Smolle J, Mair S. Alcoholic liver disease. Parenchyma to stroma relationship in fibrosis and cirrhosis as revealed by three-dimensional reconstruction and immunohisto-chemistry. *Am J Pathol* 1992; **141**: 69–83.

60. Ray MB, Mendenhall CL, French SW, Gartside PS, Veterans Administration Cooperative Study Group. Bile duct changes in alcoholic liver disease. *Liver* 1993; **13**: 36–45.

61. Nakano M, Worner TM, Lieber CS. Perivenular fibrosis in alcoholic liver injury: ultrastructure and histologic progression. *Gastroenterology* 1982; **83**: 777–785.

62. Worner TM, Lieber CS. Perivenular fibrosis as precursor lesion of cirrhosis. *JAMA* 1985; **254**: 627–630.

63. Nasrallah SM, Nassar VH, Galambos JT. Importance of terminal hepatic venule thickening. *Arch Pathol Lab Med* 1980; **104**: 84–86.

64. Van Waes L, Lieber CS. Early perivenular sclerosis in alcoholic fatty liver: an index of progressive liver injury. *Gastroenterology* 1977; **73**: 646–650.

65. Okanoue T, Burbige EJ, French SW. The role of the Ito cell in perivenular and intralobular fibrosis in alcoholic hepatitis. *Arch Pathol Lab Med* 1983; **107**: 459–463.

66. Goodman ZD, Ishak KG. Occlusive venous lesions in alcoholic liver disease. A study of 200 cases. *Gastroenterology* 1982; **83**: 786–796.

67. Burt AD, MacSween RN. Hepatic vein lesions in alcoholic liver disease: retrospective biopsy and necropsy study. *J Clin Pathol* 1986; **39**: 63–67.

68. Lefkowitch JH, Fenoglio JJ Jr. Liver disease in alcoholic cardiomyopathy: evidence against cirrhosis. *Hum Pathol* 1983; **14**: 457–463.

69. Russell RM, Boyer JL, Bagheri SA, Hruban Z. Hepatic injury from chronic hypervitaminosis A resulting in portal hypertension and ascites. *N Engl J Med* 1974; **291**: 435–440.

70. Jorens PG, Michielsen PP, Pelckmans PA et al. Vitamin A abuse: development of cirrhosis despite cessation of vitamin A. A six-year clinical and histopathologic follow-up. *Liver* 1992; **12**: 381–386.

71. Lewis D, Wainwright HC, Kew MC, Zwi S, Isaacson C. Liver damage associated with perhexiline maleate. *Gut* 1979; **20**: 186–189.

72. Pessayre D, Bichara M, Degott C, Potet F, Benhamou JP, Feldmann G. Perhexiline maleate-induced cirrhosis. *Gastroenterology* 1979; **76**: 170–177.

73. Poucell S, Ireton J, Valencia-Mayoral P et al. Amiodarone-associated phospholipidosis and fibrosis of the liver. Light, immunohistochemical, and electron microscopic studies. *Gastroenterology* 1984; **86**: 926–936.

74. Rigas B, Rosenfeld LE, Barwick KW et al. Amiodarone hepatotoxicity. A clinicopathologic study of five patients. *Ann Intern Med* 1986; **104**: 348–351.

75. Seki K, Minami Y, Nishikawa M et al. "Nonalcoholic steatohepatitis" induced by massive doses of synthetic estrogen. *Gastroenterol Japon* 1983; **18**: 197–203.

76. Orrego H, Blake JE, Blendis LM, Medline A. Prognosis of alcoholic cirrhosis in the presence and absence of alcoholic hepatitis. *Gastroenterology* 1987; **92**: 208–214.

77. Goldberg SJ, Mendenhall CL, Connell AM, Chedid A. "Nonalcoholic" chronic hepatitis in the alcoholic. *Gastroenterology* 1977; **72**: 598–604.

78. Crapper RM, Bhathaland PS, Mackay IR. Chronic active hepatitis in alcoholic patients. *Liver* 1983; **3**: 327–337.

79. Nei J, Matsuda Y, Takada A. Chronic hepatitis induced by alcohol. *Dig Dis Sci* 1983; **28**: 207–215.

80. Rosman AS, Paronetto F, Galvin K, Williams RJ, Lieber CS. Hepatitis C virus antibody in alcoholic patients. Association with the presence of portal and/or lobular hepatitis. *Arch Intern Med* 1993; **153**: 965–969.

81. Feller A, Uchida T, Rakela J. Acute viral hepatitis superimposed on alcoholic liver cirrhosis: clinical and histopathologic features. *Liver* 1985; **5**: 239–246.

82. Takase S, Takada N, Enomoto N, Yasuhara M, Takada A. Different types of chronic hepatitis in alcoholic patients: does chronic hepatitis induced by alcohol exist? *Hepatology* 1991; **13**: 876–881.

83. Caldwell SH, Jeffers LJ, Ditomaso A et al. Antibody to hepatitis C is common among patients with alcoholic liver disease with and without risk factors. *Am J Gastroenterol* 1991; **86**: 1219–1223.

84. Mendenhall CL, Seeff L, Diehl AM et al. Antibodies to hepatitis B virus and hepatitis C virus in alcoholic hepatitis and cirrhosis: their prevalence and clinical relevance. *Hepatology* 1991; **14**: 581–589.

85. Nalpos B, Thiers V, Pol S et al. Hepatitis C viremia and anti-HCV antibodies in alcoholics. *J Hepatol* 1992; **14**: 381–384.

86. Seeff LB, Cuccherini BA, Zimmerman HJ, Adler E, Benjamin S. Acetaminophen hepatotoxicity in alcoholics – a therapeutic misadventure. *Ann Intern Med* 1986; **104**: 399–404.

87. Maddrey W. Hepatic effects of acetaminophen. Enhanced toxicity in alcoholics. *J Clin Gastroenterol* 1987; **9**: 180–185.

88. Lefkowitch JH, Rushton AR, Feng-Chen KC. Hepatic fibrosis in fetal alcohol syndrome. Pathologic similarities to adult alcoholic liver disease. *Gastroenterology* 1983; **85**: 951–957.

89. Petrozza JA, Dutta SK, Latham PS, Iber FL, Gadacz TR. Prevalence and natural history of distal common bile duct stenosis in alcoholic pancreatitis. *Dig Dis Sci* 1984; **29**: 890–895.

90. Di Bisceglie AM, Paterson AC, Segal I. The liver in biliary obstruction due to chronic pancreatitis. *Liver* 1985; **5**: 189–195.

90a. Lesur G, Levy P, Flejou J-F et al. Factors predictive of liver histopathological appearance in chronic alcoholic pancreatitis with common bile duct stenosis and increased serum alkaline phosphate. *Hepatology* 1993; **18**: 1078–1081.

91. Afroudakis A, Kaplowitz N. Liver histopathology in chronic common bile duct stenosis due to chronic alcoholic pancreatitis. *Hepatology* 1981; **1**: 65–72.

92. Morgan MY, Sherlock S, Scheuer PJ. Portal fibrosis in the livers of alcoholic patients. *Gut* 1978; **19**: 1015–1021.

93. Jakobovits AW, Morgan MY, Sherlock S. Hepatic siderosis in alcoholics. *Dig Dis Sci* 1979; **24**: 305–310.

94. LeSage GD, Baldus WP, Fairbanks VF, et al. Hemochromatosis: genetic or alcohol-induced? *Gastroenterology* 1983; **84**: 1471–1477.

95. Ludwig J, Batts KP, Moyer TP, Baldus WP, Fairbanks VF. Liver biopsy diagnosis of homozygous hemochromatosis: a diagnostic algorithm. *Mayo Clin Proc* 1993; **68**: 263–267.

96. Ohnishi K, Iida S, Iwama S et al. The effect of chronic habitual alcohol intake on the development of liver cirrhosis and hepatocellular carcinoma: relation to hepatitis B surface antigen carriage. *Cancer* 1982; **49**: 672–677.

97. Hasan F, Jeffers LJ, Medina M et al. Hepatitis C-associated hepatocellular carcinoma. *Hepatology* 1990; **12**: 589–591.

98. Kiyosawa K, Sodeyama T, Tanaka E et al. Interrelationship of blood transfusion, non-A, non-B hepatitis and hepatocellular carcinoma: analysis by detection of antibody to hepatitis C virus. *Hepatology* 1990; **12**: 671–675.

99. Yamauchi M, Nakahara M, Maezawa Y et al. Prevalence of hepatocellular carcinoma in patients with alocholic cirrhosis and prior exposure to hepatitis C. *Am J Gastroenterol* 1993; **88**: 39–43.

GENERAL READING

French SW, Nash J, Shitabata P et al. Pathology of alcoholic liver disease. *Semin Liver Dis* 1993; **13**: 154–169.

Lieber CS, DeCarli LM. Hepatotoxicity of ethanol. *J Hepatol* 1991; **12**: 394–401.

de la M. Hall P. Alcoholic liver disease. In MacSween RNM, Anthony PP, Scheuer PJ, Portmann BC, Burt AD (eds): Pathology of the Liver, 3rd edn. Edinburgh: Churchill Livingstone, 1994.

DRUGS AND TOXINS

8

There are many hundreds of hepatotoxic drugs and other chemicals. Because of their large number, this chapter will be confined mainly to a description of the more important lesions seen in the liver by light microscopy, together with discussion of their differential diagnosis. Details of the lesions attributed to individual drugs can be found in several comprehensive reviews,[1,2] some of which are listed in the bibliography at the end of this chapter. Chemical injury is not confined to drugs listed in pharmacopoeias. Herbal medicines,[3–5] illicit drugs,[6–13] industrial chemicals,[2,14–17] vitamins[18] and foods[19] have all been held responsible for liver disease. Drugs suspected of causing liver damage may themselves be used for the treatment of liver disease.[20,21] Liver damage in alcohol abusers is separately discussed in Chapter 7, and the role of drugs in causing tumours and vascular lesions in Chapters 11 and 12, respectively.

GENERAL CONSIDERATIONS

In his foreword to the second edition of Stricker's *Drug-induced Hepatic Injury*,[1] Zimmerman writes: ".... virtually all known acute and chronic hepatic lesions can result from drug injury." This important observation should lead the pathologist and clinical hepatologist to consider the possibility of drug injury in many of their patients. Furthermore, the drug or combination of drugs responsible for an injury may or may not have been recorded as hepatotoxic in the literature.

Nevertheless there are certain kinds of injury, especially hepatocellular necrosis, hepatitis and cholestasis, which drugs are particularly apt to produce. Also, some groups of drugs are associated with particular kinds of injury; non-steroidal anti-inflammatory drugs (NSAID), for example, are especially associated with hepatocellular injury, while neuroleptic drugs mostly cause cholestasis.[2,22] However, these are generalizations and a drug which causes hepatocellular necrosis in one patient may cause cholestasis in another.[23]

The diagnostic pathologist should be aware of the potential of drugs and other substances to cause a wide variety of acute and chronic liver lesions and to know which lesions are most likely to be drug induced. He or she should be familiar with their likely course and outcome, and the main points of similarity and difference from other, non-drug-related liver diseases. Finally, the pathologist should know where to look up the effects of individual drugs.

Table 8.1. Examples of Liver Lesions due to Drugs and Toxins

Lesion	Example of Substance
Intrinsic hepatotoxicity	
Microvesicular steatosis	Valproate
Phospholipidosis	Amiodarone
Hepatocellular necrosis	Paracetamol (acetaminophen)
Fibrosis	Methotrexate
Cholestasis	Contraceptive steroids
Venous occlusion	Pyrrolizidine alkaloids
Angiosarcoma	Vinyl chloride
Idiosyncratic hepatotoxicity	
Hepatitis	Isoniazid
Cholestasis	Chlorpromazine
Granuloma formation	Allopurinol

CLASSIFICATION AND MECHANISMS

Drugs may be regarded as producing liver injury in two main ways (Table 8.1). **Intrinsic hepatotoxins** are those which predictably produce liver damage when taken in sufficient quantities. The type of damage is often characteristic of a particular drug; for example, the result of paracetamol (acetaminophen) overdose is always hepatocellular necrosis in patients taking a sufficiently large dose. Intrinsic hepatotoxicity can often be studied in laboratory animals. Its mechanism may be **direct**, the chemical or its metabolites causing structural damage to cells and organelles.[2] In **indirect** intrinsic hepatotoxicity, on the other hand, the chemical interferes with a specific metabolic pathway or cell component.

Most drug-related liver damage is caused by **idiosyncratic hepatotoxins**. Only a small proportion of patients on a particular drug is affected, either because of hypersensitivity or because of genetically determined differences in drug metabolism or lymphocyte reactivity.[24] Damage may follow a small dose of the offending drug and is difficult to study experimentally. With the exception of a few drugs shown to cause liver damage in patients with a particular metabolic pattern, idiosyncratic drug injury is unpredictable in the sense that the susceptibility of individuals cannot be tested before the drug is given.

Most intrinsic hepatotoxins produce liver damage within a few hours or days, whereas in the idiosyncratic type of injury there is often a latent period of weeks before liver disease becomes apparent. This period tends to shorten with repeated administration of the drug. Because of the long latent period and the tendency for idiosyncratic injury to mimic non-drug-related liver diseases, clinician and pathologist need to be alert to the possibility of idiosyncratic drug injury if diagnostic errors are to be avoided. Conclusive proof that a particular drug or combination of drugs is responsible may be impossible to obtain, although re-challenge (usually inadvertent) can provide strong circumstantial evidence. Liver injury may follow inadvertent re-challenge many years after a first episode.[25]

MORPHOLOGICAL CATEGORIES

The categories described below represent the main changes attributed to drugs and toxins, apart from alcohol-related liver damage (Chapter 7), neoplasms (Chapter 11) and vascular lesions (Chapter 12). A mixture of lesions may be found in the same liver; amiodarone, for example, produces both phospholipidosis and steatohepatitis but by

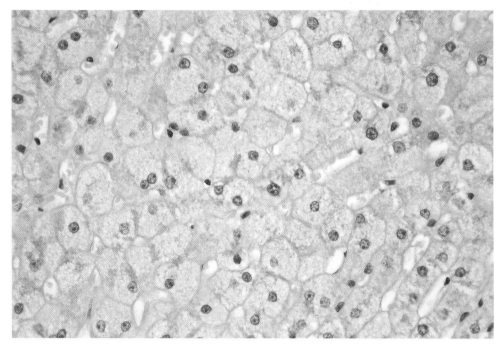

Figure 8.1. *Adaptation.* Hepatocytes in this biopsy from a patient on anti-epileptic drugs are enlarged and have abundant pale-staining cytoplasm. Needle biopsy, H & E.

different mechanisms.[26] The same drug may give rise to different forms of hepatotoxicity in different patients, an example being phenylbutazone which can cause necrosis, cholestasis, granuloma formation or combinations of these.[23]

Adaptation

Not all changes seen under the microscope necessarily represent liver damage. The increase in endoplasmic reticulum produced by long-term treatment with anti-convulsant drugs is commonly regarded as an adaptive phenomenon.[27,28] By light microscopy, this increase is seen as an abundance of pale-staining cytoplasm in hepatocytes (Fig. 8.1).

Non-hepatitic Liver-cell Damage

One of the commonest manifestations of intrinsic hepatotoxicity is **steatosis (fatty change)**. As discussed in Chapter 7, this may be macrovesicular or microvesicular. Macrovesicular steatosis, in which the nucleus of the hepatocyte is displaced by one or more fat vacuoles visible by light microscopy, is produced, for example, by chlorinated hydrocarbons and methotrexate. It is common in patients on total parenteral nutrition,[29,30] although underlying disease may also contribute to the liver changes.[31] Microvesicular steatosis is a consequence of treatment with the anti-convulsant drug valproate;[32] the fat within the hepatocytes is finely divided and may not be obvious with conventional stains, and the nuclei remain in their normal central location. There is a variable degree of associated hepatocellular necrosis.

Several drugs, among them amiodarone[26] and trimethoprim-sulphamethoxazole (co-trimoxazole),[33] are causes of acquired **phospholipidosis**. Similar changes have been reported in patients receiving total parenteral nutrition.[34] Lamellar inclusions are seen within hepatocytes and other cells by electron microscopy (Fig. 17.3, p. 284). Light microscopy of conventionally-stained sections is not diagnostic.

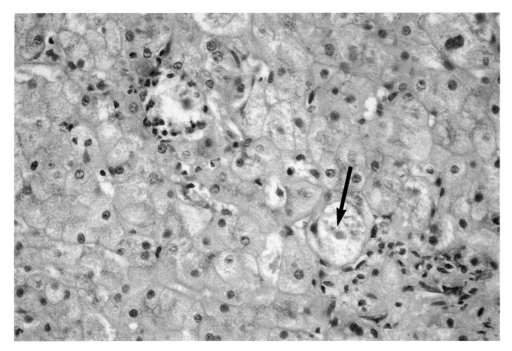

Figure 8.2. *Drug-induced steatohepatitis.* Two hepatocytes in this biopsy from a patient on amiodarone are markedly enlarged. The upper one is infiltrated by inflammatory cells, while the lower one contains Mallory bodies (arrow) in the form of irregular strands. Needle biopsy, H & E.

Steatohepatitis (fatty liver hepatitis) is also found in some patients on amiodarone,[26] synthetic oestrogens[35] or parenteral nutrition.[29] In the case of amiodarone steatosis itself may be mild or absent, but otherwise there is a close resemblance to alcoholic steatohepatitis (Fig. 8.2). Cirrhosis may develop.[36]

An unusual form of cell injury is produced by cyanamide, used in alcohol aversion therapy.[37-39] Periportal hepatocytes contain large, pale-staining **cytoplasmic inclusion bodies**, giving the cells a superficial resemblance to the ground-glass cells of chronic type B hepatitis (Fig. 9.11, p. 126). The inclusions are, however, orcein negative and diastase-PAS positive. Fibrosis and cirrhosis may eventually develop.[40]

Hepatocellular necrosis without the diffuse inflammatory lesion of hepatitis is usually a consequence of the intrinsic type of hepatotoxicity. A common example is suicidal overdose with the analgesic paracetamol (acetaminophen).[41] Jaundice develops after an interval of days, during which available glutathione, which reacts with a toxic metabolite, is used up. The necrosis, like that of shock (Fig. 12.2, p. 183), is most severe in acinar zones 3 and is accompanied by little or no inflammation (Fig. 8.3). Kupffer cells contain brown ceroid pigment. Portal tracts usually remain normal. Complete recovery is possible. While most paracetamol-induced necrosis follows suicidal overdose, it is occasionally found in habitual drinkers taking large doses in the high therapeutic range.[42] Necrosis similar to that caused by paracetamol may accompany cocaine intoxication.[6,8,9]

Acute Drug-induced Hepatitis

A large number of drugs of different chemical structure and with widely differing pharmacological actions occasionally give rise to acute hepatitis. The hepatotoxicity is of the idiosyncratic type. The histological lesion is very like that of acute viral hepatitis and usually indistinguishable from it. Incriminated drugs include the anti-tuberculous drug

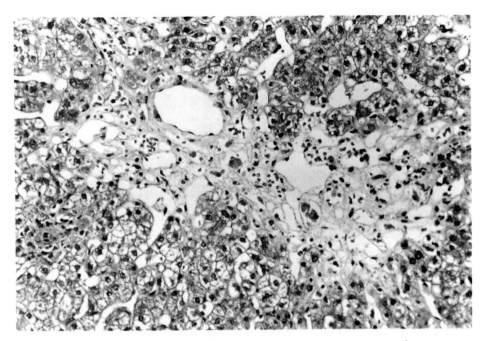

Figure 8.3. *Hepatocellular necrosis due to paracetamol (acetaminophen).* Confluent necrosis with little inflammation is seen in a perivenular area. Needle biopsy, H & E.

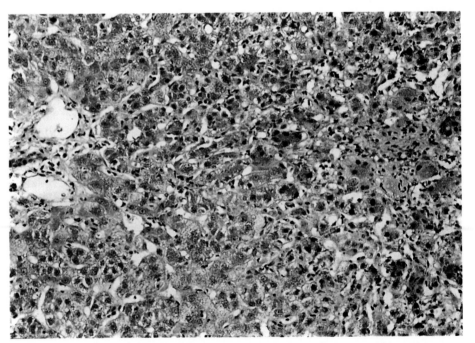

Figure 8.4. *Drug jaundice: hepatitic type.* Liver-cell plates are disrupted and the parenchyma is inflamed. The portal tract (left) shows little change. The hepatitis was attributed to isoniazid. Needle biopsy, H & E.

isoniazid (Fig. 8.4), the anaesthetic halothane (Fig. 8.5) and the NSAID indomethacin (Fig. 8.6). The latent period between exposure to the drug and clinically evident liver disease ranges from a few days to several months.[43]

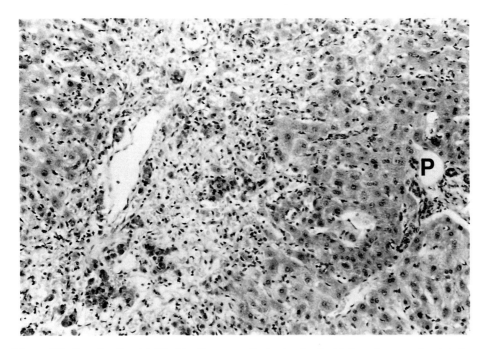

Figure 8.5. *Drug jaundice: hepatitic type.* From a patient who developed liver damage after halothane anaesthesia. Note confluent necrosis in acinar zone 3 (left) and unaffected portal tract (P). Needle biopsy, H & E.

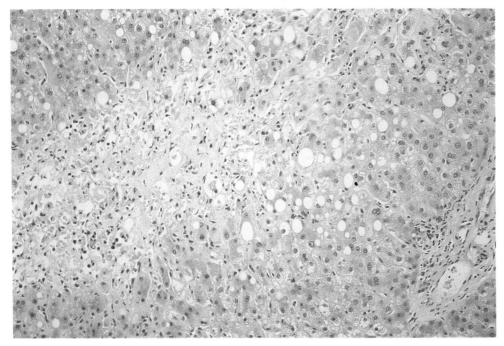

Figure 8.6. *Drug jaundice: hepatitic type.* In this acute hepatitis attributed to indomethacin, necrosis in acinar zone 3 is well demarcated from the remaining parenchyma. The latter shows steatosis. Note the very mild portal inflammation (below right). Needle biopsy, H & E.

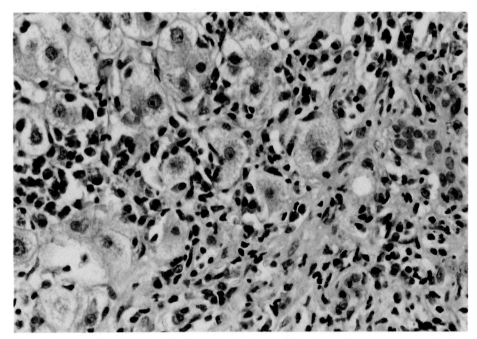

Figure 8.7. *Drug-induced chronic hepatitis.* Liver damage, here attributed to methyldopa, has taken the form of extensive piecemeal necrosis. There is a heavy lymphoplasmacytic infiltrate. Needle biopsy, H & E.

The hepatitis ranges in severity from a mild inflammatory lesion, sometimes combined with a cholestatic reaction (see under "Cholestasis", p. 110), to severe and even fatal disease.[44] In milder cases, removal of the drug usually leads to rapid improvement.

Differential Diagnosis

The possibility of drug idiosyncrasy should be considered in all patients with acute hepatitis, because in many cases the histological appearances are identical to those of viral hepatitis. A higher than usual degree of suspicion should be aroused when the hepatitis is histologically unusual. Well-demarcated zone 3 confluent necrosis (Figs. 8.5 and 8.6) is common. The portal inflammatory reaction may be poorly developed (Figs 8.4 and 8.6) or even absent (Fig. 8.5). Conversely, the portal infiltrate may be unusually rich in neutrophils or eosinophils, although the latter are neither proof of drug aetiology nor necessary for its diagnosis. The presence of epithelioid-cell granulomas increases the likelihood that drug idiosyncrasy is the correct diagnosis.

Chronic Drug-induced Hepatitis

In a few patients drug-induced hepatitis becomes chronic after prolonged or repeated exposure. The histological pattern is that of chronic hepatitis with or without cirrhosis (Fig. 8.7). In patients still taking the offending drug there is usually substantial necrosis and inflammation; inflammation confined to portal tracts is not a common pattern of drug injury. Drugs considered to be responsible for chronic hepatitis include such widely used agents as nitrofurantoin[45,46] and phenytoin.[47] The presence of autoantibodies in serum may lead to confusion with autoimmune hepatitis.[48] A high degree of suspicion of

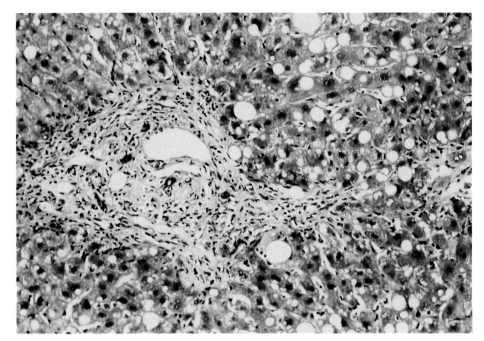

Figure 8.8. *Liver damage attributed to methotrexate.* Fibrosis extends outwards from a portal tract. The parenchyma is fatty. Needle biopsy, H & E.

possible drug aetiology is particularly important because of the possibility of improvement after withdrawal of the drug.

Differential Diagnosis

The appearances of drug-induced chronic hepatitis are indistinguishable from those of chronic hepatitis of viral or autoimmune aetiology.

Fibrosis and Cirrhosis

As already noted, cirrhosis may result from chronic drug-induced hepatitis. Progressive fibrosis and portal hypertension in a non-hepatitic setting are known complications of long-term exposure to arsenic or vinyl chloride. Cirrhosis may develop as a result of hypervitaminosis A.[18]

Pathologists are often asked to report on liver biopsies from patients given or about to receive long-term methotrexate for psoriasis or rheumatoid arthritis.[49-53] Although methotrexate was initially considered to be a potent hepatotoxin, doubt has more recently been thrown on its potential to cause serious liver disease in the absence of additional risk factors.[54] These include regular alcohol intake and obesity.[49,50] Significant liver injury is reputedly less common in patients with rheumatoid arthritis than in those with psoriasis. When cirrhosis develops, it is not rapidly progressive.[49] Histological abnormalities attributed to methotrexate include steatosis, portal fibrosis and inflammation, formation of fibrous septa extending from the portal tracts (Fig. 8.8) and cirrhosis. Minor changes such as focal necrosis and steatosis are common in baseline pre-treatment biopsies, and are presumably related to the underlying disease (e.g. psoriasis) or to additional risk factors.

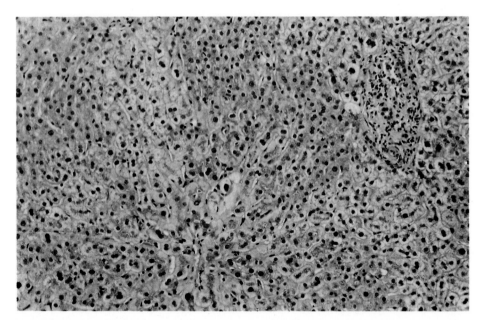

Figure 8.9. *Drug jaundice: cholestatic type.* In this patient with jaundice following chlorpromazine therapy there is mild inflammation of the portal tract (top right) and swelling of hepatocytes, especially in the perivenular area (below). Needle biopsy, H & E.

Periportal septum formation is more likely to be due to methotrexate, whereas fibrosis mainly in acinar zones 3 should lead to suspicion of alcohol abuse.

Cholestasis

Steroid-induced cholestasis lies on the borderline between intrinsic and idiosyncratic hepatotoxicity. On the one hand it is reproducible in laboratory animals, and some steroids cause biochemical abnormalities in man in a predictable and dose-dependent manner. On the other hand clinical liver disease cannot be predicted in the individual patient and is seen in only a small proportion of patients receiving anabolic or contraceptive steroids. Patients susceptible to contraceptive steroid-induced jaundice are also prone to develop cholestasis in late pregnancy.[55]

The histological picture is one of canalicular cholestasis in perivenular areas, with little or no necrosis or inflammation beyond that attributable to the cholestasis itself. Isolated hepatocytes may undergo feathery degeneration and in prolonged cholestasis liver-cell rosettes are a common finding (Fig. 4.3, p. 33). Portal tracts usually remain normal but may be minimally inflamed. Because of the lack of necrosis and inflammation, this type of lesion is sometimes known as pure or bland cholestasis. The **differential diagnosis** is from other causes of bland cholestasis such as benign recurrent cholestasis (p. 212) and is discussed in detail in Chapter 4.

Idiosyncratic drug-induced cholestasis, typified by chlorpromazine jaundice but also caused by many other drugs, differs from bland cholestasis in that portal inflammation is usually present (Figs 8.9 and 8.10). There is sometimes inflammatory infiltration of the acini and evidence of hepatocellular damage. Zimmerman and Ishak[2] therefore refer to this type of lesion as hepatocanalicular. The portal infiltrate often includes eosinophils and these are occasionally abundant, but lack of eosinophils does not exclude a diagnosis of drug-induced hepatocanalicular cholestasis. Small interlobular ducts often show minor abnormalities such as irregular distribution of epithelial cell nuclei, variation in nuclear

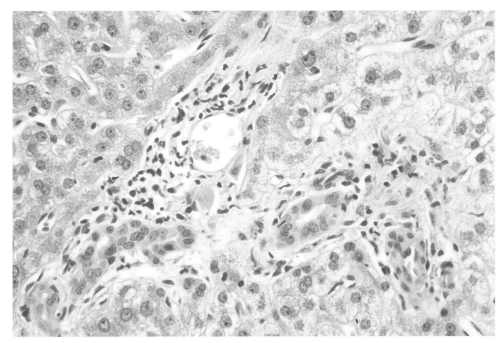

Figure 8.10. *Drug jaundice: cholestatic type.* A mildly inflamed portal tract from a patient with chlorpromazine jaundice. Eosinophils are not prominent in this example. Bile-duct epithelium is irregular and infiltrated by lymphocytes. Needle biopsy, H & E.

size and infiltration by lymphocytes (Fig. 8.10). The acinar changes are as for bland cholestasis, except for the additional element of inflammation and necrosis which is sometimes found, as mentioned above. There is therefore a spectrum of appearances in this type of cholestasis, from an almost bland cholestatic lesion to one resembling mild acute viral hepatitis. Even in the absence of necrosis and inflammation, hepatocellular changes are seen which possibly result from prolonged cholestasis itself but which may also include an element of adaptive proliferation of the smooth endoplasmic reticulum. These changes include prominent hepatocellular swelling, abundant pale-staining cytoplasm and, commonly, multinucleation (Fig. 8.11). Mitotic figures may be evident.[56]

The **differential diagnosis** of idiosyncratic drug-induced cholestasis is from bile-duct obstruction, acute viral or drug-induced hepatitis, and cholestasis of the bland type. Portal oedema, prominent neutrophils, marked bile-duct proliferation and absence of acinar inflammation favour the first. In the absence of substantial portal inflammation the distinction between idiosyncratic drug jaundice and bland steroid-induced cholestasis becomes difficult to make and requires clinical information. In such circumstances bile-duct obstruction cannot be completely ruled out. The differential diagnosis also includes other causes of bland cholestasis, such as benign recurrent cholestasis (p. 212). Severe liver-cell damage and inflammation favour viral hepatitis or the drug injury of hepatitic type already discussed.

The **clinical course** of idiosyncratic drug jaundice varies. In most patients removal of the offending drug leads to rapid improvement. Occasionally the cholestasis is slow to improve but liver biopsy shows cholestasis only, with no fibrosis or other evidence of progressive disease. In rare instances true chronic disease develops on the basis of severe bile-duct damage and duct loss, with consequent fibrosis and other features of chronic biliary disease. The clinical picture resembles primary biliary cirrhosis. This syndrome has been reported after a number of drugs including chlorpromazine,[56] prochlorperazine,[57] haloperidol,[58] ajmaline[59]; glycyrrhizin[60], and amoxycillin and flucloxacillin[60a] among

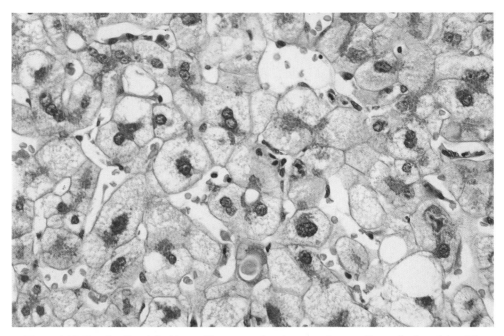

Figure 8.11. *Drug jaundice: cholestatic type.* Hepatocytes in acinar zone 3 are swollen and pale staining. There are bile thrombi in dilated canaliculi. From a patient with chlorpromazine jaundice. Needle biopsy, H & E.

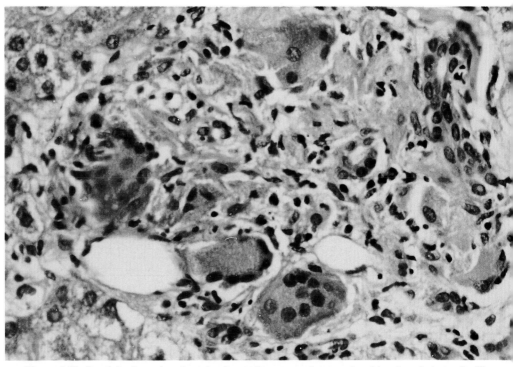

Figure 8.12. *Drug-induced granuloma formation.* A portal tract contains several multinucleated giant cells. The patient became jaundiced after taking phenylbutazone. Needle biopsy, H & E.

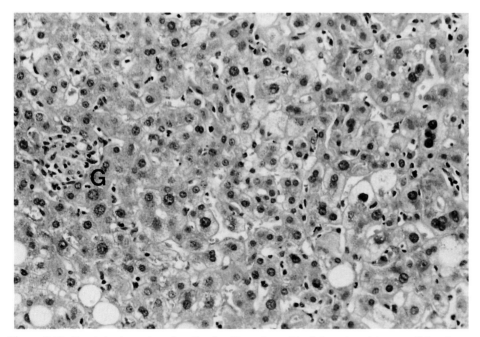

Figure 8.13. *Drug-induced granuloma formation.* In this patient with cholestasis and hepatocellular damage attributed to erythromycin estolate, cell swelling is prominent in a perivenular area (right) and a small granuloma (G) is seen to the left. There is mild steatosis. Needle biopsy, H & E.

others.[61] More acute bile duct injury is seen in poisoning with the herbicide paraquat.[62] Zimmerman and Ishak[2] designate this type of injury as ductal or cholangiodestructive, in contrast to canalicular and hepatocanalicular cholestasis.

Long-term parenteral nutrition, already noted in relation to steatosis and steatohepatitis, may be associated with a similar progressive form of liver injury, typified by cholestasis, hepatocellular damage, ductular proliferation, fibrosis and even cirrhosis.[29,30,63] Whether the parenteral nutrition itself is responsible for all these changes is not proven.[30,31] The lesion may mimic bile-duct obstruction.[64]

Granulomas

Drugs are an important cause of otherwise unexplained granulomas.[65] They are sometimes the only or main manifestation of a drug reaction, but can also form part of a cholestatic or hepatitic picture.[36] The granulomas may be portal (Fig. 8.12), parenchymal (Fig. 8.13) or both. They usually show little or no necrosis, and are infiltrated by a variety of inflammatory cells including plasma cells and eosinophils. Allopurinol has been reported to cause granulomas of the fibrin-ring type.[66] The list of drugs associated with hepatic granulomas is small compared with the list of those causing hepatitis or cholestasis, but it is nevertheless substantial.[2,67]

REFERENCES

1. Stricker BHCh. Drug-induced Hepatic Injury. Amsterdam: Elsevier, 1992.
2. Zimmerman HJ, Ishak KG. Hepatic injury due to drugs and toxins. In MacSween RNM, Anthony PP, Scheuer PJ, Portmann B, Burt AD (eds): Pathology of the Liver, 3rd edn. Edinburgh: Churchill Livingstone, 1994.

3. Katz M, Saibil F. Herbal hepatitis: subacute hepatic necrosis secondary to chaparral leaf. *J Clin Gastroenterol* 1990; **12**: 203–206.

4. Larrey D, Vial T, Pauwels A et al. Hepatitis after germander (*Teucrium chamaedrys*) administration: another instance of herbal medicine hepatotoxicity. *Ann Intern Med* 1992; **117**: 129–132.

5. Mostefa-Kara N, Pauwels A, Pines E, Biour M, Levy VG. Fatal hepatitis after herbal tea. *Lancet* 1992; **340**: 674.

6. Kanel GC, Cassidy W, Shuster L, Reynolds TB. Cocaine–induced liver cell injury: comparison of morphological features in man and in experimental models. *Hepatology* 1990; **11**: 646–651.

7. Trigueiro de Araújo MS, Gerard F, Chossegros P, Porto LC, Barlet P, Grimaud J-A. Vascular hepatotoxicity related to heroin addiction. *Virchows Arch (A)* 1990; **417**: 497–503.

8. Wanless IR, Dore S, Gopinath N et al. Histopathology of cocaine hepatotoxicity. Report of four patients. *Gastroenterology* 1990; **98**: 497–501.

9. Silva MO, Roth D, Reddy KR, Fernandez JA, Albores-Saavedra J, Schiff ER. Hepatic dysfunction accompanying acute cocaine intoxication. *J Hepatol* 1991; **12**: 312–315.

10. Mallat A, Dhumeaux D. Cocaine and the liver. *J Hepatol* 1991; **12**: 275–278.

11. McIntyre AS, Long RG. Fatal fulminant hepatic failure in a 'solvent abuser'. *Postgrad Med J* 1992; **68**: 29–30.

12. Shearman JD, Chapman RW, Satsangi J, Ryley NG, Weatherhead S. Misuse of ecstasy. *Br Med J* 1992; **305**: 309.

13. Trigueiro de Araújo MS, Gerard F, Chossegros P, Guerret S, Grimaud JA. Lack of hepatocyte involvement in the genesis of the sinusoidal dilatation related to heroin addiction: a morphometric study. *Virchows Arch (A)* 1992; **420**: 149–153.

14. Redlich CA, West AB, Fleming L, True LD, Cullen MR, Riely CA. Clinical and pathological characteristics of hepatotoxicity associated with occupational exposure to dimethylformamide. *Gastroenterology* 1990; **99**: 748–757.

15. Kahl R. Toxic liver injury. In McIntyre N, Benhamou J-P, Bircher J, Rizzetto M, Rodes J (eds): Oxford Textbook of Clinical Hepatology. Oxford: Oxford University Press, 1991, pp 905–918.

16. Kahl R. Appendix 2: liver injury in man ascribed to non-drug chemicals and natural toxins. In McIntyre N, Benhamou J-P, Bircher J, Rizzetto M, Rodes J (eds): Oxford Textbook of Clinical Hepatology. Oxford: Oxford University Press, 1991, pp 1473–1487.

17. Haratake J, Furuta A, Iwasa T, Wakasugi C, Imazu K. Submassive hepatic necrosis induced by dichloropropanol. *Liver* 1993; **13**: 123–129.

18. Jorens PG, Michielsen PP, Pelckmans PA et al. Vitamin A abuse: development of cirrhosis despite cessation of vitamin A. A six-year clinical and histopathologic follow-up. *Liver* 1992; **12**: 381–386.

19. Galler GW, Weisenberg E, Brasitus TA. Mushroom poisoning: the role of orthotopic liver transplantation. *J Clin Gastroenterol* 1992; **15**: 229–232.

20. Kassianides C, Nussenblatt R, Palestine AG, Mellow SD, Hoofnagle JH. Liver injury from cyclosporine A. *Dig Dis Sci* 1990; **35**: 693–697.

21. Silva MO, Reddy KR, Jeffers LJ, Hill M, Schiff ER. Interferon-induced chronic active hepatitis? *Gastroenterology* 1991; **101**: 840–842.

22. Rabinovitz M, Van Thiel DH. Hepatotoxicity of nonsteroidal anti-inflammatory drugs. *Am J Gastroenterol* 1992; **87**: 1696–1704.

23. Benjamin SB, Ishak KG, Zimmerman HJ, Grushka A. Phenylbutazone liver injury: a clinical-pathologic survey of 23 cases and review of the literature. *Hepatology* 1981; **1**: 255–263.

24. Larrey D, Berson A, Habersetzer F et al. Genetic predisposition to drug hepatotoxicity: role in hepatitis caused by amineptine, a tricyclic antidepressant. *Hepatology* 1989; **10**: 168–173.

25. Paiva LA, Wright PJ, Koff RS. Long-term hepatic memory for hypersensitivity to nitrofurantoin. *Am J Gastroenterol* 1992; **87**: 891–893.

26. Lewis JH, Mullick F, Ishak KG et al. Histopathologic analysis of suspected amiodarone hepatotoxicity. *Hum Pathol* 1990; **21**: 59–67.

27. Jezequel AM, Librari ML, Mosca P, Novelli G, Lorenzini I, Orlandi F. Changes induced in human liver by long-term anticonvulsant therapy. Functional and ultrastructural data. *Liver* 1984; **4**: 307–317.

28. Pamperl H, Gradner W, Fridrich L, Pointner H, Denk H. Influence of long-term anticonvulsant treatment on liver ultrastructure in man. *Liver* 1984; **4**: 294–300.

29. Klein S, Nealon WH. Hepatobiliary abnormalities associated with total parenteral nutrition. *Semin Liver Dis* 1988; **8**: 237–246.

30. Quigley EM, Marsh MN, Shaffer JL, Markin RS. Hepatobiliary complications of total parenteral nutrition. *Gastroenterology* 1993; **104**: 286–301.

31. Wolfe BM, Walker BK, Shaul DB, Wong L, Ruebner BH. Effect of total parenteral nutrition on hepatic histology. *Arch Surg* 1988; **123**: 1084–1090.

32. Zimmerman HJ, Ishak KG. Valproate-induced hepatic injury: analyses of 23 fatal cases. *Hepatology* 1982; **2**: 591–597.

33. Muñoz SJ, Martinez-Hernandez A, Maddrey WC. Intrahepatic cholestasis and phospholipidosis associated with the use of trimethoprim-sulfamethoxazole. *Hepatology* 1990; **12**: 342–347.

34. Degott C, Messing B, Moreau D et al. Liver phospholipidosis induced by parenteral nutrition: histologic, histochemical, and ultrastructural investigations. *Gastroenterology* 1988; **95**: 183–191.

35. Seki K, Minami Y, Nishikawa M et al. 'Nonalcoholic steatohepatitis' induced by massive doses of synthetic estrogen. *Gastroenterol Jpn* 1983; **18**: 197–203.

36. Harrison RF, Elias E. Amiodarone-associated cirrhosis with hepatic and lymph node granulomas. *Histopathology* 1993; **22**: 80–82.
37. Vazquez JJ, Guillen FJ, Zozaya J, Lahoz M. Cyanamide-induced liver injury. A predictable lesion. *Liver* 1983; **3**: 225–230.
38. Bruguera M, Lamar C, Bernet M, Rodes J. Hepatic disease associated with ground-glass inclusions in hepatocytes after cyanamide therapy. *Arch Pathol Lab Med* 1986; **110**: 906–910.
39. Vazquez JJ. Hepatic lesions induced by alcohol sensitizing drugs: two lesions for the price of one. *Hepatology* 1986; **6**: 748–749.
40. Moreno A, Vazquez JJ, Ruizdel-Arbol L, Guillen FJ, Colina F. Structural hepatic changes associated with cyanamide treatment: cholangiolar proliferation, fibrosis and cirrhosis. *Liver* 1984; **4**: 15–21.
41. Portmann B, Talbot IC, Day DW, Davidson AR, Murray-Lyon IM, Williams R. Histopathological changes in the liver following a paracetamol overdose: correlation with clinical and biochemical parameters. *J Pathol* 1975; **117**: 169–181.
42. Maddrey WC. Hepatic effects of acetaminophen. Enhanced toxicity in alcoholics. *J Clin Gastroenterol* 1987; **9**: 180–185.
43. Arranto AJ, Sotaniemi EA. Morphologic alterations in patients with alpha-methyldopa-induced liver damage after short- and long-term exposure. *Scand J Gastroenterol* 1981; **16**: 853–863.
44. Paterson D, Kerlin P, Walker N, Lynch S, Strong R. Piroxicam induced submassive necrosis of the liver. *Gut* 1992; **33**: 1436–1438.
45. Sharp JR, Ishak KG, Zimmerman HJ. Chronic active hepatitis and severe hepatic necrosis associated with nitrofurantoin. *Ann Intern Med* 1980; **92**: 14–19.
46. Stricker BH, Blok AP, Claas FH, Van-Parys GE, Desmet VJ. Hepatic injury associated with the use of nitrofurans: a clinicopathological study of 52 reported cases. *Hepatology* 1988; **8**: 599–606.
47. Roy AK, Mahoney HC, Levine RA. Phenytoin-induced chronic hepatitis. *Dig Dis Sci* 1993; **38**: 740–743.
48. Scully LJ, Clarke D, Barr RJ. Diclofenac induced hepatitis. 3 cases with features of autoimmune chronic active hepatitis. *Dig Dis Sci* 1993; **38**: 744–751.
49. Zachariae H, Sogaard H. Methotrexate-induced liver cirrhosis. A follow-up. *Dermatologica* 1987; **175**: 178–182.
50. Newman M, Auerbach R, Feiner H et al. The role of liver biopsies in psoriatic patients receiving long-term methotrexate treatment. Improvement in liver abnormalities after cessation of treatment. *Arch Dermatol* 1989; **125**: 1218–1224.
51. Whiting OK, Fye KH, Sack KD. Methotrexate and histologic hepatic abnormalities: a meta-analysis. *Am J Med* 1991; **90**: 711–716.
52. Themido R, Loureiro M, Pecegueiro M, Brandao M, Campos MC. Methotrexate hepatotoxicity in psoriatic patients submitted to long-term therapy. *Acta Derm Venereol (Stockh)* 1992; **72**: 361–364.
53. Walker AM, Funch D, Dreyer NA et al. Determinants of serious liver disease among patients receiving low-dose methotrexate for rheumatoid arthritis. *Arthritis and Rheumatism* 1993; **36**: 329–335.
54. Kaplan MM. Methotrexate hepatotoxicity and the premature reporting of Mark Twain's death: both greatly exaggerated. *Hepatology* 1990; **12**: 784–786.
55. Adlercreutz H, Tenhunen R. Some aspects of the interaction between natural and synthetic female sex hormones and the liver. *Am J Med* 1970; **49**: 630–648.
56. Ishak KG, Irey NS. Hepatic injury associated with the phenothiazines. Clinicopathologic and follow-up study of 36 patients. *Arch Pathol* 1972; **93**: 283–304.
57. Lok ASF, Ng IOL. Prochlorperazine-induced chronic cholestasis. *J Hepatol* 1988; **6**: 369–373.
58. Dincsoy HP, Saelinger DA. Haloperidol-induced chronic cholestatic liver disease. *Gastroenterology* 1982; **83**: 694–700.
59. Larrey D, Pessayre D, Duhamel G et al. Prolonged cholestasis after ajmaline-induced acute hepatitis. *J Hepatol* 1986; **2**: 81–87.
60. Ishii M, Miyazaki M, Yamamoto T et al. A case of drug-induced ductopenia resulting in fatal biliary cirrhosis. *Liver* 1993; **13**: 227–231.
60a. Davies MH, Harrison RF, Elias E, Hübscher SG. Antibiotic-associated acute vanishing bile duct syndrome: a pattern associated with severe, prolonged, intrahepatic cholestasis. *J Hepatol* 1994; **20**: 112–116.
61. Degott C, Feldmann G, Larrey D et al. Drug-induced prolonged cholestasis in adults: a histological semiquantitative study demonstrating progressive ductopenia. *Hepatology* 1992; **15**: 244–251.
62. Mullick FG, Ishak KG, Mahabir R, Stromeyer FW. Hepatic injury associated with paraquat toxicity in humans. *Liver* 1981; **1**: 209–221.
63. Baker AL, Rosenberg IH. Hepatic complications of total parenteral nutrition. *Am J Med* 1987; **82**: 489–497.
64. Body JJ, Bleiberg H, Bron D, Maurage H, Bigirimana V, Heimann R. Total parenteral nutrition-induced cholestasis mimicking large bile duct obstruction. *Histopathology* 1982; **6**: 787–792.
65. McMaster KR, Hennigar GR. Drug-induced granulomatous hepatitis. *Lab Invest* 1981; **44**: 61–73.
66. Vanderstigel M, Zafrani ES, Lejonc JL, Schaeffer A, Portos JL. Allopurinol hypersensitivity syndrome as a cause of hepatic fibrin-ring granulomas. *Gastroenterology* 1986; **90**: 188–190.
67. Ishak KG, Zimmerman HJ. Drug-induced and toxic granulomatous hepatitis. *Baillières Clin Gastroenterol* 1988; **2**: 463–480.

GENERAL READING

Bénichou C. Criteria of drug-induced liver disorders. Report of an international consensus meeting. *J Hepatol* 1990; **11**: 272–276.

Bircher J (ed.) Adverse drug reactions in the differential diagnosis of GI and liver disease. *Baillières Clin Gastroenterol* 1988; **2**: 259–528.

Friis H, Andreasen PB. Drug-induced hepatic injury: an analysis of 1100 cases reported to the Danish Committee on Adverse Drug Reactions between 1978 and 1987. *J Intern Med* 1992; **232**: 133–138.

Kahl R. Toxic liver injury. In McIntyre N, Benhamou J-P, Bircher J, Rizzetto M, Rodes J (eds): Oxford Textbook of Clinical Hepatology. Oxford: Oxford University Press, 1991, pp 905–918.

Kaplowitz N (ed.) Recent advances in drug metabolism and hepatotoxicity. *Semin Liver Dis* 1990; **10**: 234–338.

Pessayre D, Larrey D. Drug-induced liver injury. In McIntyre N, Benhamou J-P, Bircher J, Rizzetto M, Rodes J (eds): Oxford Textbook of Clinical Hepatology. Oxford: Oxford University Press, 1991, pp 875–902.

Sherlock S, Dooley J. Drugs and the liver. In Diseases of the Liver and Biliary System, 9th edn. Oxford: Blackwell Scientific Publications, 1993, pp 322–356.

Stricker BHCh. Drug-induced Hepatic Injury, 2nd edn. Amsterdam: Elsevier, 1992.

Zimmerman HJ, Ishak KG. Hepatic injury due to drugs and toxins. In MacSween RNM, Anthony PP, Scheuer PJ, Portmann B, Burt AD (eds): Pathology of the Liver, 3rd edn. Edinburgh: Churchill Livingstone, 1994.

CHRONIC HEPATITIS

9

DEFINITION AND CAUSES

Chronic hepatitis is universally defined as "chronic inflammation of the liver continuing without improvement for at least six months".[1] This definition has helped to make analytical and therapeutic studies comparable by establishing a border, however artificial, between acute and chronic hepatitis. In practice the border is not always easy to draw because acute hepatitis is occasionally very prolonged and because some forms of chronic hepatitis develop insidiously, without an obvious acute onset.

Applied strictly, the definition could be taken to include almost every form of chronic liver disease since many of these have an inflammatory component. In practice the diagnostic label of chronic hepatitis is usually restricted to the diseases listed in part A of Table 9.1. In part B are listed diseases which share some of the histological characteristics of chronic hepatitis, such as piecemeal necrosis, but to which the label is not normally applied.

CLASSIFICATION AND NOMENCLATURE

It is approximately a quarter of a century since the simple classification of chronic hepatitis into the small number of morphological categories in Table 9.2 was proposed.[2,3] The main reason for the separation of the categories was prognosis. While it was realized that chronic persistent hepatitis (CPH) could develop into chronic active hepatitis (CAH) in some patients, those with CPH tended to have a better prognosis than those with CAH.[4] This is still true, but it is also now apparent that prognosis and course are strongly influenced by the virus or other cause responsible for the lesion, by the extent of virus replication, by response to treatment, and by the risk factors to which the patient is exposed.[5] Furthermore, forms of necrosis other than piecemeal necrosis, the defining lesion of CAH, are thought to be important in the progression of the disease but are not incorporated into the original classification. Because the cause of a chronic hepatitis is probably the most important of these factors in clinical practice, there is a growing tendency to use this as the primary method of classification, supplemented by histological information.[6] Another reason why primary histological classification is now less popular than before is the practical difficulty experienced by pathologists in deciding between a diagnosis of CPH and one of minimal CAH. Lastly but not least important, it has become increasingly clear over the years that CPH, CAH and chronic lobular hepatitis (CLH) are not separate lesions but represent parts of a continuum.

Table 9.1. Causes of Chronic Hepatitis

A. Forms to which the label of chronic hepatitis is conventionally applied
    Hepatitis B, with or without HDV infection
    Hepatitis C
    Autoimmune hepatitis
    Drug-induced hepatitis
    Chronic hepatitis of unknown cause
B. Diseases with some histological features of chronic hepatitis but not usually so designated
    Wilson's disease
    α_1-Antitrypsin deficiency
    Primary biliary cirrhosis
    Primary sclerosing cholangitis

Table 9.2. Traditional Categories of Chronic Hepatitis[2,3]

Category	Location of Lesion
Chronic persistent hepatitis (CPH)	Portal tracts
Chronic active hepatitis (CAH) (originally called chronic aggressive hepatitis)	Portal and periportal
Chronic lobular hepatitis (CLH)	Acini (acinar component also found in CPH and CAH)

Table 9.3. Uses of Liver Biopsy in Chronic Hepatitis

Establishment of the diagnosis
Diagnosis of incidental lesions
Assessment of histological activity
Evaluation of types of necrosis
Evaluation of structural changes
Clues to aetiology and possible superinfection
Immunohistochemical assessment of viral antigens
Monitoring of therapy

For these reasons, the main histological division in this chapter will be into portal and parenchymal lesions rather than into CPH, CAH and CLH. These are, however, mentioned in the appropriate context because some pathologists and clinicians may wish to go on using the terms as a convenient shorthand. Those who opt to classify primarily by cause should specify the type and severity of the various lesions seen on biopsy. To this can be added a numerical scoring system if required.

The rapid growth of knowledge of the hepatitis viruses and the development of sophisticated serological tests has not diminished the use of liver biopsy in patients with chronic hepatitis. The many indications for biopsy include establishment of the correct diagnosis, assessment of histological activity, assessment of structural changes including cirrhosis and evaluation of therapy. In patients with multiple aetiological factors, biopsy may help to establish their relative importance. The main categories of information which can be obtained are listed in Table 9.3. In addition, the future is likely to bring an increase in the use of *in situ* hybridization for the detection of viral DNA and RNA.

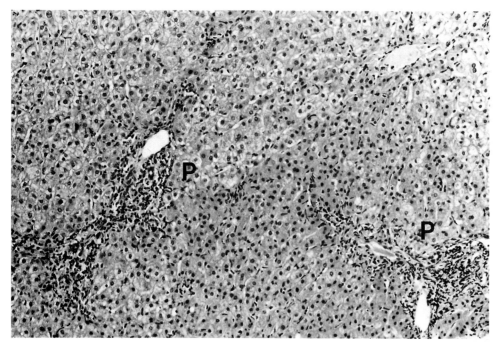

Figure 9.1. *Chronic hepatitis.* Inflammatory infiltration is here confined to the portal tracts (P), with no extension into the parenchyma. This corresponds to the original definition of chronic persistent hepatitis. Needle biopsy, H & E.

HISTOLOGICAL FEATURES OF CHRONIC HEPATITIS

Portal Changes

In most patients with chronic hepatitis the majority of the small portal tracts are infiltrated by inflammatory cells. The exception is chronic lobular hepatitis (see below). In the mildest forms of chronic hepatitis the infiltration is entirely confined to the portal tracts and the limiting plates of hepatocytes remain intact. This pattern, with or without accompanying parenchymal damage and inflammation, corresponds to the traditional category of chronic persistent hepatitis (Fig. 9.1). Stains for collagen or reticulin fibres show intact acinar architecture, with regular spacing of portal tracts and terminal hepatic venules. The portal tracts themselves are often enlarged by the inflammatory process, and short fibrous spurs may extend from them (Fig. 9.2). When they are substantially enlarged, however, this usually indicates previous periportal necrosis (chronic active hepatitis) with subsequent re-establishment of the limiting plates. Conversely, inflammation confined to portal tracts may later extend out into the acini with concomitant liver-cell necrosis, chronic persistent hepatitis thus evolving into chronic active hepatitis.[7]

The inflammatory infiltrate is mainly composed of lymphocytes. These may form aggregates or follicles with or without obvious germinal centres, especially in chronic type C hepatitis.[8–10] Plasma cells are also seen, usually when there is periportal involvement. The proportion of the various cell types and subtypes differs according to the cause of the disease.[11] The interlobular bile ducts may show focal abnormalities such as swelling of part of the wall, vacuolation of epithelial cells and infiltration by lymphocytes, as in acute hepatitis (p. 66).

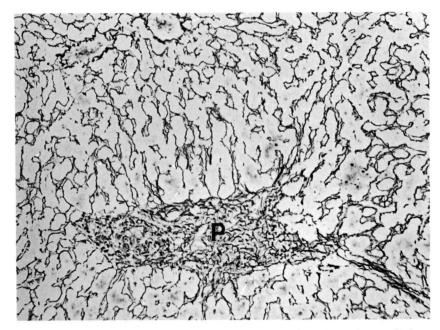

Figure 9.2. *Chronic hepatitis.* Short septa extend from the slightly enlarged portal tract (P) but normal architectural relationships are preserved. Like Figure 9.1, this corresponds to the original concept of chronic persistent hepatitis. Needle biopsy, reticulin.

Parenchymal Changes

The Periportal Lesion

In the more severe forms of chronic hepatitis the inflammatory infiltrate extends beyond the portal tracts and there is necrosis of hepatocytes (Figs 9.3 and 9.4). This necro-inflammatory process is called piecemeal necrosis, and is the defining lesion of chronic active hepatitis. An alternative name for the lesion is interface hepatitis, since it is characteristically located at the interface between a portal tract or septum and the hepatic parenchyma. The severity of this hepatitis varies greatly. In the mildest forms it is only recognized by enlargement of the affected portal tracts, slight irregularity of the interface and trapping of surviving hepatocytes within the inflammatory infiltrate (Fig. 9.5). In more severe examples the extension of the infiltrate into the acini is clearly seen at low magnification (Fig. 9.6) and there is obvious fibrosis (Fig. 9.7).[12]

Intra-acinar Changes

Deeper within the acini, the above changes may be accompanied by focal (spotty) or confluent necrosis, with or without bridging (Fig. 9.8). In biopsies with portal inflammation but no periportal necrosis the intra-acinar component is generally mild, whereas bridging necrosis is usually accompanied by piecemeal necrosis. This is not invariable, however, and there is a wide variety of patterns. The relative importance of piecemeal and bridging necrosis in the pathogenesis of cirrhosis remains a controversial issue,[13] and both probably contribute to the outcome.[14–16] Clinical exacerbations of chronic disease are characterized by a combination of piecemeal, focal and sometimes bridging necrosis.[17] Fatty change, when present, is usually mild. Cholestasis is very uncommon and its presence should raise the possibility of alternative diagnoses.

Severe intra-acinar necrosis, usually of bridging type or even panacinar, is often

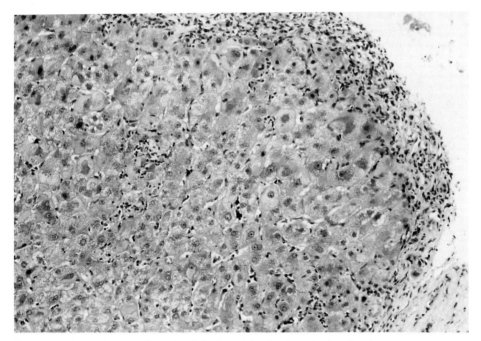

Figure 9.3. *Piecemeal necrosis*. Part of a cirrhotic nodule with irregular interface between parenchyma and connective tissue. The affected zone (right) is infiltrated by lymphocytes. Needle biopsy, H & E.

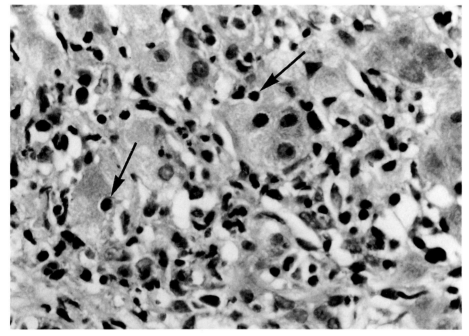

Figure 9.4. *Piecemeal necrosis*. Lymphocytes are closely apposed to hepatocytes, and some have deeply indented their cytoplasm (arrows). Needle biopsy, H & E.

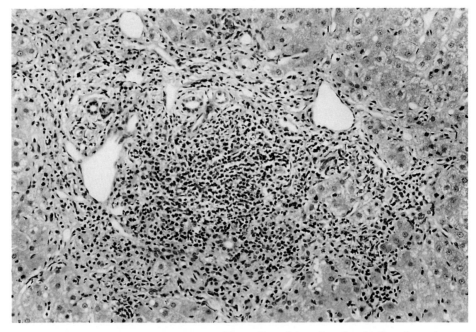

Figure 9.5. *Chronic hepatitis with piecemeal necrosis.* The outlines of the enlarged and inflamed portal tract are blurred by piecemeal necrosis. To the right, several hepatocytes have become trapped in the inflammatory infiltrate. This corresponds to mild/moderate chronic active hepatitis. Needle biopsy, H & E.

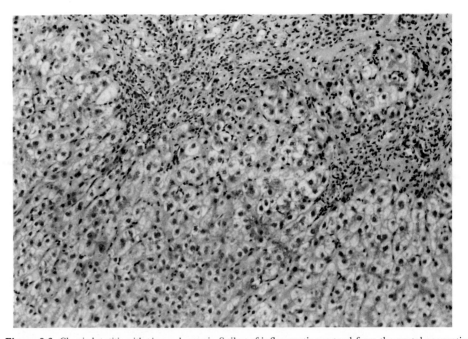

Figure 9.6. *Chronic hepatitis with piecemeal necrosis.* Spikes of inflammation extend from the portal connective tissue (above) into the parenchyma. Hepatocytes are swollen. The picture corresponds to chronic active hepatitis of moderate severity. See also Figure 9.7. Needle biopsy, H & E.

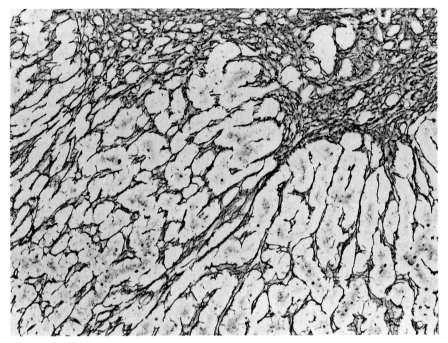

Figure 9.7. *Chronic hepatitis with piecemeal necrosis.* In this reticulin preparation of the field shown in Figure 9.6 the fibrosis is more clearly seen. Needle biopsy, reticulin.

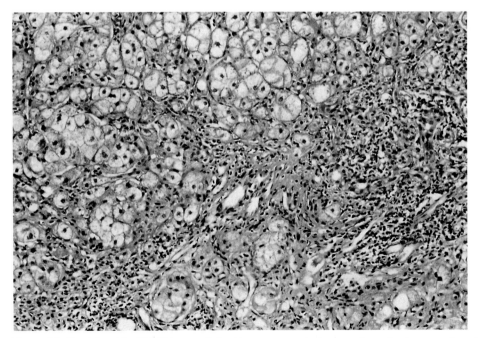

Figure 9.8. *Chronic hepatitis with bridging necrosis.* In this severe example the parenchyma has been transformed into liver-cell rosettes of hepatitic type, composed of greatly swollen hepatocytes. Curving septa extending from a portal tract (right) have resulted from bridging necrosis. Needle biopsy, H & E.

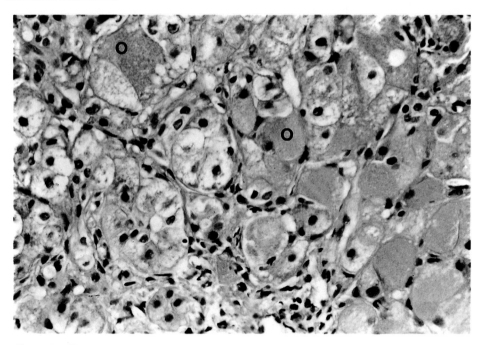

Figure 9.9. *Hepatitic rosettes and oncocytic change.* Some of the cells forming the rosettes are intensely oxyphilic and granular (O) because of abundant closely packed mitochondria. One rosette has a lumen (below left). Needle biopsy. H & E.

accompanied by the formation of small gland-like clusters of surviving hepatocytes within the inflammatory tissue. These so-called hepatitic rosettes (Fig. 9.8) are therefore surrounded by connective tissue, unlike the cholestatic rosettes described on p. 32 and illustrated in Figure 4.3. The hepatitic rosettes probably form as a result of regeneration. Some of their component cells may have a densely eosinophilic, granular cytoplasm (Fig. 9.9). The significance of such oncocytic liver cells is unclear.[18,19] Their distinction from the ground-glass hepatocytes of hepatitis B can easily be made by means of staining for the hepatitis B surface antigen.

In a few patients with severe chronic hepatitis, some of the hepatocytes fuse to form multinucleated giant cells reminiscent of neonatal hepatitis.[20,21] Giant cell hepatitis does not appear to be restricted to a single cause.[22,23] An association with paramyxovirus infection has been reported.[24]

Occasionally in the Western world and more often in the Far East,[25] acinar necrosis and inflammation are seen in the absence of a substantial portal or periportal component (Fig. 9.10). The picture then corresponds to the description of chronic lobular hepatitis[3] or, if very mild, non-specific or minimal hepatitis.[26]

INDIVIDUAL CAUSES OF CHRONIC HEPATITIS

Chronic Hepatitis B and D

The severity and pattern of chronic HBV infection differ widely from one patient to another and also at various times in the same patient. Chronic infection usually begins with a phase of high virus replication, marked by high levels of HBV-DNA and presence

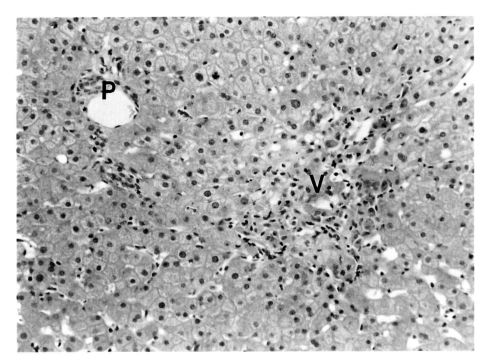

Figure 9.10. *Chronic hepatitis with predominantly lobular activity.* Liver-cell loss and inflammation are seen in a perivenular area (V) but the small portal tract (P) appears normal. This corresponds to a diagnosis of chronic lobular hepatitis. Needle biopsy, H & E.

of HBeAg in serum. At this stage of the disease histological activity may be high and both periportal and intra-acinar necrosis found on biopsy, or low. HBsAg can be demonstrated immunohistochemically. It is most abundant in the characteristic **ground-glass hepatocytes** (Fig. 9.11, and Fig. 1.7 on p. 6), but can also be seen in a membranous or submembranous location in hepatocytes without a ground-glass pattern. The ground-glass cells are typically scattered singly throughout the acini. Their name derives from a granular appearance of parts of the cytoplasm rich in endoplasmic reticulum and HBV surface material. These areas are often separated from the peripheral parts of the cell by a halo. The differential diagnosis of ground-glass hepatocytes in HBV infection is from oncocytic cells (Fig. 9.9), drug-induced hypertrophy of endoplasmic reticulum (Fig. 8.1, p. 104), cyanamide toxicity (p. 105), Lafora's disease and fibrinogen storage disease.[27] The clinical circumstances and staining for HBsAg make confusion unlikely. HBcAg is demonstrable in hepatocyte nuclei and, when activity is high, in cytoplasm (Fig. 1.8, p. 6). Hepatocyte nuclei containing abundant core particles have a pale eosinophilic appearance described as "sanded",[28] and a similar appearance has been attributed to the presence of large amounts of HDV.[29] The nuclei and cytoplasm of hepatocytes rich in HBcAg are reported to stain a reddish-violet colour with chromotrope aniline blue.[30] In addition to HBsAg and HBcAg, HBeAg can also be demonstrated by immunohistochemical methods.[31]

The phase of high virus replication is followed by seroconversion from positivity for HBeAg in serum to a low replication phase without HBeAg but with anti-HBe. This seroconversion is marked by an upsurge of histological activity.[32] In the low HBV replication phase activity is much less and inflammation minimal and more or less confined to portal tracts.[33] Ground-glass hepatocytes are now more often found in groups

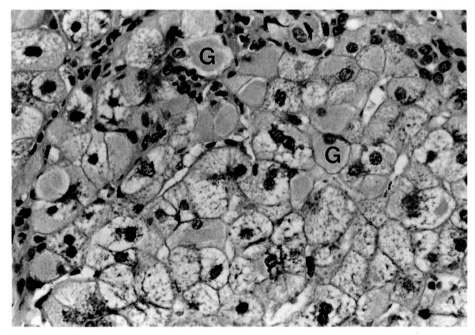

Figure 9.11. *Chronic hepatitis B with ground-glass hepatocytes.* Many of the ground-glass areas (G) are bordered by a characteristic pale-staining halo. See also Figure 1.7, p. 6. Needle biopsy, H & E.

and HBcAg is usually absent. Finally HBsAg may disappear from the serum and evidence of infection be confined to the presence of antibodies. Mild inflammation may still be seen for some time after loss of HBsAg[34] but substantial histological activity at this stage should alert the pathologist to the possibility of superinfection with another virus. There may, however, be much fibrosis or even cirrhosis as a result of previous necrosis and its consequences.

The above sequence of events represents an intentionally oversimplified picture of what may be a much more complex evolution. In patients infected with a mutant strain of virus in which expression of the e antigen is defective, for example, histological activity is sometimes high in spite of absence of HBeAg and presence of anti-HBe.[35] In immunosuppressed patients abundant HBcAg may be found in the absence of significant histological activity.[26] Both high- and low-replicative phases may be marked by periodic exacerbation and reactivation.[36] When all markers of active HBV infection have disappeared, the patient's hepatocyte nuclei may still contain HBV-DNA in integrated form.

As already noted in Chapter 6, the presence of the delta agent, HDV, is associated with relatively high histological activity. Inflammation is rarely restricted to portal tracts, and there is likely to be substantial inflammation and necrosis in periportal areas and deeper within the acini. Positive staining for HDAg denotes active infection.

Apart from the presence of ground-glass hepatocytes and HBV antigens, chronic HBV infection is often characterized by marked variation in the size and appearance of liver-cell nuclei.[26] As already noted in Chapter 6, there is close contact between hepatocytes and lymphocytes.[37] These are usually of CD8+ type, in contrast to the portal infiltrate which is rich in CD4+ lymphocytes, B lymphocytes and dendritic cells.[38] The presence of CD8+ lymphocytes in areas of necrosis correlates with expression of intercellular adhesion molecule-1 (ICAM-1) on hepatocytes but not with markers of viral replication.[39] Lymphoid follicles are occasionally found in portal tracts but are less common and less prominent than in hepatitis C.[9]

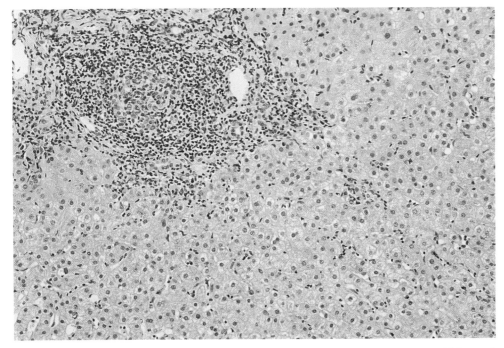

Figure 9.12. *Chronic hepatitis C.* The portal tract top left is heavily infiltrated by lymphocytes, which extend irregularly into the adjacent tissue. A lymphoid follicle with germinal centre has formed. Focal inflammation is seen deep within the parenchyma. Needle biopsy, H & E. Colour version of a half-tone figure in reference 8, with permission from the authors and Mosby-Year Book, Inc.

Table 9.4. Histological Features of Chronic Type C Hepatitis

Difficult to distinguish from acute hepatitis
Often mild but cirrhosis commonly develops
Lymphoid follicles in portal tracts
Damaged interlobular bile ducts
Acinar activity including acidophil bodies
Large-droplet fatty change
Lymphocytes in sinusoids

Chronic Hepatitis C

A chronic course is very common in post-transfusion hepatitis C[40,41] and substantial numbers of patients develop cirrhosis, often after many years or even decades. Hepatocellular carcinoma may ultimately supervene.[42,43] Other forms of transmission can also lead to chronic disease. Initially, the chronic hepatitis is often mild, with little or no periportal component and an appearance on the borderline of CPH and CAH. In periods of exacerbation there is both periportal and intra-acinar necrosis with associated inflammation (Fig. 9.12). Because of prominent portal inflammation early in the disease and acinar lesions later,[44] acute and chronic hepatitis C are sometimes very difficult to distinguish on histological grounds alone. While many patients with evidence of active HCV infection have liver disease, a carrier state with normal liver biopsy appearances has been recorded.[45] Liver histology may be abnormal in patients with normal serum alanine aminotransferase (ALT) values but with HCV-RNA in the serum.[46]

The histological features of chronic hepatitis C, although not completely diagnostic in themselves, are very characteristic (Table 9.4). The portal infiltrate is rich in lymphocytes

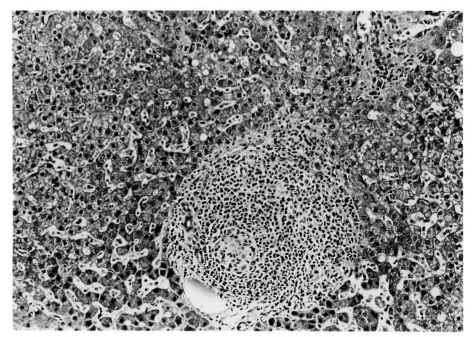

Figure 9.13. *Chronic hepatitis C.* The portal tract is greatly expanded by a lymphoid follicle with germinal centre. Needle biopsy, H & E.

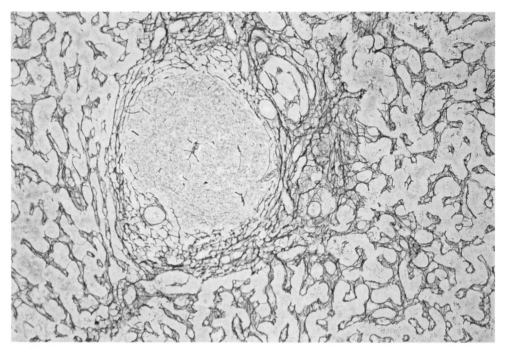

Figure 9.14. *Chronic hepatitis C.* The prominent pale area in the portal tract is the site of a lymphoid follicle. Needle biopsy, reticulin.

which often form aggregates or follicles, some of them with prominent germinal centres (Fig. 9.13).[8–10,47,48] These follicles are easily identified in reticulin preparations (Fig. 9.14).

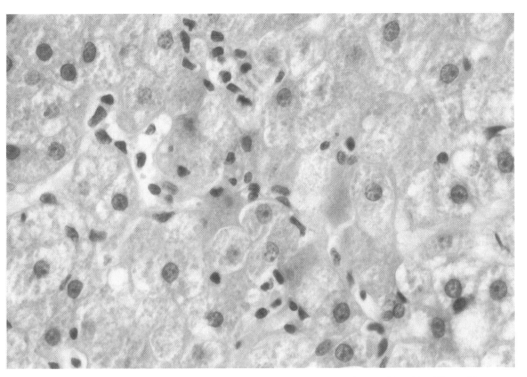

Figure 9.15. *Chronic hepatitis C: acinar component.* Several hepatocytes are abnormally acidophilic and have scalloped outlines. A few fat vacuoles are seen. There is a lymphocytic infiltrate. Needle biopsy, H & E.

Their germinal centres contain activated B cells, surrounded by follicular dendritic cells and a B cell mantle zone.[49] CD4+ cells predominate in the outer T cell zone.[50] Follicles are not restricted to hepatitis C and can also be found in hepatitis B,[9,10] autoimmune hepatitis[8] and primary biliary cirrhosis. In hepatitis C, however, they are particularly common and prominent. Within or to one side of the lymphoid infiltrates, damaged interlobular bile ducts may be seen (Fig. 6.7, p. 67). The damage takes the form of vacuolation, stratification and crowding of epithelial cells, and infiltration by lymphocytes.

The intra-acinar changes typically include acidophilic degeneration of hepatocytes (Fig. 9.15) and formation of acidophil bodies. These have already been described in Chapter 6. Large-droplet fatty change is commoner than in other forms of viral hepatitis[8,10] but because its causes are manifold its presence is rarely of diagnostic help. Clumped material somewhat like Mallory bodies has been reported in periportal hepatocytes.[10] Sinusoids are focally or diffusely infiltrated by lymphocytes. Diffuse infiltration may give rise to a bead-like appearance (Fig. 6.18, p. 76).

Viral RNA can be detected in frozen liver tissue by *in situ* hybridization.[51–53] Immunocytochemical demonstration of viral antigens has also been achieved,[53–55a] but few antibodies tried so far have given reproducible and clinically useful results in paraffin-embedded material.

Other Forms of Chronic Viral Hepatitis

As far as can be ascertained using current diagnostic methods, infection with HBV and HCV does not account for all examples of chronic viral hepatitis.[56] The existence of chronic non-A, non-B, non-C hepatitis is therefore postulated. Some of the biopsies containing paramyxovirus-like structures and showing giant-cell hepatitis[24] were from patients with chronic disease.

Autoimmune Hepatitis

Several types of autoimmune hepatitis are described, each characterized by a different antibody pattern.[57] Type 1, previously called lupoid hepatitis, is the commonest. Antinuclear antibodies and smooth muscle antibodies directed against actin typify this group. Type 2 is characterized by liver-kidney microsomal antibodies, is the commonest type to be found in children, and tends to progress rapidly to cirrhosis. A relationship to HCV infection in some patients has been postulated.[58] Further groups of patients have antibodies against a soluble liver antigen or to liver cytosol. Inability to distinguish reliably between autoimmune and cryptogenic chronic hepatitis by means of clinical, biochemical or histological features suggests that cryptogenic chronic hepatitis may sometimes represent autoimmune hepatitis without abnormal serum antibodies.[59]

Histologically the appearances are those of chronic hepatitis in general, but activity tends to be high in untreated patients. Bridging necrosis, severe piecemeal necrosis and hepatitic rosette formation are common. Giant multinucleated hepatocytes are found in some patients with acute or chronic autoimmune hepatitis.[22,23,60] In rare instances the hepatitis is fulminant.[61] The inflammatory infiltrate is mainly composed of lymphocytes and plasma cells, the latter sometimes in clusters.[8] Lymphoid follicles are occasionally present, but much less often than in hepatitis C. T helper/inducer cells predominate in the portal infiltrate.[11] Immunosuppressive treatment leads to reduction in severity of the inflammatory component and may also lessen fibrosis.[62]

As already noted in Chapter 5, there are overlap syndromes with features of both biliary disease and autoimmune chronic hepatitis. One type with the histological picture of primary biliary cirrhosis but an antibody profile like that of type 1 autoimmune hepatitis has been designated variously as immunocholangitis,[63] autoimmune cholangio-pathy[64] and autoimmune cholangitis.[65]

Drug-induced Chronic Hepatitis

This is discussed in Chapter 8 and will not be described here. It is worth bearing in mind, however, that some commonly used drugs occasionally cause chronic hepatitis and that the possibility of drug aetiology should be considered in any patient in whom the cause of a chronic hepatitis is in doubt.

SEMI-QUANTITATIVE ASSESSMENT OF LIVER BIOPSIES IN CHRONIC HEPATITIS

There is increasing need for numerical scoring of biopsy changes in chronic hepatitis, largely because of the organization of therapeutic trials. Currently the most popular system is the histological activity index (HAI) of Knodell and colleagues.[66,67] In this system four variables are assessed and given scores as follows: periportal and bridging necrosis (0–10), intralobular degeneration and focal necrosis (0–4), portal inflammation (0–4) and fibrosis or cirrhosis (0–4). Readers should refer to the original paper for details of the scoring. Many observers now separate the fibrosis/cirrhosis score from the rest, because it represents the effects of the necro-inflammatory process rather than the process itself. The widespread use of the Knodell system has established a helpful degree of comparability between different therapeutic trials of anti-viral agents. Some pathologists have modified the Knodell system or have devised different scoring systems to suit local needs.[5,68] The main requirements of any semi-quantitative scoring system are that it should give clinically useful information, that it should be simple to apply, and that it should be reproducible by one or more observers.[69,70]

DIFFERENTIAL DIAGNOSIS

In biopsies with inflammation confined to portal tracts, other possibilities to be considered include **resolving acute hepatitis, non-specific inflammation near a focal lesion, primary biliary cirrhosis and lymphoma**. The nature of the infiltrate and involvement of most or all portal tracts in chronic hepatitis should resolve the issue in most cases, but clinical information is also required.

More severe chronic hepatitis needs to be distinguished from **acute hepatitis**, which is sometimes difficult. As discussed on p. 70, staining for elastic fibres may enable recently formed bridges to be distinguished from old fibrous septa. Canalicular cholestasis, common in acute hepatitis, is not often found in chronic hepatitis. In HBV infection the presence of HBsAg-containing ground-glass hepatocytes indicates chronic disease.

Other diseases to be considered in the more severe forms include **chronic biliary tract disorders**, especially primary biliary cirrhosis and primary sclerosing cholangitis, α_1-**antitrypsin deficiency, Wilson's disease and lymphoma**. Partial or complete loss of small and medium-sized bile ducts indicates biliary tract disease rather than chronic hepatitis. α_1-Antitrypsin deficiency can be diagnosed by appropriate staining (p. 206), while Wilson's disease should be established principally by clinical features and biochemical findings. The infiltrates of various lymphomas are usually extensive and irregular, and there may be areas of necrosis within them. As in all forms of liver disease, coordination of clinical and histological information reduces the risk of diagnostic error.

REFERENCES

1. Leevy CM, Popper H, Sherlock S (eds). Diseases of the Liver and Biliary Tract. Standardization of Nomenclature, Diagnostic Criteria, and Diagnostic Methodology. Washington: US Government Printing Office, 1976, p 9.
2. De Groote J, Desmet VJ, Gedigk P et al. A classification of chronic hepatitis. *Lancet* 1968; **ii**: 626–628.
3. Popper H, Schaffner F. The vocabulary of chronic hepatitis. *N Engl J Med* 1971; **284**: 1154–1156.
4. Becker MD, Scheuer PJ, Baptista A, Sherlock S. Prognosis of chronic persistent hepatitis. *Lancet* 1970; **i**: 53–57.
5. Scheuer PJ. Classification of chronic viral hepatitis: a need for reassessment. *J Hepatol* 1991; **13**: 372–374.
6. Ludwig J. The nomenclature of chronic active hepatitis: an obituary. *Gastroenterology* 1993; **105**: 274–278.
7. Fattovich G, Brollo L, Alberti A et al. Chronic persistent hepatitis type B can be a progressive disease when associated with sustained virus replication. *J Hepatol* 1990; **11**: 29–33.
8. Bach N, Thung SN, Schaffner F. The histological features of chronic hepatitis C and autoimmune chronic hepatitis: a comparative analysis. *Hepatology* 1992; **15**: 572–577.
9. Scheuer PJ, Ashrafzadeh P, Sherlock S, Brown D, Dusheiko GM. The pathology of hepatitis C. *Hepatology* 1992; **15**: 567–571.
10. Lefkowitch JH, Schiff ER, Davis GL et al. Pathological diagnosis of chronic hepatitis C: a multicenter comparative study with chronic hepatitis B. *Gastroenterology* 1993; **104**: 595–603.
11. Senaldi G, Portmann B, Mowat AP, Mieli-Vergani G, Vergani D. Immunohistochemical features of the portal tract mononuclear cell infiltrate in chronic aggressive hepatitis. *Arch Dis Child* 1992; **67**: 1447–1453.
12. Takahara T, Nakayama Y, Itoh H et al. Extracellular matrix formation in piecemeal necrosis: immunoelectron microscopic study. *Liver* 1992; **12**: 368–380.
13. Combes B. The initial morphologic lesion in chronic hepatitis, important or unimportant? *Hepatology* 1986; **6**: 518–522.

14. Cooksley WGE, Bradbear RA, Robinson W et al. The prognosis of chronic active hepatitis without cirrhosis in relation to bridging necrosis. *Hepatology* 1986; **6**: 345–348.

15. Chen T-J, Liaw Y-F. The prognostic significance of bridging hepatic necrosis in chronic type B hepatitis: a histopathologic study. *Liver* 1988; **8**: 10–16.

16. Mattsson L, Weiland O, Glaumann H. Application of a numerical scoring system for assessment of histological outcome in patients with chronic posttransfusion non-A, non-B hepatitis with or without antibodies to hepatitis C. *Liver* 1990; **10**: 257–263.

17. Villari D, Raimondo G, Brancatelli S, Longo G, Rodino G, Smedile V. Histological features in liver biopsy specimens of patients with acute reactivation of chronic type B hepatitis. *Histopathology* 1991; **18**: 73–77.

18. Lefkowitch JH, Arborgh BA, Scheuer PJ. Oxyphilic granular hepatocytes. Mitochondrion-rich liver cells in hepatic disease. *Am J Clin Pathol* 1980; **74**: 432–441.

19. Gerber MA, Thung SN. Hepatic oncocytes. Incidence, staining characteristics, and ultrastructural features. *Am J Clin Pathol* 1981; **75**: 498–503.

20. Richey J, Rogers S, Van Thiel DH, Lester R. Giant multinucleated hepatocytes in an adult with chronic active hepatitis. *Gastroenterology* 1977; **73**: 570–574.

21. Thaler H. Post-infantile giant cell hepatitis. *Liver* 1982; **2**: 393–403.

22. Devaney K, Goodman ZD, Ishak KG. Postinfantile giant-cell transformation in hepatitis. *Hepatology* 1992; **16**: 327–333.

23. Lau JYN, Koukoulis G, Mieli-Vergani G, Portmann BC, Williams R. Syncytial giant-cell hepatitis – a specific disease entity? *J Hepatol* 1992; **15**: 216–219.

24. Phillips MJ, Blendis LM, Poucell S et al. Syncytial giant-cell hepatitis. Sporadic hepatitis with distinctive pathological features, a severe clinical course, and paramyxoviral features. *N Engl J Med* 1991; **324**: 455–460.

25. Liaw YF, Chu CM, Chen TJ, Lin DY, Chang-Chien CS, Wu CS. Chronic lobular hepatitis: a clinicopathological and prognostic study. *Hepatology* 1982; **2**: 258–262.

26. Bianchi L, Gudat F. Chronic hepatitis. In MacSween RNM, Anthony PP, Scheuer PJ, Portmann B, Burt AD (eds): Pathology of the Liver, 3rd edn. Edinburgh: Churchill Livingstone, 1994.

27. Callea F, de Vos R, Togni R, Tardanico R, Vanstapel MJ, Desmet VJ. Fibrinogen inclusions in liver cells: a new type of ground-glass hepatocyte. Immune light and electron microscopic characterization. *Histopathology* 1986; **10**: 65–73.

28. Bianchi L, Gudat F. Sanded nuclei in hepatitis B: eosinophilic inclusions in liver cell nuclei due to excess in hepatitis B core antigen formation. *Lab Invest* 1976; **35**: 1–5.

29. Moreno A, Ramón y Cajal S, Marazuela M et al. Sanded nuclei in delta patients. *Liver* 1989; **9**: 367–371.

30. Ozeki T, Mizuno S, Sanefuzi H et al. Localization of hepatitis B core antigens in chronic active hepatitis using immunoperoxidase and chromotrope aniline blue staining. *Br J Exp Pathol* 1987; **68**: 605–612.

31. Chu CM, Liaw YF. Immunohistological study of intrahepatic expression of hepatitis B core and E antigens in chronic type B hepatitis. *J Clin Pathol* 1992; **45**: 791–795.

32. Liaw Y-F, Yang S-S, Chen T-J, Chu C-M. Acute exacerbation in hepatitis B e antigen positive chronic type B hepatitis. *J Hepatol* 1985; **1**: 227–233.

33. Chu CM, Karayiannis P, Fowler MJ, Monjardino J, Liaw YF, Thomas HC. Natural history of chronic hepatitis B virus infection in Taiwan: studies of hepatitis B virus DNA in serum. *Hepatology* 1985; **5**: 431–434.

34. Perrillo RP, Brunt EM. Hepatic histologic and immunohistochemical changes in chronic hepatitis B after prolonged clearance of hepatitis B e antigen and hepatitis B surface antigen. *Ann Intern Med* 1991; **115**: 113–115.

35. Naoumov NV, Schneider R, Grötzinger T et al. Precore mutant hepatitis B virus infection and liver disease. *Gastroenterology* 1992; **102**: 538–543.

36. Davis GL, Hoofnagle JH. Reactivation of chronic type B hepatitis presenting as acute viral hepatitis. *Ann Intern Med* 1985; **102**: 762–765.

37. Dienes HP, Popper H, Arnold W, Lobeck H. Histologic observations in human hepatitis non-A, non-B. *Hepatology* 1982; **2**: 562–571.

38. van den Oord JJ, De Vos R, Facchetti F, Delabie J, De Wolf Peeters C, Desmet VJ. Distribution of non-lymphoid, inflammatory cells in chronic HBV infection. *J Pathol* 1990; **160**: 223–230.

39. Horiike N, Onji M, Kumon I, Kanaoka M, Michitaka K, Ohta Y. Intercellular adhesion molecule-1 expression on the hepatocyte membrane of patients with chronic hepatitis B and C. *Liver* 1993; **13**: 10–14.

40. Tremolada F, Casarin C, Alberti A et al. Long-term follow-up of non-A, non-B (type C) post-transfusion hepatitis. *J Hepatol* 1992; **16**: 273–281.

41. Verbaan H, Widell A, Lindgren S, Lindmark B, Nordenfelt E, Eriksson S. Hepatitis C in chronic liver disease: an epidemiological study based on 566 consecutive patients undergoing liver biopsy during a 10-year period. *J Int Med* 1992; **232**: 33–42.

42. Gerber MA. Relation of hepatitis C virus to hepatocellular carcinoma. *Hepatology* 1993; **17**(Suppl 3): S108–S111.

43. Tsukuma H, Hiyama T, Tanaka S et al. Risk factors for hepatocellular carcinoma among patients with chronic liver disease. *N Engl J Med* 1993; **328**: 1797–1801.

44. Roberts JM, Searle JW, Cooksley WGE. Histological patterns of prolonged hepatitis C infection. *Gastroenterol Jpn* 1993; **28** (Suppl. 5): 37–41.

45. Brillanti S, Foli M, Gaiani S, Masci C, Miglioli M, Barbara L. Persistent hepatitis C viraemia without liver disease. *Lancet* 1993; **341**: 464–465.

46. Alberti A, Morsica G, Chemello L et al. Hepatitis C viraemia and liver disease in symptom-free individuals with anti-HCV. *Lancet* 1992; **340**: 697–698.

47. Gerber MA, Krawczynski K, Alter MJ, Sampliner RE, Margolis HS. Sentinel Counties Chronic Non-A Non-B Hepatitis Study Team. Histopathology of community acquired chronic hepatitis C. *Modern Pathol* 1992; **5**: 483–486.

48. Kobayashi K, Hashimoto E, Ludwig J, Hisamitsu T, Obata H. Liver biopsy features of acute hepatitis C compared with hepatitis A, B, and non-A, non-B, non-C. *Liver* 1993; **13**: 69–73.

49. Mosnier J-F, Degott C, Marcellin P, Hénin D, Erlinger S, Benhamou J-P. The intraportal lymphoid nodule and its environment in chronic active hepatitis C: an immunohistochemical study. *Hepatology* 1993; **17**: 366–371.

50. Hino K, Okuda M, Konishi T et al. Analysis of lymphoid follicles in liver of patients with chronic hepatitis C. *Liver* 1992; **12**: 387–391.

51. Haruna Y, Hayashi N, Hiramatsu N et al. Detection of hepatitis C virus RNA in liver tissues by an in situ hybridization technique. *J Hepatol* 1993; **18**: 96–100.

52. Tanaka Y, Enomoto N, Kojima S et al. Detection of hepatitis C virus RNA in the liver by *in situ* hybridization. *Liver* 1993; **13**: 203–208.

53. Yamada G, Nishimoto H, Endou H et al. Localization of hepatitis C viral RNA and capsid protein in human liver. *Dig Dis Sci* 1993; **38**: 882–887.

54. Hiramatsu N, Hayashi N, Haruna Y et al. Immunohistochemical detection of hepatitis C virus-infected hepatocytes in chronic liver disease with monoclonal antibodies to core, envelope and NS3 regions of the hepatitis C virus genome. *Hepatology* 1992; **16**: 306–311.

55. Krawczynski K, Beach MJ, Bradley DW et al. Hepatitis C virus antigen in hepatocytes: immunomorphologic detection and identification. *Gastroenterology* 1992; **103**: 622–629.

55a. González-Peralta RP, Fang JWS, Davis GL et al. Optimization for the detection of hepatitis C virus antigens in the liver. *J Hepatol* 1994; **20**: 143–147.

56. Chemello L, Cavalletto D, Pontisso P et al. Patterns of antibodies to hepatitis C virus in patients with chronic non-A, non-B hepatitis and their relationship to viral replication and liver disease. *Hepatology* 1993; **17**: 179–182.

57. Johnson PJ, McFarlane IG, Eddleston ALWF. The natural course and heterogeneity of autoimmune-type chronic active hepatitis. *Semin Liver Dis* 1991; **11**: 187–196.

58. Michel G, Ritter A, Gerken G, Meyer zum Büschenfelde KH, Decker R, Manns MP. Anti-GOR and hepatitis C virus in autoimmune liver diseases. *Lancet* 1992; **339**: 267–269.

59. Czaja AJ, Carpenter HA, Santrach PJ, Moore SB, Homburger HA. The nature and prognosis of severe cryptogenic chronic active hepatitis. *Gastroenterology* 1993; **104**: 1755–1761.

60. Lefkowitch JH, Apfelbaum TF, Weinberg L, Forester G. Acute liver biopsy lesions in early autoimmune ("lupoid") chronic active hepatitis. *Liver* 1984; **4**: 379–386.

61. Porta G, Gayotto LCC, Alvarez F. Anti-liver-kidney microsome antibody-positive autoimmune hepatitis presenting as fulminant liver failure. *J Pediatr Gastroenterol Nutr* 1990; **11**: 138–140.

62. Schvarcz R, Glaumann H, Weiland O. Survival and histological resolution of fibrosis in patients with autoimmune chronic active hepatitis. *J Hepatol* 1993; **18**: 15–23.

63. Brunner G, Klinge O. Ein der chronisch-destruierenden nicht-eitrigen Cholangitis ähnliches Krankheitsbild mit antinukleären Antikörpern (Immuncholangitis). *Dtsch Med Wochenschr* 1987; **112**: 1454–1458.

64. Ben-Ari Z, Dhillon AP, Sherlock S. Autoimmune cholangiopathy: part of the spectrum of autoimmune chronic active hepatitis. *Hepatology* 1993; **18**: 10–15.

65. Michieletti P, Wanless IR, Katz A et al. Are patients with antimitochondrial antibody negative primary biliary cirrhosis a distinct syndrome of autoimmune cholangitis? *Gut* 1994; **35**: 260–265.

66. Knodell RG, Ishak KG, Black WC et al. Formulation and application of a numerical scoring system for assessing histological activity in asymptomatic chronic active hepatitis. *Hepatology* 1981; **1**: 431–435.

67. Lindh G, Weiland O, Glaumann H. The application of a numerical scoring system for evaluating the histological outcome in patients with chronic hepatitis B followed in long term. *Hepatology* 1988; **8**: 98–103.

68. Lok ASF, Lindsay I, Scheuer PJ, Thomas HC. Clinical and histological features of delta infection in chronic hepatitis B virus carriers. *J Clin Pathol* 1985; **38**: 530–533.

69. Goldin R, Patel N, Goldin J et al. Comparison of liver biopsies in chronic hepatitis: Knodell or Scheuer? *J Pathol* 1993; **169** (Suppl) (Abstract).

70. Patel N, Goldin R, Hubscher S et al. Reporting chronic viral hepatitis: intraobserver variation when using the Knodell and Scheuer systems. *J Pathol* 1993; **170** (Suppl) (Abstract).

GENERAL READING

Bianchi L, Gudat F. Chronic hepatitis. In MacSween RNM, Anthony PP, Scheuer PJ, Portmann B, Burt AD (eds): Pathology of the Liver, 3rd edn. Edinburgh: Churchill Livingstone, 1994.

Carman WF, Thomas HC. Genetic variation in hepatitis B virus. *Gastroenterology* 1992; **102**: 711–719.

Colombari R, Dhillon AP, Piazzola E et al. Chronic hepatitis in multiple virus infection: histopathological evaluation. *Histopathology* 1993; **22**: 319–325.

Czaja AJ, Carpenter HA. Sensitivity, specificity, and predictability of biopsy interpretations in chronic hepatitis. *Gastroenterology* 1993; **105**: 1824–1832.

Desmet VJ. Immunopathology of chronic viral hepatitis. *Hepato-gastroenterol* 1991; **38**: 14–21.

Gerber MA. Chronic hepatitis C: the beginning of the end of a time-honored nomenclature? *Hepatology* 1992; **15**: 733–734.

Johnson PJ, McFarlane IG, Eddleston ALWF. The natural course and heterogeneity of autoimmune-type chronic active hepatitis. *Semin Liver Dis* 1991; **11**: 187–196.

Scheuer PJ. Classification of chronic viral hepatitis: a need for reassessment. *J Hepatol* 1991; **13**: 372–374.

10

CIRRHOSIS

Cirrhosis is a diffuse process in which the normal acini are replaced by nodules separated by fibrous tissue.[1,2] The nodules, which are most commonly the result of regenerative hyperplasia following hepatocellular injury, are functionally less efficient than normal hepatic parenchyma and there is a profound disturbance of vascular relationships.

Several different kinds of information can be obtained about the cirrhotic liver by means of liver biopsy (Table 10.1). The most important functions of biopsy are to establish a diagnosis, to assess the cause of the cirrhosis as far as possible and to detect hepatocellular carcinoma.

THE DIAGNOSIS OF CIRRHOSIS BY LIVER BIOPSY

The ease with which the pathologist can diagnose cirrhosis from a biopsy specimen depends on the sample as well as on the criteria used. The sample may be sufficiently large, and the nodules sufficiently small, to make the diagnosis obvious. On the other hand a slender core from within a large cirrhotic nodule can be difficult to identify as such. There are occasions when the pathologist can do no more than hint at the possibility of cirrhosis.

The type of biopsy needle used also influences the ease of diagnosis. Very narrow needles may be adequate to obtain tumour samples but inadequate for the accurate diagnosis of medical conditions. Some clinicians prefer to use the Trucut type of needle when cirrhosis is suspected in order to lessen the risk of fragmentation but suitable samples can usually be obtained with needles of the aspiration type.[3,4] Transjugular biopsy is used when there is a risk of haemorrhage by other routes, and provides samples which, though often small, are usually adequate for the diagnosis of cirrhosis.[5] The combination of biopsy with laparoscopy has been advocated.[6] Operative wedge biopsies of cirrhotic liver give an accurate idea of the relative proportions of parenchyma and stroma in the liver as a whole.[7]

The histological criteria for a diagnosis of cirrhosis are outlined in Table 10.2. The two fundamental criteria, nodularity and fibrosis, reflect the definition of cirrhosis. When there are well-defined rounded nodules surrounded by fibrous septa the diagnosis is easily established. The only likely confusion is with recent bridging necrosis, a problem which can be resolved by examination of stains for elastic fibres, as discussed on p. 70, and by attention to clinical data. Occasionally, a nodular appearance just deep to the liver

Table 10.1. Main Information from Liver Biopsy in Cirrhosis

Diagnosis of cirrhosis
Assessment of cause
Stage of development
Histological activity
Diagnosis of hepatocellular carcinoma

Table 10.2. Cirrhosis: Diagnostic Criteria

A. Fundamental
    Nodularity
    Fibrosis
B. Relative
    Fragmentation
    Abnormal structure
    Hepatocellular changes
        Regenerative hyperplasia
        Pleomorphism
        Large-cell dysplasia
        Small-cell dysplasia
        Excess copper-associated protein

capsule is not representative of the whole liver but has resulted from transection of a tongue or peninsula extending from the main bulk of the parenchyma.

In many patients the relative criteria listed in Table 10.2 are equally important. They enable a tentative diagnosis of cirrhosis to be reached, readily convertible to a firm diagnosis when correlated with other data. These include the consistency of the liver when penetrated by the biopsy needle.

Fragmentation

Fragmentation of the specimen, either at the time of biopsy or during processing in the laboratory, should itself suggest the possibility of cirrhosis (Fig. 10.1). The specimen is more likely to break into fragments when needles of the aspiration type (e.g. Menghini) are used, and when biopsy is by the transjugular route.

Abnormal Structure

Structural changes should be assessed by means of a reticulin preparation, preferably not counterstained. This may show two features not readily seen with other stains. First, although nodules are readily cored out of the dense fibrous stroma of a cirrhotic liver during aspiration biopsy, a thin layer of connective tissue tends to adhere to the nodules over much of their surface (Fig. 10.2). This layer may be difficult to see even with the help of collagen stains and is easily missed in haematoxylin and eosin-stained sections (Fig. 10.3). Secondly, minor alterations of structure become apparent even in those nodules which closely mimic normal liver. Such alterations include abnormal orientation of reticulin fibres resulting from different patterns and rates of growth in different areas (Fig. 10.4), and approximation of portal tracts and terminal venules. The number of venules may be abnormally large in relation to the number of portal tracts (Fig. 10.5),

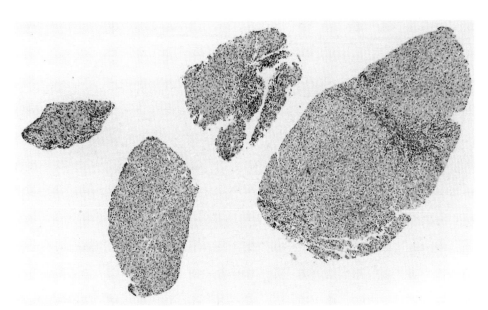

Figure 10.1. *Cirrhosis: fragmented sample*. A specimen obtained by the aspiration biopsy method has broken into several pieces. Needle biopsy, H & E.

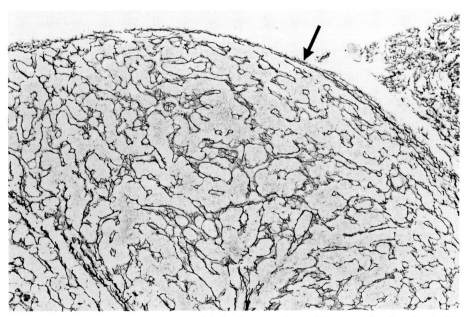

Figure 10.2. *Cirrhosis: selective sampling*. A nodule has been cored out of the connective tissue by the biopsy procedure but a thin layer of connective tissue (arrow) has adhered to the nodule margin. Needle biopsy, reticulin.

and the latter are sometimes abnormally small and poorly formed (Fig. 1.4, p. 4). A more obvious structural abnormality in cirrhosis is the presence of septa linking terminal hepatic venules to portal tracts. These septa must be distinguished from recently formed necrotic bridges, as discussed on p. 70.

In wedge biopsies, excess fibrous tissue in and near the capsule and crowding of vessels

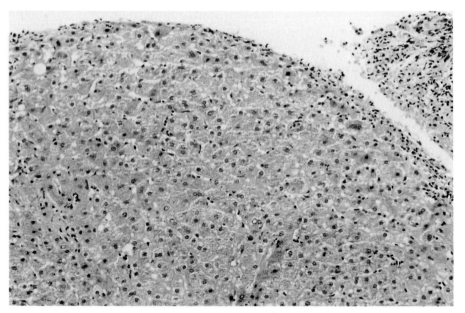

Figure 10.3. *Cirrhosis: selective sampling.* Same field as in Figure 10.2. In a haematoxylin and eosin preparation the thin layer of connective tissue is not easily seen. Needle biopsy, H & E.

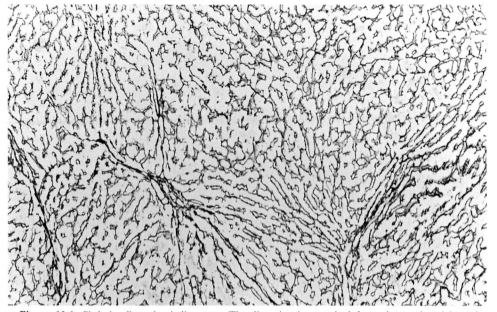

Figure 10.4. *Cirrhosis: distorted reticulin pattern.* The distortion has resulted from abnormal and irregular hepatocyte growth patterns. Needle biopsy, reticulin.

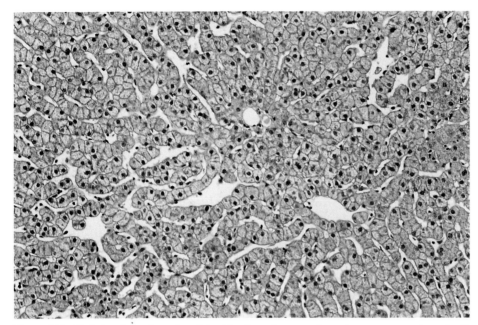

Figure 10.5. *Cirrhosis: abnormal vascular relationships.* Several venous channels are seen near to each other. Wedge biopsy, H & E.

must be distinguished from the changes of cirrhosis. The latter extend through the specimen whereas the former are confined to the capsular and immediately subcapsular area.[8] Very occasionally a wedge biopsy of part of a large well-differentiated regeneration nodule fails to show the histological features of cirrhosis.

Hepatocellular Changes

In some biopsies from cirrhotic livers the hepatocytes are normal in appearance and arrangement, so that diagnosis rests on the structural changes discussed above. In others there are more or less obvious abnormalities of growth.

Regeneration is indicated by thickening of the liver-cell plates (Fig. 10.6). In any liver an oblique plane of sectioning will cause a few plates to appear more than one cell thick but widespread double-cell plates are seen when there is active growth. Hepatocytes in hyperplastic areas contain little or no lipofuscin pigment even near terminal venules. Regeneration is not always evident in cirrhosis because it is not a continuous process. Its absence does not therefore exclude the diagnosis. Conversely its presence does not prove cirrhosis, because it is found also in other circumstances, for example, after an acute hepatitis.

A very characteristic feature of cirrhosis is the presence of adjacent populations of hepatocytes growing at different rates and having different cell and nuclear characteristics (Fig. 10.7). This **pleomorphism** gives rise to the abnormalities of reticulin pattern already mentioned, notably a tendency for reticulin fibres in the different growth areas to lie in different directions.

In a minority of cirrhotic livers the hepatocytes show structural atypia of a degree sufficient to warrant a label of **dysplasia**. Two types of dysplasia have been described.[9] In the large-cell form, the cells are enlarged and their nuclei hyperchromatic and

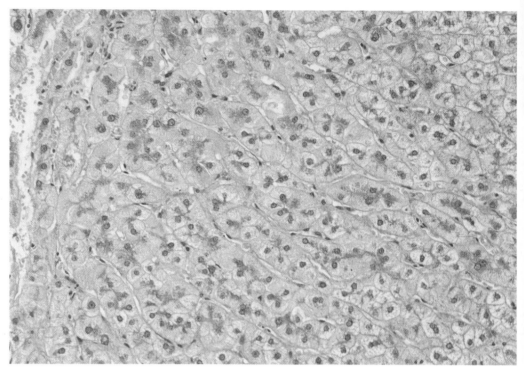

Figure 10.6. *Cirrhosis: hepatocellular regeneration.* Liver-cell plates are two or more cells thick, indicating active growth. Needle biopsy, H & E.

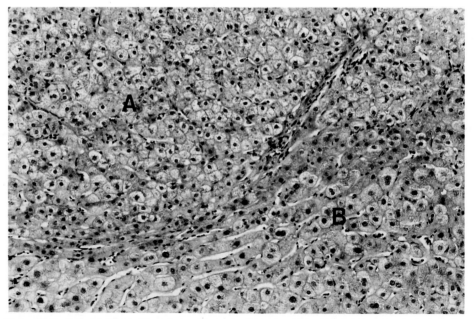

Figure 10.7. *Cirrhosis: different cell populations.* The parenchyma in area A has compressed area B, the cells of which are larger. Wedge biopsy, H & E.

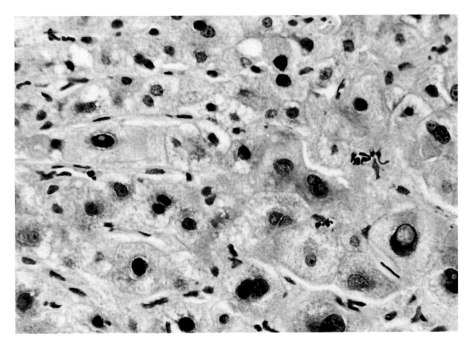

Figure 10.8. *Cirrhosis: large-cell dysplasia.* The nuclei of the enlarged hepatocytes below right are irregular in shape and vary greatly in size and staining intensity. Compare with the normal hepatocytes above. Wedge biopsy, H & E.

irregular in shape, with prominent nucleoli (Fig. 10.8). Nuclear–cytoplasmic ratio is normal or only moderately increased.[10] This type of dysplasia was first described in an African population with a high incidence of hepatocellular carcinoma.[11] There is some evidence that it is associated with an increased risk of development of this cancer independently of other risk factors.[12] Large-cell dysplasia is mainly found in patients with HBV infection but is not restricted to them.[13] In small-cell dysplasia the nuclear–cytoplasmic ratio is increased but the overall size of the affected cells is less than normal (Fig. 10.9).[9] Zones of dysplastic hepatocytes of either type support a diagnosis of cirrhosis and are regarded by some clinicians as an indication for increased monitoring for hepatocellular carcinoma.

Differential Diagnosis

When there is nodularity and evidence of regeneration but little or no fibrosis, **nodular regenerative hyperplasia** (p. 155) should be considered. In **congenital hepatic fibrosis** (p. 201) the acinar architecture remains intact and the ductal plate malformation is seen. In **chronic hepatitis** with fibrosis and structural abnormalities, the differential diagnosis is between active cirrhosis and chronic hepatitis which has not yet reached the stage of cirrhosis. This problem cannot always be resolved on the basis of a liver biopsy. Similar doubt may arise in alcoholic liver disease. The presence of substantial quantities of copper and copper-associated protein in non-cholestatic chronic liver disease supports a diagnosis of cirrhosis.[14] Cirrhotic nodules can usually be distinguished from well-differentiated **hepatocellular carcinoma**. In the latter the cell plate architecture is more abnormal, reticulin may be scanty or absent and the cells have malignant cytological characteristics (p. 160).

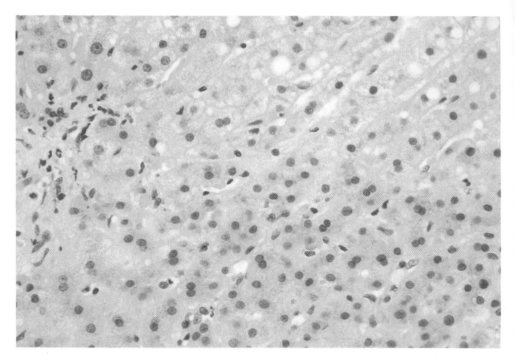

Figure 10.9. *Cirrhosis: small-cell dysplasia.* The hepatocytes below and to the right have normal-sized nuclei, but their overall size is reduced. Nuclear–cytoplasmic ratios are therefore increased. Needle biopsy, H & E.

ASSESSMENT OF CAUSE

Biopsy may help to establish the cause of a cirrhosis. In some of the categories listed in Table 10.3 the histological appearances are diagnostic. The term "cryptogenic" should only be applied when full clinical and laboratory investigations have been completed and the features listed in Table 10.4 have been assessed. This can be achieved by means of a small range of routine stains.

Table 10.3. Main Causes of Cirrhosis

Viral hepatitis (B, C, D)
Alcohol abuse
Biliary disease
Metabolic disorders
   Haemochromatosis
   Wilson's disease
   α_1-Antitrypsin deficiency, etc.
Venous outflow obstruction
Drugs and toxins
Autoimmune disease

Pattern of Nodules and Fibrosis

Irregularly shaped nodules suggest the possibility of a biliary cause, especially if there is perinodular oedema, ductular proliferation and chronic cholestasis (p. 34). In a pre-

Table 10.4. Cirrhosis: Assessment of Cause

Pattern of nodules and fibrosis
Bile ducts
Blood vessels
Steatohepatitis
Evidence of viral infection
Abnormal deposits
Iron
Copper, copper-associated protein
α_1-Antitrypsin globules

cirrhotic stage of venous outflow obstruction (p. 188) there is regular fibrosis in acinar zones 3, and normal portal tracts and dilated sinusoids are seen within the "nodules".

Bile Ducts

Assessment of bile duct numbers in cirrhosis is very important. The number of ducts should approximately equal the number of arteries of similar size and location. Definite duct loss almost always indicates primary biliary cirrhosis or primary sclerosing cholangitis. In children or young adults, other ductopenic syndromes should also be considered. Typical bile-duct lesions of primary biliary cirrhosis, with or without granulomas, are still sometimes found at a stage of cirrhosis. Periductal fibrosis may be very prominent in primary sclerosing cholangitis. Ductular proliferation is a non-specific finding, but when severe and focal it often reflects biliary disease. Following extensive hepatocellular damage in cirrhosis, for example, after variceal haemorrhage, there is sometimes very extensive proliferation of duct-like structures which can be mistaken for cholangiocarcinoma.

Blood Vessels

Occluded, narrowed or recanalized veins suggest that the cirrhosis may be the result of venous outflow block, but are also found in cirrhosis from other causes.[15] Recognition of venous lesions is often difficult without the help of stains for collagen or elastic fibres.

Steatohepatitis (Fatty Liver Hepatitis)

This is found in alcohol abusers (p. 89) and occasionally in the obese, in diabetic subjects and as a feature of drug toxicity. In amiodarone toxicity (p. 105) the fatty change is usually absent. Steatohepatitis must be distinguished from chronic cholestasis, in which there are also swollen hepatocytes containing Mallory bodies (p. 34).

Evidence of Viral Infection

Features of chronic hepatitis, notably piecemeal necrosis and lymphocytic infiltration, are often but by no means always due to infection with one of the hepatitis viruses. Liver-cell dysplasia also favours a viral cause. Ground-glass hepatocytes and viral antigens help in the diagnosis of hepatitis B virus infection, but are not always present or detectable. Lymphoid aggregates or follicles should suggest the possibility of hepatitis C (Fig. 10.10). More than one virus or other causal agent may be responsible for a patient's cirrhosis.

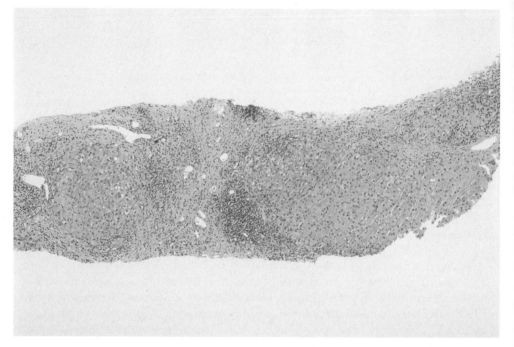

Figure 10.10. *Cirrhosis following hepatitis C virus infection.* Lymphoid aggregates are still visible. Needle biopsy, H & E.

Abundant plasma cells raise the possibility of autoimmune hepatitis (p. 130) but are also sometimes found in viral hepatitis.

Abnormal Deposits

Severe siderosis should always raise the possibility of genetic haemochromatosis, even when another cause is also evident. In pure genetic haemochromatosis the nodules are sometimes irregular as in biliary cirrhosis.

Copper and copper-associated protein can often be detected in cirrhosis, whatever its cause.[14] Large amounts at the edges of nodules suggest biliary disease while staining of entire nodules is seen in Wilson's disease. Other nodules may be negative. In some stages of the disease the copper is not histochemically demonstrable, so that negative staining does not exclude the diagnosis. Abundant copper and Mallory bodies are also features of Indian childhood cirrhosis.[16]

α_1-Antitrypsin bodies (p. 206) should always be looked for in cirrhosis. Immunocytochemical staining is more sensitive than diastase-PAS.

ANATOMICAL TYPE

Because of possible sampling error, the pathologist cannot confidently assess nodule size in the rest of the liver on the basis of a biopsy specimen. This is of little consequence to the patient. Primary classification of cirrhosis by nodule size is no longer appropriate, because aetiology is clinically much more important.

However, nodule size does influence ease of histological diagnosis. When nodules are of

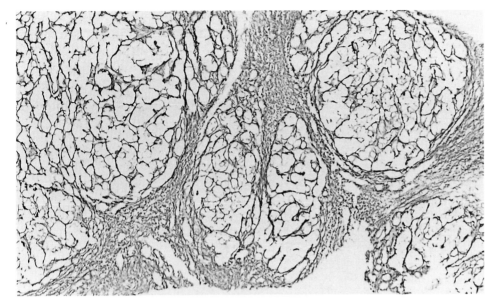

Figure 10.11. *Cirrhosis: micronodular pattern.* Nodules are of acinar size or smaller. Needle biopsy, reticulin.

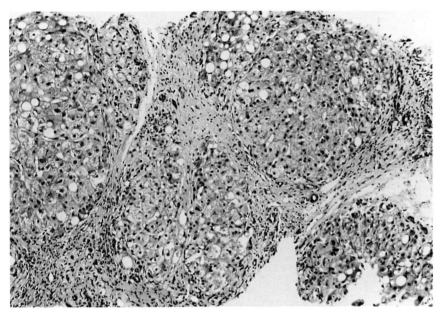

Figure 10.12. *Cirrhosis: micronodular pattern.* Same field as in Figure 10.11. There is steatosis. Needle biopsy, H & E.

the size order of the acini from which they are derived, several nodules are usually seen in one biopsy and diagnosis is easy (Figs 10.11 and 10.12). When nodules are larger (Figs 10.13 and 10.14), more subtle diagnostic criteria need to be considered. The most difficult anatomical type to recognize is **incomplete septal cirrhosis**. This is characterized by indistinct nodularity, slender septa some of which end blindly, poorly formed small portal tracts and abnormal relationships between portal tracts and efferent venules (Fig.

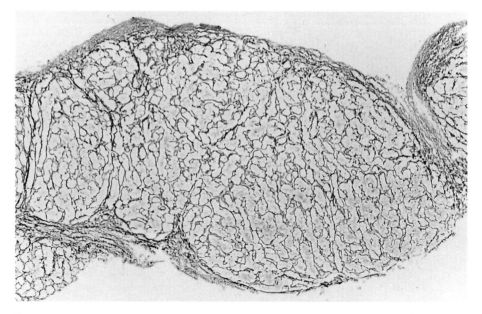

Figure 10.13. *Cirrhosis: macronodular pattern.* Nodules are larger than in Figures 10.11 and 10.12. The magnification is slightly smaller. Needle biopsy, reticulin.

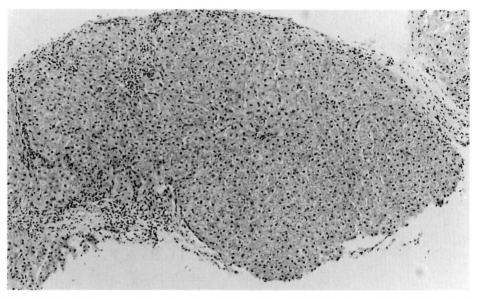

Figure 10.14. *Cirrhosis: macronodular pattern.* Same field as in Figure 10.13. The diagnosis is less obvious than in the reticulin preparation. Needle biopsy, H & E.

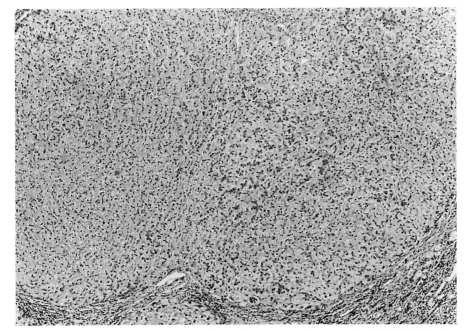

Figure 10.15. *Cirrhosis: incomplete septal pattern.* No portal tracts or venules are seen in this field. Wedge biopsy, H & E.

10.15).[17] There is evidence of hepatocytic hyperplasia, giving rise to crowding of reticulin fibres in adjacent areas. Sinusoidal dilatation is common, while inflammation and necrosis are generally modest or absent. A reticulin preparation is important for diagnosis because the slender septa are easily missed (Figs 10.15 and 10.16). The diagnosis is more easily made in wedge biopsies than in needle specimens. A relationship with various forms of non-cirrhotic portal hypertension has been postulated.[17,18]

STAGE OF DEVELOPMENT

In some patients cirrhosis is obvious and appears mature, in the sense that the well-demarcated nodules and dense fibrosis give an impression of long-standing disease. In others there is doubt as to whether there is cirrhosis or merely fibrosis. An impression may be gained that cirrhosis is incipient or at an early stage of development (Figs 10.17 and 10.18). When doubt is unresolved, a report of "developing cirrhosis" is sometimes appropriate. Once cirrhosis is fully established, reversion to a normal acinar pattern is unlikely.

Paradoxically, there may be confusion between mild chronic hepatitis and an inactive well-established cirrhosis. This reflects difficulty in diagnosing some examples of late cirrhosis by needle biopsy, because of a tendency for nodule size to increase with time.

HISTOLOGICAL ACTIVITY

Activity is a convenient term to describe the rate of progression of the cirrhosis. It is usually taken to mean the various forms of liver-cell damage and inflammation typical of

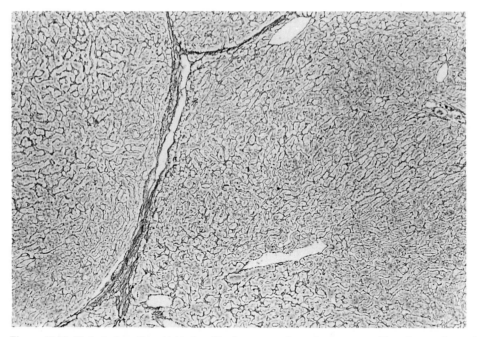

Figure 10.16. *Cirrhosis: incomplete septal pattern.* Slender septa and vessels are present. There is a small portal tract on the right, towards the top of the figure. Wedge biopsy, reticulin.

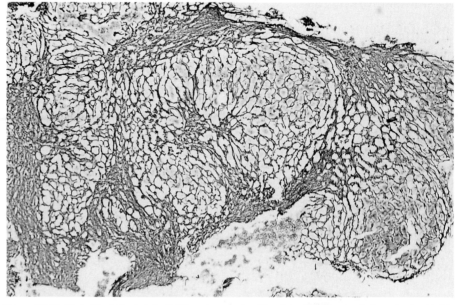

Figure 10.17. *Early (developing) cirrhosis.* There is extensive fibrosis and architectural distortion in this biopsy from an alcohol abuser. Nodules are beginning to form but are not yet clearly defined. Needle biopsy, reticulin.

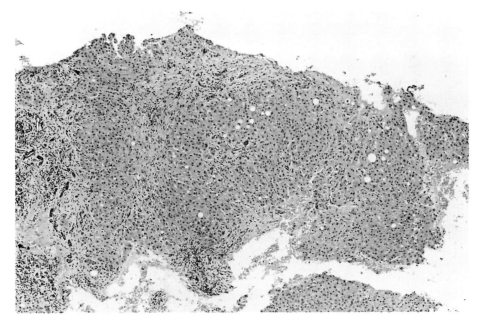

Figure 10.18. *Early (developing) cirrhosis.* Same field as in Figure 10.17. Structural changes are more difficult to assess than in the reticulin preparation. There is mild steatosis. Needle biopsy, H & E.

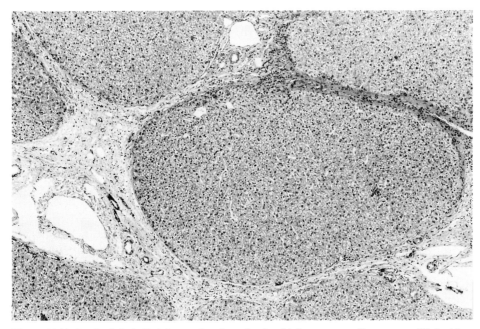

Figure 10.19. *Inactive cirrhosis.* Nodules are sharply outlined and inflammatory cells are scanty. Wedge biopsy, H & E.

chronic viral hepatitis. In cirrhosis following steatohepatitis, however, the severity of the latter should also be taken into account.

In an inactive cirrhosis the interface between septa and nodules is sharply defined (Fig. 10.19). Cellular infiltration is mild and may be confined to the septa. There is little or no

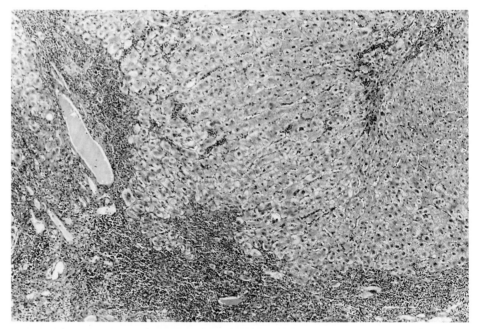

Figure 10.20. *Active cirrhosis.* The outline of the nodule is blurred by piecemeal necrosis and there is a heavy inflammatory infiltrate. Wedge biopsy, H & E.

focal necrosis or intranodular inflammation. In an active, rapidly progressive cirrhosis on the other hand the interface is blurred by hepatocellular damage and inflammation (Fig. 10.20). Isolated hepatocytes or groups of cells may be seen within the inflamed septa. There is hepatocellular damage and inflammation deep within the nodules.

Histological activity often varies in severity from one part of the liver to another. Comparison of activity in multiple biopsies from an individual patient should therefore be made with caution and with reference to clinical and biochemical data.

COMPLICATIONS

Hypoperfusion leads to coagulative necrosis involving whole nodules or their centres.[19] This is sometimes referred to as **nodular infarction**.

One or more nodules of a cirrhotic liver may enlarge disproportionately to form **macroregenerative nodules**. The term adenomatous hyperplasia is used for the same process. The nodules are defined either by their size or by their different macroscopic appearance.[20–23] Histologically there may be little or no difference from other nodules, or there may be hepatocellular dysplasia. The importance of macroregenerative nodules lies in their possible relationship to **hepatocellular carcinoma**.[21a,23] This commonly arises in cirrhotic liver. Both macroregenerative nodules and hepatocellular carcinoma are discussed in detail in Chapter 11.

REFERENCES

1. Anthony PP, Ishak KG, Nayak NC, Poulsen HE, Scheuer PJ, Sobin LH. The morphology of cirrhosis: definition, nomenclature, and classification. *Bull World Health Organ* 1977; **55**: 521–540.

2. Anthony PP, Ishak KG, Nayak NC, Poulsen HE, Scheuer PJ, Sobin LH. The morphology of cirrhosis. Recommendations on definition, nomenclature, and classification by a working group sponsored by the World Health Organization. *J Clin Pathol* 1978; **31**: 395–414.
3. Bateson MC, Hopwood D, Duguid HL, Bouchier IA. A comparative trial of liver biopsy needles. *J Clin Pathol* 1980; **33**: 131–133.
4. Littlewood ER, Gilmore IT, Murray-Lyon IM, Stephens KR, Paradinas FJ. Comparison of the Trucut and Surecut liver biopsy needles. *J Clin Pathol* 1982; **35**: 761–763.
5. Sawyerr AM, McCormick PA, Tennyson GS et al. A comparison of transjugular and plugged-percutaneous liver biopsy in patients with impaired coagulation. *J Hepatol* 1993; **17**: 81–85.
6. Orlando R, Lirussi F, Okolicsanyi L. Laparoscopy and liver biopsy: further evidence that the two procedures improve the diagnosis of liver cirrhosis. A retrospective study of 1,003 consecutive examinations. *J Clin Gastroenterol* 1990; **12**: 47–52.
7. Imamura H, Kawasaki S, Bandai Y, Sanjo K, Idezuki Y. Comparison between wedge and needle biopsies for evaluating the degree of cirrhosis. *J Hepatol* 1993; **17**: 215–219.
8. Petrelli M, Scheuer PJ. Variation in subcapsular liver structure and its significance in the interpretation of wedge biopsies. *J Clin Pathol* 1967; **20**: 743–748.
9. Crawford JM. Pathologic assessment of liver cell dysplasia and benign liver tumors: differentiation from malignant tumors. *Sem Diagnostic Pathol* 1990; **7**: 115–128.
10. Roncalli M, Borzio M, Tombesi MV, Ferrari A, Servida E. A morphometric study of liver cell dysplasia. *Hum Pathol* 1988; **19**: 471–474.
11. Anthony PP, Vogel CL, Barker LF. Liver cell dysplasia: a premalignant condition. *J Clin Pathol* 1973; **26**: 217–223
12. Borzio M, Bruno S, Roncalli M et al. Liver cell dysplasia and risk of hepatocellular carcinoma in cirrhosis: a preliminary report. *Br Med J* 1991; **302**: 1312.
13. Lefkowitch JH, Apfelbaum TF. Liver cell dysplasia and hepatocellular carcinoma in non–A, non–B hepatitis. *Arch Pathol Lab Med* 1987; **111**: 170–173.
14. Guarascio P, Yentis F, Cevikbas U, Portmann B, Williams R. Value of copper-associated protein in diagnostic assessment of liver biopsy. *J Clin Pathol* 1983; **36**: 18–23.
15. Nakanuma Y, Ohta G, Doishita K. Quantitation and serial section observations of focal venocclusive lesions of hepatic veins in liver cirrhosis. *Virchows Arch (A)* 1985; **405**: 429–438.
16. Mehrotra R, Pandey RK, Nath P. Hepatic copper in Indian childhood cirrhosis. *Histopathology* 1981; **5**: 659–665.
17. Sciot R, Staessen D, Van Damme B et al. Incomplete septal cirrhosis: histopathological aspects. *Histopathology* 1988; **13**: 593–603.
18. Lopez JI. Does incomplete septal cirrhosis link non-cirrhotic nodulations with cirrhosis? *Histopathology* 1989; **15**: 318–320.
19. Henrion J, Colin L, Schmitz A, Schapira M, Heller FR. Ischemic hepatitis in cirrhosis. Rare but lethal. *J Clin Gastroenterol* 1993; **16**: 35–39.
20. Theise ND, Schwartz M, Miller C, Thung SN. Macroregenerative nodules and hepatocellular carcinoma in forty-four sequential adult liver explants with cirrhosis. *Hepatology* 1992; **16**: 949–955.
21. Nakanuma Y, Terada T, Ueda K, Terasaki S, Nonomura A, Matsui O. Adenomatous hyperplasia of the liver as a precancerous lesion. *Liver* 1993; **13**: 1–9.
22. Ferrell LD, Crawford JM, Dhillon AP, Scheuer PJ, Nakanuma Y. Proposal for standardized criteria for the diagnosis of benign, borderline, and malignant hepatocellular lesions arising in chronic advanced liver disease. *Am J Surg Pathol* 1993; **17**: 1113–1123.
23. Terada T, Terasaki S, Nakanuma Y. A clinicopathologic study of adenomatous hyperplasia of the liver in 209 consecutive cirrhotic livers examined by autopsy. *Cancer* 1993; **72**: 1551–1556.

GENERAL READING

Millward-Sadler GH. Cirrhosis. In MacSween RNM, Anthony PP, Scheuer PJ, Portmann B, Burt AD (eds): Pathology of the Liver, 3rd edn. Edinburgh: Churchill Livingstone, 1994.

NEOPLASMS AND NODULES

11

This chapter is intended to provide a working overview of the tumours and tumour-like nodular lesions that the pathologist will encounter with some frequency in every-day practice. The majority of these can be classified according to the indigenous cells of the liver (hepatocytes, bile-duct epithelium and endothelium) from which they arise (Table 11.1). Neoplastic and nodular lesions of children are covered at the end of the chapter. The reader is encouraged to consult the references and general reading list for additional details and coverage of some of the rarer tumours.

NEOPLASMS AND NODULES IN ADULTS

Benign Lesions

Liver-cell Adenoma

Liver-cell adenomas are solitary or occasionally multiple tumours composed of hepatocytes. Macroscopically they are well-defined but often not encapsulated. The cells of the tumour closely resemble normal hepatocytes (Fig. 11.1). Nuclei are small and regular, and mitoses are almost never seen. These features are evident in fine-needle aspiration biopsies.[1] The cells are arranged in normal or thickened trabeculae interspersed with prominent arteries and thin-walled blood vessels. Small liver-cell rosettes (acini) with a central bile-filled or empty lumen may be seen, as in cholestatic liver. In addition to bile, adenomas may contain fat or even show steatohepatitis with Mallory bodies.[2] Non-necrotizing granulomas within adenomas have also been described.[3] In adenomas, reticulin is normal or reduced, but extensive loss is in most cases confined to areas of necrosis or haemorrhage. The latter are characteristically found in adenomas in oral contraceptive users, and are responsible for pain and for the serious complication of haemoperitoneum. They probably also explain the fibrous scars which are sometimes found in the lesions. Regular septa, portal tracts and bile ducts are, however, absent; this distinguishes liver-cell adenomas both from non-neoplastic liver and from macroregenerative nodules in cirrhosis as well as focal nodular hyperplasia (see below). The distinction from hepatocellular carcinoma is occasionally difficult, but can usually be made confidently on the basis of trabecular pattern, retention of normal amounts of reticulin and appearance of the tumour cells.

Most liver-cell adenomas arise in women of child-bearing age, usually after prolonged use of oral contraceptives.[4] Adenomatosis, in which multiple tumours are seen throughout the liver, is much less common, and is found in either sex,[5,6] sometimes in patients taking

Table 11.1. Classification of Liver Tumours and Nodular Lesions

Cell of Origin	Benign	Malignant
Hepatocyte	Liver-cell adenoma MRN FNH NRH PNT	Hepatocellular carcinoma Fibrolamellar carcinoma Hepatoblastoma
Bile-duct epithelium	Bile-duct adenoma Cystadenoma Adenofibroma	Cholangiocarcinoma Cystadenocarcinoma
Mixed liver-cell and bile-duct cell	Mesenchymal hamartoma	Combined hepatocellular-cholangiocarcinoma
Endothelial cell	Haemangioma Infantile haemangioendothelioma*	Angiosarcoma Epithelioid haemangioendothelioma

MRN, macroregenerative nodule; FNH, focal nodular hyperplasia; NRH, nodular regenerative hyperplasia; PNT, partial nodular transformation.
*Some cases may behave more aggressively and are capable of metastasis.

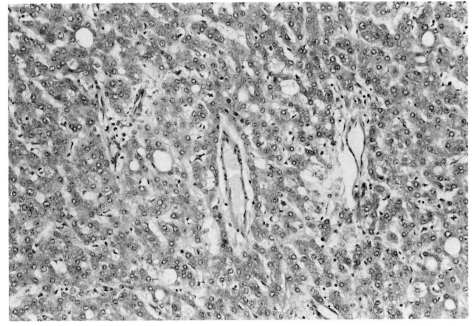

Figure 11.1. *Hepatocellular adenoma.* Liver cells appear normal or contain fat vacuoles. Blood vessels but no portal tracts are seen within the lesion. Operative specimen, H & E.

anabolic/androgenic steroids.[7] Anabolic/androgenic steroid-related hepatocellular tumours[8] in children or adults sometimes appear malignant histologically but do not necessarily behave in a malignant manner, and may therefore be regarded as adenomas rather than carcinomas.[9,10] They may contain areas of peliosis, blood-filled spaces with an incomplete endothelial lining. Liver cell adenomas may also arise in patients with diabetes[11] or type I glycogen storage disease,[12] and in children or young adults not receiving steroid hormones (see "Neoplasms and nodules in children", p. 171).

Macroregenerative Nodules

The macroregenerative nodule (MRN) is an unusually large regenerative nodule measuring 0.8 cm or more in diameter which develops in cirrhosis or other chronic liver disease[13–25] (Fig. 11.2). MRNs are particularly common in macronodular cirrhosis.[26] In addition to size, they can grossly be discerned by their colour and texture which differ from the surrounding liver.[13,16,26] The cirrhotic liver may harbour several macroregenerative nodules.

As mentioned in Chapter 10, the macroregenerative nodule is synonymous with adenomatous hyperplasia. The MRN histologically shows hyperplastic liver parenchyma arranged in plates 2–3 cells thick, which is typical of cirrhosis. The nodule contains portal tracts and fibrous septa with bile ducts, hepatic arteries and portal vein branches. Steatosis, hemosiderin, bile plugs and Mallory bodies may be present.[13] Japanese investigators[26] have characterized two types of MRNs. The type I (ordinary or typical) macroregenerative nodule is structurally quite similar, except for its size, to surrounding cirrhotic nodules and shows no cellular atypia. Type II MRNs (atypical adenomatous hyperplasia) are histologically disturbing because of varied degrees of large and small cell dysplasia, increased cellularity, and foci where the liver cords are less cohesive or pseudoacini have formed.[13,14] These atypical MRNs should be classified as borderline lesions.[14] The major diagnostic concern is to distinguish the MRN from hepatocellular carcinoma. The presence of intranodular portal tracts and maintenance of an orderly liver-cell plate arrangement with well-defined reticulin fibres are characteristic of the former, while loss of reticulin, formation of broad trabeculae and an infiltrative margin are features of carcinoma.[13,14,16,17] From a conceptual standpoint regarding the development of hepatocellular carcinoma, macroregenerative nodules may coexist with carcinoma elsewhere in the liver, they may contain foci of carcinoma and they may represent a precursor lesion.

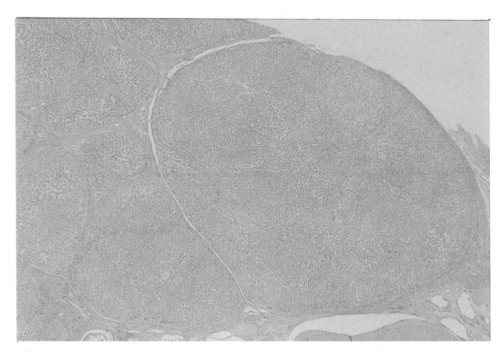

Figure 11.2. *Macroregenerative nodule.* This low magnification view demonstrates the increased size of the nodule at right compared to the cirrhotic nodules at left. Operative specimen, H & E. Illustration kindly provided by Dr Kamal Ishak, Washington, DC.

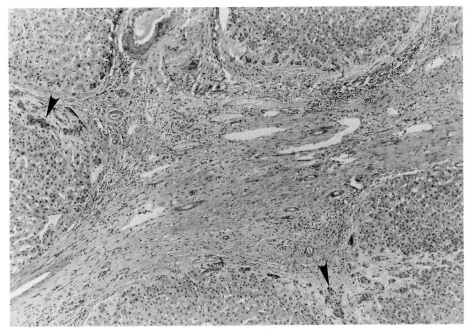

Figure 11.3. *Focal nodular hyperplasia.* Part of a central scar containing blood vessels and small bile duct-like structures (arrowheads). The parenchyma is nodular. Operative specimen, H & E.

Focal Nodular Hyperplasia (FNH)

This is a fairly common lesion, seen in either sex and at any age. Its nature and pathogenesis are still controversial, but Wanless and colleagues suggest that it may represent a hyperplastic response to an abnormal blood supply.[27] FNH, unlike liver-cell adenoma, does not appear to be caused by oral contraceptives, although these may cause an increase in size and vascularity.[28] Bleeding and rupture are rare. Features of focal nodular hyperplasia and adenoma are only very occasionally seen in the same tumour, and the occurrence of the two lesions in the same liver may be coincidental.[29] There may be multiple FNH in the same patient, and these individuals often have other lesions, including vascular anomalies (hepatic haemangioma, telangiectasis of the brain, berry aneurysm, dysplastic systemic arteries, portal vein atresia) and central nervous system neoplasms (meningioma, astrocytoma).[30,31]

Macroscopically the nodules are well demarcated from the normal hepatic parenchyma. They are usually pale and are dissected by fibrous septa into nodules, giving them an appearance very like that of cirrhosis. There may be a prominent central fibrous scar (Fig. 11.3). Histologically the appearance is also very like that of an inactive cirrhosis. The dense fibrous septa contain large thick-walled and sometimes narrowed arteries, as well as bile duct-like structures probably derived by metaplasia from liver-cell plates.[32] The presence of bile duct cells in fine-needle aspiration cytology of FNH is helpful in distinguishing this lesion from hepatocellular carcinoma.[33]

Nodular Regenerative Hyperplasia (NRH)

In this condition multiple hyperplastic parenchymal nodules with thickened liver-cell plates are seen, but fibrosis is absent or slight (Fig. 11.4). This distinguishes the lesion from cirrhosis. In some cases perisinusoidal fibrosis is found in the compressed liver tissue between nodules. Portal tracts may be found at the centres of the nodules but this is not

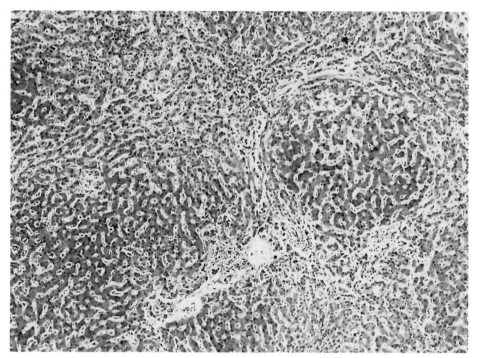

Figure 11.4. *Nodular regenerative hyperplasia.* This abnormal growth pattern is not accompanied by the formation of fibrous septa. The condition is therefore different from cirrhosis. Post-mortem liver, H & E.

invariable. Diagnosis is often difficult in needle biopsy specimens. The nodularity may be more clearly seen in reticulin preparations. A wedge liver biopsy may be required to establish the diagnosis firmly and to exclude an important differential, incomplete septal cirrhosis.

NRH is associated with a wide range of conditions, mainly rheumatic diseases, myeloproliferative disorders and chronic venous congestion.[34-36] Patients with NRH may have received therapeutic drugs, including corticosteroids, anabolic steroids, oral contraceptives, anti-neoplastics, anti-convulsants and immunosuppressive agents.[34,37,38] NRH has also been associated with the toxic oil syndrome,[39] Behçet's disease,[40] early histological stages of primary biliary cirrhosis,[41] livers containing metastatic neuroendocrine tumours[42] and non-cirrhotic liver in which hepatocellular carcinoma has developed.[43] Some patients with NRH have portal hypertension. Serum alkaline phosphatase and gamma glutamyl transpeptidase may be elevated.[36,41]

Wanless and co-workers have postulated that the basic lesion is portal venous thrombosis, leading to atrophy and compensatory hyperplasia.[44] Arterial lesions, particularly arteriosclerosis of ageing, may also contribute to these changes.[36] Portal venous thrombosis has also been invoked in the pathogenesis of the rare **partial nodular transformation**, in which somewhat larger nodules are found, often localized to the perihilar region.[45] Nodular regenerative hyperplasia, focal nodular hyperplasia and partial nodular transformation share the common feature of liver-cell hyperplastic growth in the form of nodules; they have accordingly been grouped under the umbrella heading of "nodular transformation" by Wanless.[46] The main features of the various non-cirrhotic nodular conditions so far discussed are summarized in Table 11.2.

Table 11.2. Non-cirrhotic Parenchymal Nodules

Type	Number	Involvement of Liver	Structure	Relation to Other Conditions and Drugs	Portal Hypertension
Focal nodular hyperplasia	Solitary or few	Focal	Mixed	—	No
Liver-cell adenoma	Solitary or few; rarely many	Focal	Liver cells	Probable relation to oral contraceptives	No
Nodular regenerative hyperplasia	Many	Diffuse	Liver cells	Myeloproliferative disorders, rheumatoid diseases, drugs, toxins, congestion, etc.	Sometimes
Partial nodular transformation	Several	Perihilar	Liver cells, some fibrous tissue	Thickened portal veins	Usually

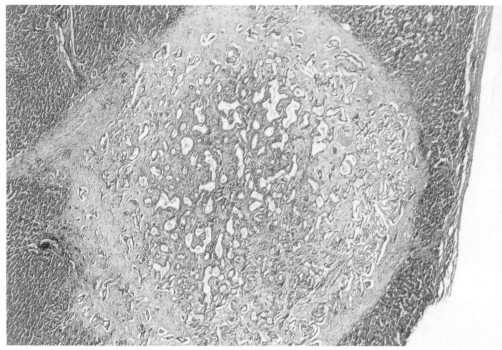

Figure 11.5. *Bile-duct adenoma.* This subcapsular tumour consists of closely packed bile ducts set in a dense fibrous stroma. The capsule is at right. Operative specimen, H & E.

Bile-duct Adenoma

Bile-duct adenomas are small grey–white, usually subcapsular nodules measuring from 1 to 20 mm in diameter.[47] They are more often solitary than multiple. Histologically they are composed of small well-formed ducts embedded in a stroma of mature fibrous tissue which may contain chronic inflammatory cells[47–49] (Fig. 11.5). Their chief importance is that they may be mistaken for metastatic carcinoma, both macroscopically and microscopically. They differ from microhamartomas (von Meyenburg complexes; p. 202) in that the ducts are smaller and more numerous, are usually not dilated and do not contain bile.[47,50] PAS-positive, diastase-resistant globules of α_1-antitrypsin within the bile-duct epithelium of multiple adenomas were described in a patient with heterozygous α_1-antitrypsin deficiency.[51] The bile-duct adenoma should also be distinguished from the rare **biliary adenofibroma**, a much larger tumour composed of tubulocystic bile-duct structures with apocrine metaplasia and intraluminal bile embedded in fibrous stroma, resembling fibroadenoma of the breast.[52]

Biliary Cystadenoma

This is a multilocular tumour, the cystic spaces of which contain mucoid fluid and are lined by columnar, mucin-secreting epithelium which may form papillary projections. A variant with subepithelial **mesenchymal stroma** containing myofibroblasts occurs in women.[53,54] Malignant change is common.[55]

Haemangioma

The cavernous haemangioma is the most common benign tumour of the liver, found incidentally at autopsy or operation and occasionally seen in biopsy material.[56] A few

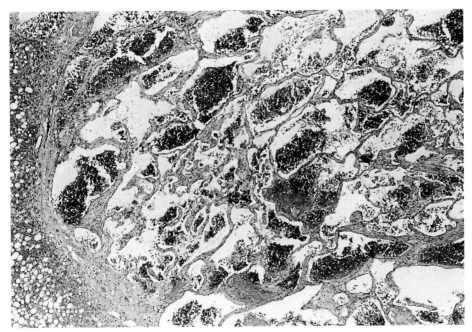

Figure 11.6. *Haemangioma.* Blood-filled spaces are separated by fibrous septa. Liver tissue (left) is fatty. Operative specimen, H & E.

reach a large and clinically significant size. As in other sites, the lesions are composed of endothelium-lined channels supported by a fibrous stroma (Fig. 11.6). Complications include thrombosis, sclerosis and calcification.[57] Spontaneous rupture is recorded but uncommon. A distinction should be made between cavernous haemangiomas and peliosis (p. 186); the latter lacks the complete endothelial layer and fibrous trabeculae. **Lymphangioma** of the liver has been reported as part of multiorgan lymphangiomatosis or as a solitary hepatic lesion,[58] but is very rare. The endothelial-lined channels of this neoplasm are empty or contain lymph with occasional leucocytes. It should not be mistaken for mesenchymal hamartoma (see "Neoplasms and nodules in children", p. 171).

Mesenchymal and Neural Tumours

Connective-tissue elements, adipocytes and smooth muscle of the liver, nerve sheaths of intrahepatic nerves and other mesenchymal cells may give rise to rare tumours, including lipomas, myelolipomas, angiomyelolipomas,[59,60] schwannomas and neurofibromas[61,62] and chondromas.[63] **Angiomyolipomas** resemble their commoner renal counterparts, and contain blood vessels, smooth muscle and fat.[64] Muscle cells may be partly of epithelioid type, with finely granular eosinophilic cytoplasm and pleomorphic nuclei.[65,66] These may be mistaken for hepatocytes or malignant cells. Megakaryocytes and other bone marrow elements are commonly present. **Pseudolipomas**[67] probably represent separated nodules of peritoneal fat which become embedded in the liver capsule.

Inflammatory Pseudotumour

This is an inflammatory lesion of unknown cause, which may be mistaken histologically for a malignant neoplasm.[68–71] The various components include vimentin-positive[70] spindle cells which may be arranged in bundles or whorls, plasma cells, lymphocytes, eosinophils and foamy histiocytes. There is fibrosis both within and around the mass. Granulomas and partly obliterated blood vessels may be present.

Malignant Lesions

Hepatocellular Carcinoma (HCC)

Advances in molecular biology have enhanced our understanding of the pathogenesis of hepatocellular carcinoma, one of the most common cancers in man. While hepatitis B virus infection worldwide remains a major risk factor, our perspective now includes roles for hepatitis C virus infection,[72-75] liver damage in haemochromatosis and aflatoxin exposure, cellular growth factors and oncogenes.[76] Chronic necrosis and inflammation of the liver in and of itself may drive the multistep process of hepatocarcinogenesis.[76,77] Studies of oval cells, a periportal stem-cell population with features of both hepatocytes and bile-duct epithelium, hold out the possibility that these cells are progenitors of hepatocellular carcinoma.[78,79]

The majority of hepatocellular carcinomas develop in cirrhotic liver.[80] The non-neoplastic liver tissue may show varying degrees of **liver-cell dysplasia**, especially in hepatitis B virus carriers, but this varies according to the population studied.[81] The **large cell** form of liver-cell dysplasia, the type most often observed, shows cell and nuclear enlargement, nuclear pleomorphism, increased multinucleation and increased nuclear staining (Fig. 10.8, p. 141). The **small cell** form shows enlarged, hyperchromatic nuclei within small hepatocytes (increased nuclear–cytoplasmic ratio) arranged in crowded clusters[82] (Fig. 10.9, p. 142). The significance of large cell versus small cell dysplasia in the development of hepatocellular carcinoma remains unsettled,[80,83,84] although the large cell variant is usually aneuploid[85] and has for several decades been stressed as a pre-neoplastic lesion. Other cellular changes have been cited as indicators of pre-malignancy, such as the presence of intracytoplasmic Mallory bodies[86] and iron-negative foci in siderotic macroregenerative nodules.[87]

The cirrhosis associated with carcinoma is often macronodular in pattern. It is usually inactive, although inflammation and necrosis may be seen near the tumour itself. Hepatocellular carcinoma sometimes develops in the livers of hepatitis B virus carriers in the absence of cirrhosis.[88,89] Intrahepatic tumour spread is both portal (via portal-vein branches) and acinar.[90]

The outstanding histological features of hepatocellular carcinoma are the resemblance of the tumour cells to normal hepatocytes, and of their arrangement to the trabeculae of normal liver (Fig. 11.7). However, the trabeculae are for the most part thicker and reticulin is often scanty or even absent (Fig. 11.8). In exceptional cases where there may be an increase in reticulin, other histological features and/or the clinical behaviour of the tumour must be used as diagnostic criteria of malignancy. Between the trabeculae there is a network of sinusoids lined by endothelium which is positive with immunostains for factor VIII-related antigen and *Ulex europaeus* lectin.[91] The absence of portal tracts and a cohesive connective tissue framework in the tumour results in a characteristic fragmentation of needle biopsy specimens with separation of tumour trabeculae that is readily observed at low magnification. Although connective tissue stroma is uncommon except in **fibrolamellar carcinoma** (described below), focal areas of fibrosis may follow tumour necrosis. A form of HCC designated as **sclerosing carcinoma**[92] is often associated with hypercalcaemia; some of these tumours appear to be of bile-duct rather than hepatocellular origin. The **adenoid** (acinar) variant of hepatocellular carcinoma (Fig. 11.9) should not be confused with adenocarcinoma of the biliary tree. Bile-duct carcinomas are usually scirrhous, mucin-secreting tumours, whereas the characteristic secretion of hepatocellular

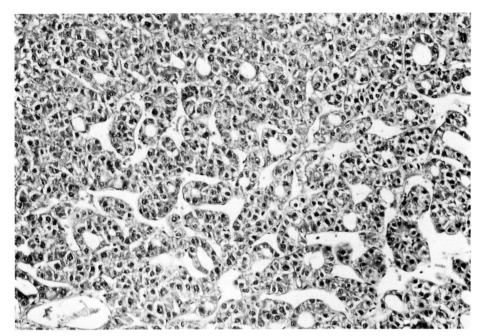

Figure 11.7. *Hepatocellular carcinoma.* Note the trabecular-sinusoidal structure and resemblance of the tumour cells to normal hepatocytes. Needle biopsy, H & E.

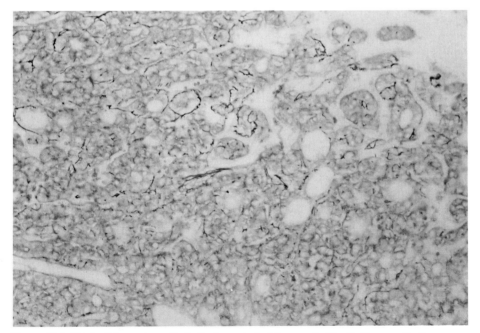

Figure 11.8. *Hepatocellular carcinoma.* Reticulin is scanty in this example. Needle biopsy, reticulin.

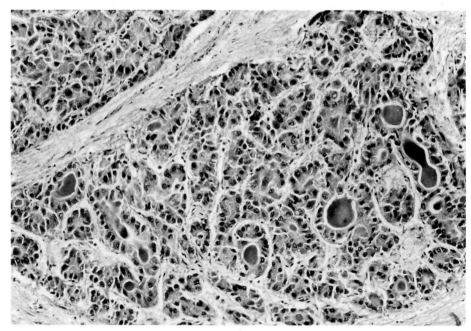

Figure 11.9. *Hepatocellular carcinoma.* Adenoid pattern. Other areas of this tumour showed a more typical trabecular structure. Post-mortem liver, H & E.

carcinomas is bile, seen in a minority of tumours in spaces homologous with normal bile canaliculi. In hepatitis B-positive patients, the varied histological expression of HCC may be related to different patterns of viral DNA integration.[93]

At a cellular level, variants include giant-cell forms with multinucleated tumour cells (Fig. 11.10), spindle-cell or sarcomatoid tumours[94,95] and clear-cell carcinomas. The latter must be distinguished from metastatic renal adenocarcinoma.[96,97] Grading of hepatocellular carcinoma appears to have little value in establishing prognosis. Fine-needle aspiration yields diagnostic material in a high proportion of patients.[98–101]

When there is doubt about the hepatocellular origin of a carcinoma, further evidence can sometimes be gained from the characteristics of the tumour cells. In hepatocellular carcinoma these often contain fat and glycogen, and may also contain α_1-antitrypsin globules (p. 208) even in patients without genetic α_1-antitrypsin deficiency. Mallory bodies are commonly found in the cytoplasm of the tumour cells.[102] Bile canaliculi sometimes stain positively with polyclonal antibody to carcinoembryonic antigen (CEA).[103] Evidence of hepatocellular origin is also provided when immunohistochemical stains of paraffin sections are positive for albumin, fibrinogen, liver-cell cytokeratins (8 and 18), α_1-antitrypsin or α_1-antichymotrypsin.[104–108] The monoclonal antibody Hep Par 1 (Hepatocyte Paraffin 1), with high specificity for hepatocyte staining, also holds promise.[108a] α-Fetoprotein is an unreliable immunohistochemical marker for HCC, in contrast to hepatoblastoma where most cases stain positively. Tumour cells are negative with monoclonal anti-CEA[104] and with AE1 cytokeratin[106] stains. More aggressive carcinomas show diminished staining for extracellular matrix proteins collagen type IV and laminin.[109]

Fibrolamellar Carcinoma

This tumour usually develops in non-cirrhotic liver in older children and adults and carries a better prognosis (because of its resectability[110]) than typical hepatocellular carcinoma.[111–113] The lesions are solitary or multiple, and occasionally resemble focal

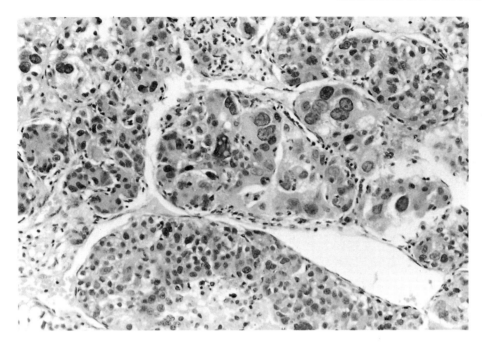

Figure 11.10. *Hepatocellular carcinoma.* Giant multinucleated tumour cells (centre) contrast with the smaller cells below. Needle biopsy, H & E.

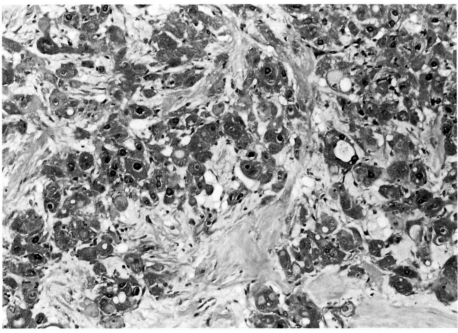

Figure 11.11. *Hepatocellular carcinoma: fibrolamellar type.* Groups of large, densely stained tumour cells are surrounded by pale fibrous septa. Many of the tumour cells contain vacuoles or inclusions. Needle biopsy, H & E.

nodular hyperplasia macroscopically in having a central fibrous scar.[114] The unique histological features distinguish this tumour from routine hepatocellular carcinoma. Fibrous lamellae are arranged in parallel separate groups of large, densely eosinophilic tumour cells[113,115] (Fig. 11.11). The eosinophilia is due to the presence of abundant

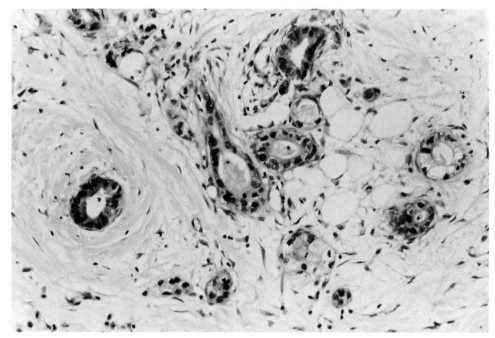

Figure 11.12. *Bile-duct carcinoma.* There are islands of adenocarcinoma in the connective tissue. The appearances are different from those of the hepatocellular carcinoma of adenoid pattern shown in Figure 11.9. Operative specimen, H & E.

mitochondria.[112,116] Tumour cells commonly contain eosinophilic, diastase-PAS negative globules which stain immunohistochemically for C-reactive protein, fibrinogen and α_1-antitrypsin, as well as cytoplasmic "pale bodies" which are reactive for fibrinogen.[113] Additional features include bile production (as in other forms of hepatocellular carcinoma), copper and copper-associated protein within tumour cells,[117,118] and stainable carcinoembryonic antigen in bile canaliculi.[119] Some fibrolamellar carcinomas have neuroendocrine features[120,121] and in some cases the tumour shows features of both fibrolamellar and typical hepatocellular carcinoma. Despite isolated reports such as the association of Fanconi anaemia with fibrolamellar carcinoma,[122] the pathogenesis of this tumour is uncertain and risk factors are not apparent.

Bile-duct Carcinoma

Carcinoma of the bile ducts can arise anywhere between the papilla of Vater and the smaller branches of the biliary tree within the liver. It is not usually associated with cirrhosis. Carcinoma of the hepatic ducts is an important cause of biliary obstruction which may be missed at laparotomy unless the intrahepatic bile ducts are explored or visualized. The commonest known predisposing factors to bile-duct cancer are infestation with oriental flukes, ulcerative colitis[123] (presumably on the basis of primary sclerosing cholangitis) and congenital cystic lesions of the biliary tree.[124] Of these, Caroli's disease and choledochal cysts are important precursors, but carcinoma may also arise in von Meyenburg complexes (bile-duct microhamartomas).[125] Tumours arising from bile ducts within the liver are often referred to as **cholangiocarcinomas**.[126] Intrahepatic cholangiocarcinoma is a known consequence of hepatolithiasis in Japan.[127]

Microscopically, bile-duct carcinomas are mucin-secreting adenocarcinomas with a fibrous stroma (Fig. 11.12). They are composed of cuboidal or columnar cells and may have a papillary pattern. Adenosquamous, squamous, mucinous and anaplastic

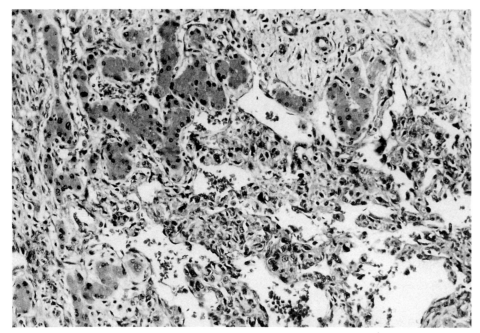

Figure 11.13. *Angiosarcoma.* Elongated tumour cells surround islands of hepatocytes in this highly vascular tumour. Operative specimen, H & E.

histological types are less common.[128] Intra- and perineural invasion are common. The presence of free stromal mucin, small groups and isolated tumour cells in fibrous stroma and the concurrence of apparently normal epithelium and abnormal tumour cells within a duct-like structure all help to distinguish cholangiocarcinoma from metastatic tumour.[129] Cholangiocarcinoma must be distinguished from the acinar type of hepatocellular carcinoma, a distinction usually made with confidence on the basis of mucin or bile secretion, respectively. In difficult cases positive staining for epithelial membrane antigen,[130] tissue polypeptide antigen,[131] biliary cytokeratins[105] (7 and 19), Lewis^x and Lewis^y blood group-related antigens,[132] and α-amylase[133] helps to exclude hepatocellular carcinoma. Truly mixed tumours are rare, and are sometimes fibrolamellar in type.[134] The differential diagnosis of bile-duct cancer includes epithelioid haemangioendothelioma (p. 166). Bile-duct tumours are very occasionally of neuroendocrine type, with characteristic neurosecretory granules in their cytoplasm.

Cystadenocarcinomas are rare malignant tumours which sometimes develop from benign cystadenomas.[53,55] Although these have been considered distinct from the more aggressive carcinomas arising from pre-existing congenital cystic lesions,[135] occasional tumours with features of cystadenocarcinoma develop in fibropolycystic disease.[136]

Angiosarcoma

This uncommon, highly malignant tumour forms multiple or less often solitary haemorrhagic masses. Predisposing factors include treatment with arsenic,[137] injection of the radioactive contrast medium thorotrast[138–140] and industrial exposure to vinyl chloride.[141] Other postulated factors include copper-containing vineyard sprays,[142] steroid hormones,[143–145] phenelzine[146] and urethane.[147] Positive staining of tumour cells for factor VIII-related antigen and other endothelial markers is evidence of their endothelial origin.[148,149] Their growth is characteristically along sinusoids and around surviving, hyperplastic hepatocytes (Fig. 11.13). The presence of the latter may lead to confusion

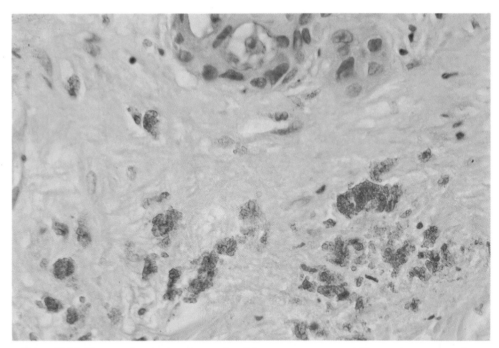

Figure 11.14. *Thorotrast.* Green refractile granules of thorotrast are present within portal tract macrophages. This patient had developed cholangiocarcinoma, seen at top. Operative specimen, H & E.

with hepatocellular carcinoma, with which angiosarcoma, however, occasionally co-exists. Infiltration of sinusoids beyond the main tumour mass makes the outlines of the tumour indistinct. Both cavernous and solid areas may be present. Other features include islands of haemopoietic cells, and areas of thrombosis and infarction.

The non-neoplastic liver tissue is usually not cirrhotic, but may show fibrosis and other changes attributable to the predisposing factors listed above, including deposits of refractile thorotrast granules in macrophages (Fig. 11.14). Features seen irrespective of the cause include focal dilatation of sinusoids, hyperplasia of hepatocytes, sinusoid-lining cells and perisinusoidal cells, and increased perisinusoidal reticulin.[150] These changes may precede the development of the tumour.[151]

Epithelioid Haemangioendothelioma

This endothelial tumour of soft tissues or the lung (intravascular bronchioloalveolar tumour) may uncommonly present as a primary liver tumour. In the liver it is seen in patients from the second to eighth decades of life with women more commonly affected.[152,153] Its prognosis varies very widely, some patients surviving for decades while others die within months of diagnosis.[154] Histologically it may be confused with adenocarcinoma or with veno-occlusive disease. Its causes are unknown, but a relation-ship to oral contraceptive use has been postulated.[155]

The lesion consists of proliferated endothelial cells with pleomorphic nuclei, arranged in clusters or singly, some of them with rounded lumens (Fig. 11.15). Ishak and colleagues[152] have described two types of tumour cell, dendritic and epithelioid, the latter giving rise to the adenocarcinoma-like appearance. Most cases show positive staining of tumour cells for factor VIII-related antigen and other endothelial markers. Further evidence of vascular differentiation is seen ultrastructurally where Weibel–Palade bodies in tumour cells and a tumour tissue component of pericytes have been noted.[156] Vascular

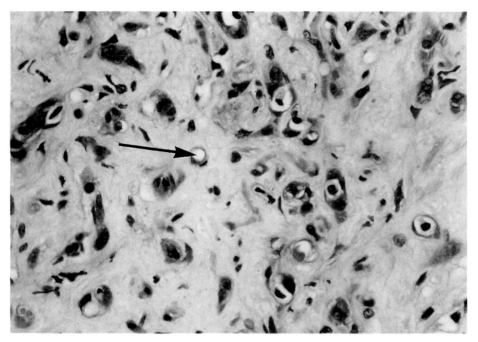

Figure 11.15. *Epithelioid haemangioendothelioma.* Individual tumour cells and small groups are set in a dense fibrous stroma. Some of the tumour cells have formed vascular lumens (arrow). Operative specimen, H & E.

occlusion by dense fibrous tissue containing tumour cells, a characteristic feature, is seen in both portal and hepatic vein branches. This is best seen with connective tissue stains. The problem of confusion with veno-occlusive disease is compounded by the fact that the tumour sometimes has a zonal distribution, affecting zones 3 and 2 of each acinus in a more or less regular fashion (Fig. 11.16).

EXTRAHEPATIC MALIGNANCY AND THE LIVER

Patients with extrahepatic tumour may have biochemical evidence of hepatic dysfunction in the absence of liver metastases, particularly when the tumour is a renal adenocarcinoma. Liver biopsies in such patients have shown Kupffer-cell proliferation, hepatocellular swelling, focal necrosis, fatty change and mild inflammation.[157,158] Granulomas are occasionally found, and there may be cholestasis, especially in Hodgkin's disease (p. 169).

Metastatic Tumour

Blind percutaneous needle biopsy may reveal metastatic tumour but the yield of correct diagnoses is increased if the needle is guided by means of an imaging method. Multiple punctures may be needed to sample the tumour. Guided fine-needle aspiration is a helpful diagnostic procedure,[159,160] and cytological examination of aspiration fluid and touch preparations of biopsy specimens increase the yield of positive results.[161] Step sections of biopsy specimens should be examined if tumour is suspected clinically but initial sections are negative. The primary site of a tumour can sometimes be determined histologically. Some metastases, notably from renal adenocarcinoma, can mimic hepatocellular carci-

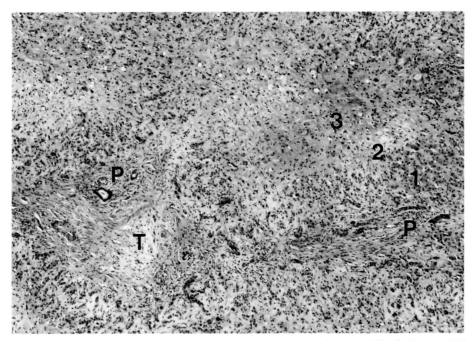

Figure 11.16. *Epithelioid haemangioendothelioma.* In this example the tumour has a zonal distribution, mimicking the fibrosis of venous outflow obstruction. The tumour stroma is predominantly seen in acinar zones 3 and 2, while zone 1 hepatocytes survive near a portal tract (*P*) below and to the right. A portal vein branch in another portal tract (*P*) is blocked by tumour (*T*). Operative specimen, H & E.

noma and metastatic tumour may invade liver-cell plates, giving a false impression of primary carcinoma arising within them (Fig. 11.17).

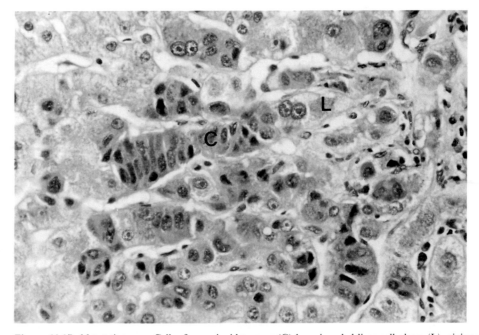

Figure 11.17. *Metastatic tumour.* Cells of a carcinoid tumour (C) have invaded liver-cell plates (L), giving a false impression of origin from the latter. Needle biopsy, H & E.

Biopsy specimens from the vicinity of a metastasis typically show portal oedema, proliferation of bile ducts and infiltration by neutrophils, as well as focal sinusoidal dilatation[162] (Fig. 1.5, p. 4). The proliferated ducts sometimes have abnormal epithelium with atypical, hyperchromatic nuclei. The portal changes are reminiscent of those seen in biliary obstruction.

Lymphomas and Leukaemias

Hodgkin's Disease

Liver biopsy plays an important part in staging; wedge biopsies are more likely than multiple needle biopsies to reveal deposits and either may be positive in spite of normal macroscopic appearances of the liver at laparotomy.[163] Negative biopsy does not rule out liver involvement. Hepatic involvement by Hodgkin's disease is usually associated with splenic involvement.[164] Step sections of initially negative small biopsies should be examined because the infiltrates of Hodgkin's disease are unevenly distributed and may be sparse. Correct diagnosis of an infiltrate may be difficult because Reed–Sternberg cells are often very scanty, so that the correct diagnosis must be suspected on the basis of other features. These include an abnormal population of cells with deeply stained angular nuclei or vesicular nuclei with prominent nucleoli (Fig. 11.18), irregular infiltration beyond portal tracts with destruction of hepatocytes and abundant reticulin fibres. There is a variable component of reactive lymphoid cells, eosinophils and histiocytes. The differential diagnosis of Hodgkin's disease in the liver includes reactive infiltrates and other lymphomas, especially of the T-cell type.

A variety of non-specific changes may be seen in parts of the liver adjacent to the malignant deposits. Even in the absence of malignant deposits there may be acinar lymphoid aggregates with some degree of cellular atypia[165] or epithelioid-cell

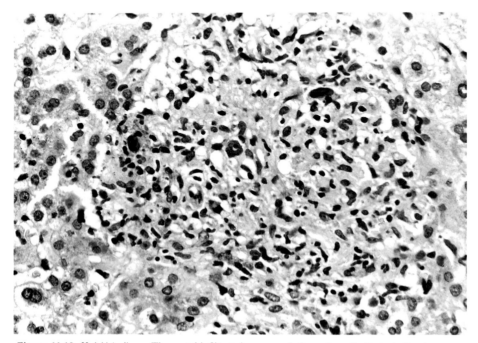

Figure 11.18. *Hodgkin's disease.* The portal infiltrate is composed of a variety of cells, including large tumour cells with angular, hyperchromatic nuclei. Needle biopsy, H & E.

granulomas.[166] Sinusoidal dilatation with or without Hodgkin's infiltrates in the liver has been reported, most often in patients with general symptoms.[167] The lesion is most severe in acinar zones 2 and 3. **Cholestasis** in Hodgkin's disease is uncommon, seen in the absence of hepatic infiltration in some patients,[168] but more often as a feature of advanced disease. In some cases cholestasis is explained by destruction of interlobular bile ducts (ductopenia) related directly to the malignant infiltrates or resembling that seen in ductopenic rejection after liver transplantation.[169,170] Hodgkin's disease may also develop in patients with primary sclerosing cholangitis.[170a]

Non-Hodgkin's Lymphoma and Other Haemopoietic Malignancies

Non-Hodgkin's lymphomas primarily involve portal tracts, but may spread to periportal parenchyma and sinusoids. Predominantly sinusoidal infiltration is also recognized.[171] Tumour deposits and fibrosis may cause portal hypertension[172] and, rarely, massive infiltration presents clinically as liver failure.[173] Malignant infiltrates can usually be distinguished from inflammatory ones by their dense and homogeneous appearance, and by the total or near-total involvement of portal tracts (Fig. 11.19). Immunohistochemical stains are important in establishing the type of lymphoma.[174] The disease is usually systemic, with involvement of lymphoid tissues as well as liver. **Primary hepatic lymphoma** is quite rare, representing less than 1% of extranodal lymphomas.[175–177] Both B- and T-cell hepatic lymphomas are seen, with the former predominating.[176,178] Peripheral T-cell lymphoma with hepatic sinusoidal infiltration and splenic involvement has also been described.[179,180] Primary hepatic lymphomas present as solitary or multiple masses, as diffuse hepatic involvement with hepatomegaly, or as liver failure with elevated serum lactate dehydrogenase activity.[176]

The liver may be diffusely or focally infiltrated in **multiple myeloma**.[181] In **macroglobulinaemia**[182] mononuclear cells, some with pyroninophilic cytoplasm, may be found in portal tracts and sinusoids. Both diseases are sometimes complicated by amyloid deposition. In **systemic mast cell disease** with liver involvement, infiltration

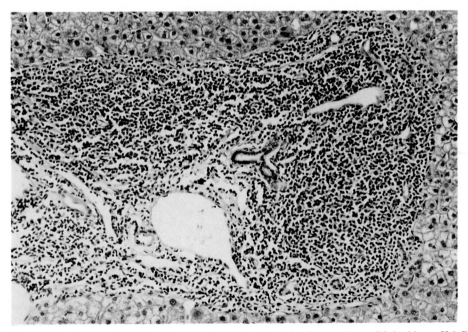

Figure 11.19. *Lymphocytic lymphoma.* Tumour cells are seen throughout the portal tract. Wedge biopsy, H & E.

of portal tracts by mast cells is associated with fibrosis.[183] Parenchymal infiltrates are also seen. The infiltrating cells may be rounded, histiocyte-like or spindle-shaped. Their nature may not be suspected on routine stains of paraffin sections; plastic sections or special mast cell stains make the diagnosis clear.

The infiltrates of various **leukaemias** are often seen in the liver. Schwartz and co-workers[184] reported hepatic involvement in nearly all cases of **chronic lymphocytic leukaemia** examined, and noted marked widening of portal tracts with portal–portal linking and a variable degree of fibrosis. In **hairy cell leukaemia** the hepatic sinusoids are infiltrated by the leukaemic cells, often identifiable by the halo-like clear cytoplasm around rounded or indented nuclei.[185] However, these are not always present.[186] Another histological characteristic is the formation of angiomatous lesions, in which vascular channels in portal tracts or acini are lined by leukaemic cells rather than by endothelium. Endothelial disruption with communication of sinusoids with the perisinusoidal space of Disse is seen by electron microscopy.[187] Staining for tartrate-resistant acid phosphatase in paraffin sections has sometimes been helpful in diagnosis.[188]

NEOPLASMS AND NODULES IN CHILDREN

Benign Lesions

Liver cell adenoma rarely may develop spontaneously in children with no underlying disease or exposure to hormones.[189] The vast majority pursue a benign course but transformation to hepatocellular carcinoma after many years of observation has been reported.[190] The identification of **focal nodular hyperplasia** in infancy as well as adulthood has been taken as additional evidence that it is a tumour-like malformation rather than a true neoplasm. **Nodular regenerative hyperplasia** is unusual in childhood. It occurs as early as 7 months of age and shows the same histological features as in adults.[191] Hepatosplenomegaly and portal hypertension may be present and in some patients there is a history of prior chemotherapy or anti-convulsant medication.

Mesenchymal Hamartoma

This is an uncommon lesion of infancy and childhood, rarely seen in older subjects. Loose, oedematous connective tissue rich in blood vessels contains lymphangioma-like cystic spaces, bile ducts and hepatocytes (Fig. 11.20).[192,193] Haemopoietic cells are often present. The edge of the lesion is irregular, gradually merging with adjacent normal liver.

Infantile Haemangioendothelioma

This solitary or multicentric tumour is composed of capillary-like vascular channels lined by plump endothelium which, with time undergo progressive maturation, scarring and eventual involution.[60,194] Central portions of the tumour may show increased fibrous stroma, and thrombosis and dystrophic calcification are sometimes present. The margin of the tumour often merges into adjacent liver parenchyma (Fig. 11.21). Dehner and Ishak[194] described Type I tumours with cytologically bland endothelium and Type II tumours capable of aggressive behaviour and metastasis, with atypical, hyperchromatic endothelium and intravascular budding. Most cases present in the first 6 months of life with hepatomegaly, abdominal mass or diffuse abdominal enlargement.[60,194,195] There may be high-output cardiac failure due to shunting through the tumour, liver failure or tumour rupture. The possibility that some of these tumours will pursue a malignant course should be kept in mind in evaluating the histopathology of individual cases.

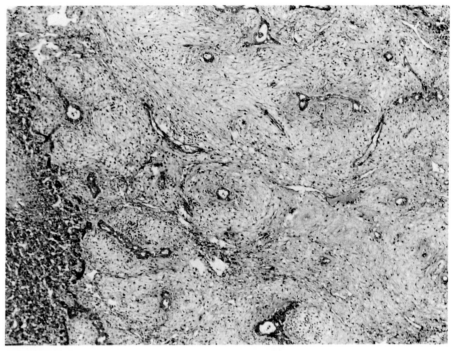

Figure 11.20. *Mesenchymal hamartoma.* Loose connective tissue contains bile ducts and blood vessels. Operative specimen, H & E.

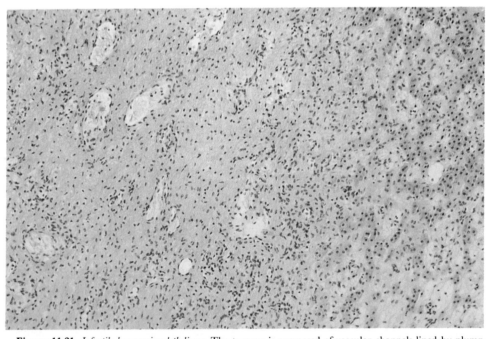

Figure 11.21. *Infantile haemangioendothelioma.* The tumour is composed of vascular channels lined by plump endothelium. A dense fibrous stroma is seen at left, while at right the tumour margin extends into adjacent cords of hepatocytes. Operative specimen, H & E.

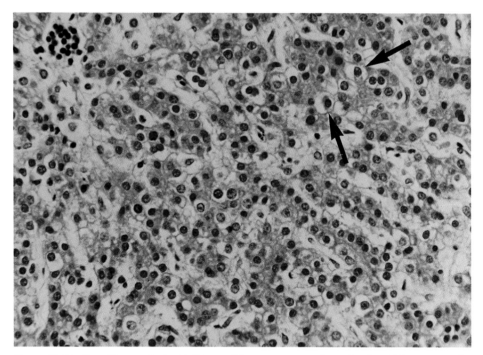

Figure 11.22. *Hepatoblastoma, fetal epithelial type.* The tumour grows in cords of small hepatocytes. Some tumour cells (arrows) have a clear cytoplasm due to increased glycogen content. A focus of extramedullary haemopoiesis, characteristically only found in regions of fetal epithelium, is seen at upper left. Operative specimen, H & E.

Malignant Lesions

Hepatoblastoma

Hepatoblastoma is the most common liver tumour in childhood, usually presenting under 2 years of age. The prognosis depends on surgical resectability and histological type. These tumours are usually solitary and histologically classified as **epithelial**, **mixed epithelial–mesenchymal** and **anaplastic (undifferentiated)** types.[196–199]
The epithelial type consists of fetal or embryonal liver cells, or both. Fetal cells somewhat resemble adult hepatocytes in appearance but are smaller (Fig. 11.22). The fat and glycogen content in some fetal cells gives them a pale appearance, thereby rendering a "light-and-dark" pattern to fetal areas at low magnification. These areas are also characterized by foci of extramedullary haemopoiesis and an absence of mitoses. By histological pattern, the purely fetal type has the best prognosis.[200] Embryonal cells have less cytoplasm, higher nuclear–cytoplasmic ratios, poorly defined cellular margins and mitotic activity (Fig. 11.23). They may form rosettes, acini or tubules. Squamous differentiation may be present in epithelial hepatoblastomas. The anaplastic type shows sheets of cells resembling neuroblastoma cells with little cytoplasm, hyperchromatic nuclei and no mitoses. Gonzalez-Crussi et al[201] described a **"macrotrabecular"** pattern reminiscent of hepatocellular carcinoma, but containing fetal or embryonal cells. Anaplastic and macrotrabecular variants have the worst prognosis.[196] Mixed epithelial–mesenchymal hepatoblastomas contain mesenchymal elements such as osteoid and cartilage in addition to epithelium. Staining for α-fetoprotein is common in hepatoblastoma, and depending on the type of histological differentiation immunohistochemistry may also be positive for α_1-antitrypsin, cytokeratins, vimentin and carcinoembryonic antigen.[202]

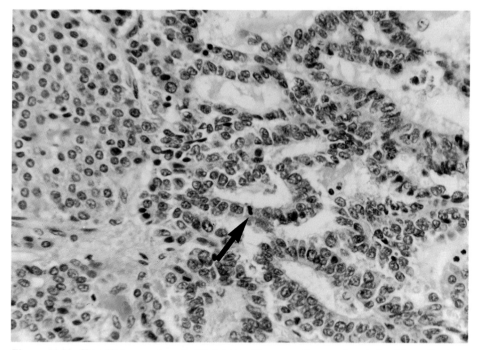

Figure 11.23. *Hepatoblastoma, embryonal epithelial type.* Tumour cells grow in tubules. The cells show an increased nuclear–cytoplasmic ratio and mitotic activity (arrow). At left, part of the tumour shows a fetal epithelial pattern. Operative specimen, H & E.

Sarcoma and Lymphoma

Undifferentiated sarcomas with a poor prognosis occasionally develop in the liver in children.[203] Epithelium trapped within the tumour may give rise to confusion. Light microscopic and ultrastructural features suggest malignant fibrous histiocytoma[204,205] or myoblastic differentiation.[205] Immunohistochemical results are inconsistent, with reports of staining for histiocytic markers, desmin, vimentin and even cytokeratin.[205,206] Another form of sarcoma, arising in the biliary tract, is the **embryonal rhabdomyosarcoma** or **sarcoma botryoides**.[200] Exceptionally rare **primary non-Hodgkin's lymphoma** in the liver has been reported in childhood.[207]

Hepatocellular Carcinoma

This resembles the adult type histologically, but cirrhosis is usually absent.[200] Predisposing causes include tyrosinaemia and type I glycogenosis. The fibrolamellar type of carcinoma has been described in older children, with better prognosis than hepatocellular carcinoma in general.[112]

REFERENCES

1. Tao L-C. Oral contraceptive-associated liver cell adenoma and hepatocellular carcinoma. Cytomorphology and mechanism of malignant transformation. *Cancer* 1991; **68**: 341–347.
2. Heffelfinger S, Irani DR, Finegold MJ. "Alcoholic hepatitis" in a hepatic adenoma. *Hum Pathol* 1987; **18**: 751–754.
3. Le Bail B, Jouhanole H, Deugnier Y et al. Liver adenomatosis with granulomas in two patients on long-term oral contraceptives. *Am J Surg Pathol* 1992; **16**: 982–987.

4. Rooks JB, Ory HW, Ishak KG et al. Epidemiology of hepatocellular adenoma. The role of oral contraceptive use. *JAMA* 1979; **242**: 644–648.

5. Lui AF, Hiratzka LF, Hirose FM. Multiple adenomas of the liver. *Cancer* 1980; **45**: 1001–1004.

6. Flejou JF, Barge J, Menu Y et al. Liver adenomatosis. An entity distinct from liver adenoma? *Gastroenterology* 1985; **89**: 1132–1138.

7. Kahn H, Manzarbeitia C, Theise N, Schwartz M, Miller C, Thung SN. Danazol-induced hepatocellular adenomas. *Arch Pathol Lab Med* 1991; **115**: 1054–1057.

8. Søe KL, Søe M, Gluud C. Liver pathology associated with the use of anabolic-androgenic steroids. *Liver* 1992; **12**: 73–79.

9. Anthony PP. Hepatoma associated with androgenic steroids. *Lancet* 1975; **1**: 685–686.

10. Chandra RS, Kapur SP, Kelleher J Jr, Luban N, Patterson K. Benign hepatocellular tumors in the young. A clinicopathologic spectrum. *Arch Pathol Lab Med* 1984; **108**: 168–171.

11. Foster JH, Donohue TA, Berman MM. Familial liver-cell adenomas and diabetes mellitus. *N Engl J Med* 1978; **299**: 239–241.

12. Coire CI, Qizilbash AH, Castelli MF. Hepatic adenomata in type Ia glycogen storage disease. *Arch Pathol Lab Med* 1987; **111**: 166–169.

13. Nakanuma Y, Terada T, Ueda K, Terasaki S, Nonomura A, Matsui O. Adenomatous hyperplasia of the liver as a precancerous lesion. *Liver* 1993; **13**: 1–9.

14. Ferrell LD, Crawford JM, Dhillon AP, Scheuer PJ, Nakanuma Y. Proposal for standardized criteria for the diagnosis of benign, borderline, and malignant hepatocellular lesions arising in chronic advanced liver disease. *Am J Surg Pathol* 1993; **17**: 1113–1123.

15. Terada T, Ueda K, Nakanuma Y. Histopathological and morphometric analysis of atypical adenomatous hyperplasia of human cirrhotic livers. *Virchows Archiv (A)* 1993; **422**: 381–388.

16. Ferrell L, Wright T, Lake J, Roberts J, Ascher N. Incidence and diagnostic features of macroregenerative nodules vs. small hepatocellular carcinoma in cirrhotic livers. *Hepatology* 1992; **16**: 1372–1381.

17. Theise ND, Schwartz M, Miller C, Thung SN. Macroregenerative nodules and hepatocellular carcinoma in forty-four sequential adult liver explants with cirrhosis. *Hepatology* 1992; **16**: 949–955.

18. Eguchi A, Nakashima O, Okudaira S, Sugihara S, Kojiro M. Adenomatous hyperplasia in the vicinity of small hepatocellular carcinoma. *Hepatology* 1992; **15**: 843–848.

19. Wada K, Kondo F, Kondo Y. Large regenerative nodules and dysplastic nodules in cirrhotic livers: a histopathologic study. *Hepatology* 1988; **8**: 1684–1688.

20. Sakamoto M, Hirohashi S, Shimosata Y. Early stages of multistep hepatocarcinogenesis: adenomatous hyperplasia and early hepatocellular carcinoma. *Hum Pathol* 1991; **22**: 172–178.

21. Hoso M, Nakanuma Y. Cytophotometric DNA analysis of adenomatous hyperplasia in cirrhotic livers. *Virchows Archiv (A)* 1991; **418**: 401–404.

22. Orsatti G, Theise ND, Thung SN, Paronetto F. DNA image cytometric analysis of macroregenerative nodules (adenomatous hyperplasia) of the liver: evidence in support of their preneoplastic nature. *Hepatology* 1993; **17**: 621–627.

23. Terada T, Kitani S, Ueda K, Nakanuma Y, Kitagawa K, Masuda S. Adenomatous hyperplasia of the liver resembling focal nodular hyperplasia in patients with chronic liver disease. *Virchows Archiv (A)* 1993; **422**: 247–252.

24. Haratake J, Hisaoka M, Yamamoto O. An ultrastructural comparison of sinusoids in hepatocellular carcinoma, adenomatous hyperplasia, and fetal liver. *Arch Pathol Lab Med* 1992; **116**: 67–70.

25. Ueda K, Terada T, Nakanuma Y, Matsui O. Vascular supply in adenomatous hyperplasia of the liver and hepatocellular carcinoma: a morphometric study. *Hum Pathol* 1992; **23**: 619–626.

26. Furuya K, Nakamura M, Yamamoto Y et al. Macroregenerative nodule of the liver. A clinicopathologic study of 345 autopsy cases of chronic liver disease. *Cancer* 1988; **61**: 99–105.

27. Wanless IR, Mawdsley C, Adams R. On the pathogenesis of focal nodular hyperplasia of the liver. *Hepatology* 1985; **5**: 1194–1200.

28. Nime F, Pickren JW, Vana J, Aronoff BL, Baker HW, Murphy GP. The histology of liver tumors in oral contraceptive users observed during a national survey by the American College of Surgeons Commission on Cancer. *Cancer* 1979; **44**: 1481–1489.

29. Friedman LS, Gang DL, Hedberg SE, Isselbacher KJ. Simultaneous occurrence of hepatic adenoma and focal nodular hyperplasia: report of a case and review of the literature. *Hepatology* 1984; **4**: 536–540.

30. Wanless IR, Albrecht S, Bilbao J et al. Multiple focal nodular hyperplasia of the liver associated with vascular malformations of various organs and neoplasia of the brain: a new syndrome. *Modern Pathol* 1989; **2**: 456–462.

31. Portmann B, Stewart S, Higenbottam TW, Clayton PT, Lloyd JK, Williams R. Nodular transformation of the liver associated with portal and pulmonary arterial hypertension. *Gastroenterology* 1993; **104**: 616–621.

32. Butron Vila MM, Haot J, Desmet VJ. Cholestatic features in focal nodular hyperplasia of the liver. *Liver* 1984; **4**: 387–395.

33. Ruschenburg I, Droese M. Fine needle aspiration cytology of focal nodular hyperplasia of the liver. *Acta Cytologica* 1989; **33**: 857–860.

34. Stromeyer FW, Ishak KG. Nodular transformation (nodular "regenerative" hyperplasia) of the liver. A clinicopathologic study of 30 cases. *Hum Pathol* 1981; **12**: 60–71.

35. Thorne C, Urowitz MB, Wanless I, Roberts E, Blendis LM. Liver disease in Felty's syndrome. *Am J Med* 1982; **73**: 35–40.

36. Wanless IR. Micronodular transformation (nodular regenerative hyperplasia) of the liver: a report of 64

cases among 2,500 autopsies and a new classification of benign hepatocellular nodules. *Hepatology* 1990; **11**: 787–797.

37. Paradinas FJ, Bull TB, Westaby D, Murray-Lyon IM. Hyperplasia and prolapse of hepatocytes into hepatic veins during longterm methyltestosterone therapy: possible relationships of these changes to the development of peliosis hepatis and liver tumours. *Histopathology* 1977; **1**: 225–246.

38. Baker BL, Axiotis C, Hurwitz ES, Leavitt R, Di Bisceglie AM. Nodular regenerative hyperplasia of the liver in idiopathic hypereosinophilic syndrome. *J Clin Gastroenterol* 1991; **13**: 452–456.

39. Solis-Herruzo JA, Vidal JV, Colina F, Santalla F, Castellano G. Nodular regenerative hyperplasia of the liver associated with the toxic oil syndrome: report of five cases. *Hepatology* 1986; **6**: 687–693.

40. Bloxham CA, Henderson DC, Hampson J, Burt AD. Nodular regenerative hyperplasia of the liver in Behçet's disease. *Histopathology* 1992; **20**: 452–454.

41. Colina F, Pinedo F, Solís A, Moreno D, Nevado M. Nodular regenerative hyperplasia of the liver in early histological stages of primary biliary cirrhosis. *Gastroenterology* 1992; **102**: 1319–1324.

42. Minato H, Nakanuma Y. Nodular regenerative hyperplasia of the liver associated with metastases of pancreatic endocrine tumour: report of two autopsy cases. *Virchows Archiv (A)* 1992; **421**: 171–174.

43. Kobayashi S, Saito K, Nakanuma Y. Nodular regenerative hyperplasia of the liver in hepatocellular carcinoma. *J Clin Gastroenterol* 1993; **16**: 155–159.

44. Wanless IR, Godwin TA, Allen F, Feder A. Nodular regenerative hyperplasia of the liver in hematologic disorders: a possible response to obliterative portal venopathy. A morphometric study of nine cases with an hypothesis on the pathogenesis. *Medicine* 1980; **59**: 367–379.

45. Wanless IR, Lentz JS, Roberts EA. Partial nodular transformation of liver in an adult with persistent ductus venosus. Review with hypothesis on pathogenesis. *Arch Pathol Lab Med* 1985; **109**: 427–432.

46. Wanless IR. Vascular disorders. In MacSween RNM, Anthony PP, Scheuer PJ, Portmann BC, Burt AD (eds): Pathology of the Liver, 3rd edn. Edinburgh: Churchill Livingstone, 1994.

47. Allaire GS, Rabin L, Ishak KG, Sesterhenn IA. Bile duct adenoma. A study of 152 cases. *Am J Surg Pathol* 1988; **12**: 708–715.

48. Cho C, Rullis I, Rogers LS. Bile duct adenomas as liver nodules. *Arch Surg* 1978; **113**: 272–274.

49. Gold JH, Guzman IJ, Rosai J. Benign tumors of the liver. Pathologic examination of 45 cases. *Am J Clin Pathol* 1978; **70**: 6–17.

50. Govindarajan S, Peters RL. The bile duct adenoma. A lesion distinct from Meyenburg complex. *Arch Pathol Lab Med* 1984; **108**: 922–924.

51. Scheele PM, Bonar MJ, Zumwalt R, Ray MB. Bile duct adenomas in heterozygous (MZ) deficiency of α1-protease inhibitor. *Arch Pathol Lab Med* 1988; **112**: 945–947.

52. Tsui WMS, Loo KT, Chow LTC, Tse CCH. Biliary adenofibroma. A heretofore unrecognized benign biliary tumor of the liver. *Am J Surg Pathol* 1993; **17**: 186–192.

53. Wheeler DA, Edmondson HA. Cystadenoma with mesenchymal stroma (CMS) in the liver and bile ducts. A clinicopathologic study of 17 cases, 4 with malignant change. *Cancer* 1985; **56**: 1434–1445.

54. Gourley WK, Kumar D, Bouton MS, Fish JC, Nealon W. Cystadenoma and cystadenocarcinoma with mesenchymal stroma of the liver. Immunohistochemical analysis. *Arch Pathol Lab Med* 1992; **116**: 1047–1050.

55. Ishak KG, Willis GW, Cummins SD, Bullock AA. Biliary cystadenoma and cystadenocarcinoma: report of 14 cases and review of the literature. *Cancer* 1977; **39**: 322–338.

56. Tung GA, Cronan JJ. Percutaneous needle biopsy of hepatic cavernous hemangioma. *J Clin Gastroenterol* 1993; **16**: 117–122.

57. Berry CL. Solitary "necrotic nodule" of the liver: a probable pathogenesis. *J Clin Pathol* 1985; **38**: 1278–1280.

58. Van Steenbergen W, Joosten E, Marchal G et al. Hepatic lymphangiomatosis. Report of a case and review of the literature. *Gastroenterology* 1985; **88**: 1968–1972.

59. Peters WM, Dixon MF, Williams NS. Angiomyelolipoma of the liver. *Histopathology* 1983; **7**: 99–106.

60. Goodman ZD. Benign tumors of the liver. In Okuda K, Ishak KG (eds): Neoplasms of the Liver. Tokyo: Springer-Verlag, 1990, pp 105–126.

61. Hytiroglou P, Linton P, Klion F, Schwartz M, Miller C, Thung SN. Benign schwannoma of the liver. *Arch Pathol Lab Med* 1993; **117**: 216–218.

62. Lederman SM, Martin EC, Laffey KT, Lefkowitch JH. Hepatic neurofibromatosis, malignant schwannoma and angiosarcoma in von Recklinghausen's disease. *Gastroenterology* 1989; **92**: 234–239.

63. Fried RH, Wardzala A, Willson RA, Sinanan MN, Marchioro TL, Haggitt R. Benign cartilaginous tumor (chondroma) of the liver. *Gastroenterology* 1992; **103**: 678–680.

64. Nonomura A, Mizukami Y, Isobe M, Kurachi M, Matsubara F. Smallest angiomyolipoma of the liver in the oldest patient. *Liver* 1993; **13**: 51–53.

65. Pounder DJ. Hepatic angiomyolipoma. *Am J Surg Pathol* 1982; **6**: 677–681.

66. Goodman ZD, Ishak KG. Angiomyolipomas of the liver. *Am J Surg Pathol* 1984; **8**: 745–750.

67. Karhunen PJ. Hepatic pseudolipoma. *J Clin Pathol* 1985; **38**: 877–879.

68. Chen KT. Inflammatory pseudotumor of the liver. *Hum Pathol* 1984; **15**: 694–696.

69. Anthony PP, Telesinghe PU. Inflammatory pseudotumour of the liver. *J Clin Pathol* 1986; **39**: 761–768.

70. Shek TWH, Ng IOL, Chan KW. Inflammatory pseudotumor of the liver. Report of four cases and review of the literature. *Am J Surg Pathol* 1993; **17**: 231–238.

71. Nakajima T, Sugano I, Matsuzaki O et al. Hepatic inflammatory lesions manifested as a pseudotumor. Report of two cases with different characteristics. *Arch Pathol Lab Med* 1993; **117**: 157–159.

72. Kaklamani E, Trichopoulos D, Tzonou A et al . Hepatitis B and C-viruses and their interaction in the origin of hepatocellular carcinoma. *JAMA* 1991; **265**: 1974–1976.

73. Yu M-W, You S-L, Chang AS et al. Association between hepatitis C virus antibodies and hepatocellular carcinoma in Taiwan. *Cancer Res* 1991; **51**: 5621–5625.

74. Di Bisceglie AM, Order SE, Klein JL et al. The role of chronic viral hepatitis in hepatocellular carcinoma in the United States. *Am J Gastroenterol* 1991; **86**: 335–338.

75. Tsukuma H, Hiyama T, Tanaka S et al. Risk factors for hepatocellular carcinoma among patients with chronic liver disease. *N Engl J Med* 1993; **328**: 1797–1801.

76. Schirmacher P, Rogler CE, Dienes HP. Current pathogenetic and molecular concepts in viral liver carcinogenesis. *Virchows Archiv (B)* 1993; **63**: 71–89.

77. Popper H, Thung SN, McMahon BJ, Lanier AP, Hawkins I, Alberts SR. Evolution of hepatocellular carcinoma associated with chronic hepatitis B virus infection in Alaskan eskimos. *Arch Pathol Lab Med* 1988; **112**: 498–504.

78. Hsia CC, Evarts RP, Nakatsukasa H, Marsden ER, Thorgeirsson SS. Occurrence of oval-type cells in hepatitis B virus-associated human hepatocarcinogenesis. *Hepatology* 1992; **16**: 1327–1333.

79. Desmet V, De Vos R. Ultrastructural characteristics of novel epithelial cell types identified in human pathologic liver specimens with chronic ductular reaction. *Am J Pathol* 1992; **140**: 1441–1450.

80. Anthony PP. Tumours and tumour-like lesions of the liver and biliary tract. In MacSween RNM, Anthony PP, Scheuer PJ, Portmann BC, Burt AD (eds): Pathology of the Liver, 3rd edn. Edinburgh: Churchill Livingstone, 1994.

81. Paterson AC, Kew MC, Dusheiko GM, Isaacson C. Liver cell dysplasia accompanying hepatocellular carcinoma in southern Africa. *J Hepatol* 1989; **8**: 241–248.

82. Watanabe S, Okita K, Harada T et al. Morphologic studies of the liver cell dysplasia. *Cancer* 1983; **51**: 2197–2205.

83. Cohen C, Berson SD. Liver cell dysplasia in normal, cirrhotic, and hepatocellular carcinoma patients. *Cancer* 1986; **57**: 1535–1538.

84. Roncalli M, Borzio M, De Biagi G, Ferrari AR, Macchi R, Tombesi VM. Liver cell dysplasia in cirrhosis. A serologic and immunohistochemical study. *Cancer* 1986; **57**: 1515–1521.

85. Thomas RM, Berman JJ, Yetter RA, Moore W, Hutchins GM. Liver cell dysplasia: a DNA aneuploid lesion with distinct morphologic features. *Hum Pathol* 1992; **23**: 496–503.

86. Terada T, Hoso M, Nakanuma Y. Mallory body clustering in adenomatous hyperplasia in human cirrhotic livers. *Hum Pathol* 1989; **20**: 886–890.

87. Terada T, Nakanuma Y. Iron-negative foci in siderotic macroregenerative nodules in human cirrhotic liver. *Arch Pathol Lab Med* 1989; **113**: 916–920.

88. Shikata T, Yamazaki S, Uzawa T. Hepatocellular carcinoma and chronic persistent hepatitis. *Acta Pathol Japon* 1977; **27**: 297–304.

89. Tabarin A, Bioulac-Sage P, Boussarie L, Balabaud C, de Mascarel A, Grimaud JA. Hepatocellular carcinoma developed on noncirrhotic livers. *Arch Pathol Lab Med* 1987; **111**: 174–180.

90. Kondo Y, Wada K. Intrahepatic metastasis of hepatocellular carcinoma: a histopathologic study. *Hum Pathol* 1991; **22**: 125–130.

91. Dhillon AP, Colombari R, Savage K, Scheuer PJ. An immunohistochemical study of the blood vessels within primary hepatocellular tumours. *Liver* 1992; **12**: 311–318.

92. Omata M, Peters RL, Tatter D. Sclerosing hepatic carcinoma: relationship to hypercalcemia. *Liver* 1981; **1**: 33–49.

93. Hsu H-C, Chiou T-J, Chen J-Y, Lee C-S, Lee P-H, Peng S-Y. Clonality and clonal evolution of hepatocellular carcinoma with multiple nodules. *Hepatology* 1991; **13**: 923–928.

94. Kakizoe S, Kojiro M, Nakashima T. Hepatocellular carcinoma with sarcomatous change. *Cancer* 1987; **59**: 310–316.

95. Haratake J, Horie A. An immunohistochemical study of sarcomatoid liver carcinomas. *Cancer* 1991; **68**: 93–97.

96. Buchanan TF Jr., Huvos AG. Clear-cell carcinoma of the liver. A clinicopathologic study of 13 patients. *Am J Clin Pathol* 1974; **61**: 529–539.

97. Wu PC, Lai CL, Lam KC, Lok AS, Lin HJ. Clear cell carcinoma of liver. An ultrastructural study. *Cancer* 1983; **52**: 504–507.

98. Ajdukiewicz A, Crowden A, Hudson E, Pyne C. Liver aspiration in the diagnosis of hepatocellular carcinoma in the Gambia. *J Clin Pathol* 1985; **38**: 185–192.

99. Noguchi S, Yamamoto R, Tatsuta M et al. Cell features and patterns in fine-needle aspirates of hepatocellular carcinoma. *Cancer* 1986; **58**: 321–328.

100. Pedio G, Landolt U, Zöbeli L, Gut D. Fine needle aspiration of the liver. Significance of hepatocytic naked nuclei in the diagnosis of hepatocellular carcinoma. *Acta Cytologica* 1988; **32**: 437–442.

101. Bottles K, Cohen MB, Holly EA et al. A step-wise logistic regression analysis of hepatocellular carcinoma. An aspiration biopsy study. *Cancer* 1988; **62**: 558–563.

102. Nakanuma Y, Ohta G. Expression of Mallory bodies in hepatocellular carcinoma in man and its significance. *Cancer* 1986; **57**: 81–86.

103. Ma CK, Zarbo RJ, Frierson HF, Lee MW. Comparative immunohistochemical study of primary and metastatic carcinomas of the liver. *Am J Clin Pathol* 1993; **99**: 551–557.

104. Hurlimann J, Gardiol D. Immunohistochemistry in the differential diagnosis of liver carcinomas. *Am J Surg Pathol* 1991; **15**: 280–288.

105. Van Eyken P, Sciot R, Paterson A, Callea F, Kew MC, Desmet VJ. Cytokeratin expression in hepatocellular carcinoma: an immunohistochemical study. *Hum Pathol* 1988; **19**: 562–568.

106. Lai Y-S, Thung SN, Gerber MA, Chen M-L, Schaffner F. Expression of cytokeratins in normal and diseased livers and in primary liver carcinomas. *Arch Pathol Lab Med* 1989; **113**: 134–138.

107. Thung SN, Gerber MA, Sarno E, Popper H. Distribution of five antigens in hepatocellular carcinoma. *Lab Invest* 1979; **41**: 101–105.

108. Ordonez NG, Manning JT Jr. Comparison of alpha-1-antitrypsin and alpha-1-antichymotrypsin in hepatocellular carcinoma: an immunoperoxidase study. *Am J Gastroenterol* 1984; **79**: 959–963.

108a. Wennerberg AE, Nalesnik MA, Coleman WB, Hepatocyte Paraffin 1: a monoclonal antibody that reacts with hepatocytes and can be used for differential diagnosis of hepatic tumors. *Am. J. Pathol* 1993; **143**: 1050–1054.

109. Grigioni WF, Garbisa S, D'Errico A et al. Evaluation of hepatocellular carcinoma aggressiveness by a panel of extracellular matrix antigens. *Am J Pathol* 1991; **138**: 647–654.

110. Nagorney DM, Adson MA, Weiland LH, Knight CD, Jr, Smalley SR. Fibrolamellar hepatoma. *Am J Surg* 1985; **149**: 113–119.

111. Berman MM, Libbey NP, Foster JH. Hepatocellular carcinoma. Polygonal cell type with fibrous stroma – an atypical variant with a favorable prognosis. *Cancer* 1980; **46**: 1448–1455.

112. Craig JR, Peters RL, Edmondson HA, Omata M. Fibrolamellar carcinoma of the liver: a tumor of adolescents and young adults with distinctive clinico-pathologic features. *Cancer* 1980; **46**: 372–379.

113. Berman MA, Burnham JA, Sheahan DG. Fibrolamellar carcinoma of the liver: an immunohistochemical study of nineteen cases and a review of the literature. *Hum Pathol* 1988; **19**: 784–794.

114. Vecchio FM, Fabiano A, Ghirlanda G, Manna R, Massi G. Fibrolamellar carcinoma of the liver: the malignant counterpart of focal nodular hyperplasia with oncocytic change. *Am J Clin Pathol* 1984; **81**: 521–526.

115. Vecchio FM. Fibrolamellar carcinoma of the liver: a distinct entity within the hepatocellular tumors. A review. *Appl Pathol* 1988; **6**: 139–148.

116. Farhi DC, Shikes RH, Silverberg SG. Ultrastructure of fibrolamellar oncocytic hepatoma. *Cancer* 1982; **50**: 702–709.

117. Lefkowitch JH, Muschel R, Price JB, Marboe C, Braunhut S. Copper and copper-binding protein in fibrolamellar liver cell carcinoma. *Cancer* 1983; **51**: 97–100.

118. Vecchio FM, Federico F, Dina MA. Copper and hepatocellular carcinoma. *Digestion* 1986; **35**: 109–114.

119. Teitelbaum DH, Tuttle S, Carey LC, Clausen KP. Fibrolamellar carcinoma of the liver. Review of three cases and the presentation of a characteristic set of tumor markers defining this tumor. *Ann Surg* 1985; **202**: 36–41.

120. Payne CM, Nagle RB, Paplanus SH, Graham AR. Fibrolamellar carcinoma of liver: a primary malignant oncocytic carcinoid? *Ultrastruc Pathol* 1986; **10**: 539–552.

121. Subramony C, Herrera GA, Lockard V. Neuroendocrine differentiation in hepatic neoplasms: report of four cases. *Surg Pathol* 1993; **5**: 17–33.

122. LeBrun DP, Silver MM, Freedman MH, Phillips MJ. Fibrolamellar carcinoma of the liver in a patient with Fanconi anemia. *Hum Pathol* 1991; **22**: 396–398.

123. Case records of the Massachusetts General Hospital. Case 29-1987. *N Engl J Med* 1987; **317**: 153–160.

124. Bloustein PA. Association of carcinoma with congenital cystic conditions of the liver and bile ducts. *Am J Gastroenterol* 1977; **67**: 40–46.

125. Burns CD, Kuhns JG, Wieman J. Cholangiocarcinoma in association with multiple biliary microhamartomas. *Arch Pathol Lab Med* 1990; **114**: 1287–1289.

126. Schlinkert RT, Nagorney DM, Van Heerden JA, Adson MA. Intrahepatic cholangiocarcinoma: clinical aspects, pathology and treatment. *HPB Surg* 1992; **5**: 95–102.

127. Nakanuma Y, Yamaguchi K, Ohta G, Terada T, The Japanese Hepatolithiasis Study Group. Pathologic features of hepatolithiasis in Japan. *Hum Pathol* 1988; **19**: 1181–1186.

128. Nakajima T, Knodo Y, Miyazaki M, Okui K. A histopathologic study of 102 cases of intrahepatic cholangiocarcinoma: histologic classification and modes of spreading. *Hum Pathol* 1988; **19**: 1228–1234.

129. Weinbren K, Mutum SS. Pathological aspects of cholangiocarcinoma. *J Pathol* 1983; **139**: 217–238.

130. Bonetti F, Chilosi M, Pisa R, Novelli P, Zamboni G, Menestrina F. Epithelial membrane antigen expression in cholangiocarcinoma. An useful immunohistochemical tool for differential diagnosis with hepatocarcinoma. *Virchows Archiv A Pathol Anat Histopathol* 1983; **401**: 307–313.

131. Pastolero GC, Wakabayashi T, Oka T, Mori S. Tissue polypeptide antigen – a marker antigen differentiating cholangiolar tumors from other hepatic tumors. *Am J Clin Pathol* 1987; **87**: 168–173.

132. Jovanovic R, Jagirdar J, Thung SN, Paronetto F. Blood-group-related antigen Lewis-X and Lewis-Y in the differential diagnosis of cholangiocarcinoma and hepatocellular carcinoma. *Arch Pathol Lab Med* 1989; **113**: 139–142.

133. Terada T, Nakanuma Y. An immunohistochemical survey of amylase isoenzymes in cholangiocarcinoma and hepatocellular carcinoma. *Arch Pathol Lab Med* 1993; **117**: 160–162.

134. Goodman ZD, Ishak KG, Langloss JM, Sesterhenn IA, Rabin L. Combined hepatocellular-cholangiocarcinoma. A histologic and immunohistochemical study. *Cancer* 1985; **55**: 124–135.

135. Azizah N, Paradinas FJ. Cholangiocarcinoma coexisting with developmental liver cysts: a distinct entity different from liver cystadenocarcinoma. *Histopathology* 1980; **4**: 391–400.

136. Theise ND, Miller F, Worman HJ et al. Biliary cystadenocarcinoma arising in a liver with fibropolycystic disease. *Arch Pathol Lab Med* 1993; **117**: 163–165.

137. Lander JJ, Stanley RJ, Sumner HW, Boswell DC, Aach RD. Angiosarcoma of the liver associated with Fowler's solution (potassium arsenite). *Gastroenterology* 1975; **68**: 1582–1586.

138. Horta JS. Late effects of thorotrast on the liver and spleen, and their efferent lymph nodes. *Ann New York Acad Sci* 1967; **145**: 676–699.

139. Visfeldt J, Poulsen H. On the histopathology of liver and liver tumours in thorium-dioxide patients. *Acta Pathol Microbiol Scand A* 1972; **80**: 97–108.

140. Winberg CD, Ranchod M. Thorotrast induced hepatic cholangiocarcinoma and angiosarcoma. *Hum Pathol* 1979; **10**: 108–112.

141. Thomas LB, Popper H, Berk PD, Selikoff I, Falk H. Vinyl-chloride-induced liver disease. From idiopathic portal hypertension (Banti's syndrome) to angiosarcomas. *N Engl J Med* 1975; **292**: 17–22.

142. Pimentel JC, Menezes AP. Liver disease in vineyard sprayers. *Gastroenterology* 1977; **72**: 275–283.

143. Hoch-Ligeti C. Angiosarcoma of the liver associated with diethylstilbestrol. *JAMA* 1978; **240**: 1510–1511.

144. Falk H, Thomas LB, Popper H, Ishak KG. Hepatic angiosarcoma associated with androgenic-anabolic steroids. *Lancet* 1979; **2**: 1120–1123.

145. Monroe PS, Riddell RH, Siegler M, Baker AL. Hepatic angiosarcoma. Possible relationship to long-term oral contraceptive ingestion. *JAMA* 1981; **246**: 64–65.

146. Daneshmend TK, Scott GL, Bradfield JW. Angiosarcoma of liver associated with phenelzine. *Br Med J* 1979; **1**: 1679.

147. Cadranel JF, Legendre C, Desaint B, Delamarre N, Florent C, Levy VG. Liver disease from surreptitious administration of urethane. *J Clin Gastroenterol* 1993; **17**: 52–56.

148. Fortwengler HP Jr, Jones D, Espinosa E, Tamburro CH. Evidence for endothelial cell origin of vinyl chloride-induced hepatic angiosarcoma. *Gastroenterology* 1981; **80**: 1415–1419.

149. Manning JT Jr, Ordonez NG, Barton JH. Endothelial cell origin of thorium oxide-induced angiosarcoma of liver. *Arch Pathol Lab Med* 1983; **107**: 456–458.

150. Popper H, Thomas LB, Telles NC, Falk H, Selikoff IJ. Development of hepatic angiosarcoma in man induced by vinyl chloride, thorotrast, and arsenic. Comparison with cases of unknown etiology. *Am J Pathol* 1978; **92**: 349–369.

151. Tamburro CH, Makk L, Popper H. Early hepatic histologic alterations among chemical (vinyl monomer) workers. *Hepatology* 1984; **4**: 413–418.

152. Ishak KG, Sesterhenn IA, Goodman ZD, Rabin L, Stromeyer FW. Epithelioid hemangioendothelioma of the liver: a clinicopathologic and follow-up study of 32 cases. *Hum Pathol* 1984; **15**: 839–852.

153. Ishak KG. Malignant mesenchymal tumors of the liver. In Okuda K, Ishak KG (eds): Neoplasms of the Liver. Tokyo: Springer-Verlag, 1987, pp 159-176.

154. Ekfors TO, Joensuu K, Toivio I, Laurinen P, Pelttari L. Fatal epithelioid haemangioendothelioma presenting in the lung and liver. *Virchows Archiv A Pathol Anat Histopathol* 1986; **410**: 9–16.

155. Dean PJ, Haggitt RC, O'Hara CJ. Malignant epithelioid hemangioendothelioma of the liver in young women. Relationship to oral contraceptive use. *Am J Surg Pathol* 1985; **9**: 695–704.

156. Scoazec J-Y, Degott C, Reynes M, Benhamou J-P, Feldmann G. Epithelioid hemangioendothelioma of the liver: an ultrastructural study. *Hum Pathol* 1989; **20**: 673–681.

157. Utz DC, Warren MM, Gregg JA, Ludwig J, Kelalis PP. Reversible hepatic dysfunction associated with hypernephroma. *Mayo Clin Proc* 1970; **45**: 161–169.

158. Strickland RC, Schenker S. The nephrogenic hepatic dysfunction syndrome: a review. *Am J Dig Dis* 1977; **22**: 49–55.

159. Tao LC, Donat EE, Ho CS, McLoughlin MJ. Percutaneous fine-needle aspiration biopsy of the liver. Cytodiagnosis of hepatic cancer. *Acta Cytologica* 1979; **23**: 287–291.

160. Axe SR, Erozan YS, Ermatinger SV. Fine-needle aspiration of the liver. A comparison of smear and rinse preparations in the detection of cancer. *Am J Clin Pathol* 1986; **86**: 281–285.

161. Atterbury CE, Enriquez RE, Desuto-Nagy GI, Conn HO. Comparison of the histologic and cytologic diagnosis of liver biopsies in hepatic cancer. *Gastroenterology* 1979; **76**: 1352–1357.

162. Gerber MA, Thung SN, Bodenheimer HC Jr, Kapelman B, Schaffner F. Characteristic histologic triad in liver adjacent to metastatic neoplasm. *Liver* 1986; **6**: 85–88.

163. Glees JP, Thomas M, Redding WH, Hefney M, Gazet JC. Liver biopsy at lymphoma laparotomy. *Lancet* 1978; **1**: 210–211.

164. Kim H, Dorfman RF, Rosenberg SA. Pathology of malignant lymphomas of the liver: application in staging. In Popper H, Schaffner F (eds): Progress in Liver Diseases, Vol. V. New York: Grune and Stratton, 1976, pp 683–698.

165. Leslie KO, Colby TV. Hepatic parenchymal lymphoid aggregates in Hodgkin's disease. *Hum Pathol* 1984; **15**: 808–809.

166. Abt AB, Kirschner RH, Belliveau RE et al. Hepatic pathology associated with Hodgkin's disease. *Cancer* 1974; **33**: 1564–1571.

167. Bruguera M, Caballero T, Carreras E, Aymerich M, Rodes J, Rozman C. Hepatic sinusoidal dilatation in Hodgkin's disease. *Liver* 1987; **7**: 76–80.

168. Perera DR, Greene ML, Fenster LF. Cholestasis associated with extrabiliary Hodgkin's disease. Report of three cases and review of four others. *Gastroenterology* 1974; **67**: 680–685.

169. Hubscher SG, Lumley MA, Elias E. Vanishing bile duct syndrome: a possible mechanism for intrahepatic cholestasis in Hodgkin's lymphoma. *Hepatology* 1993; **17**: 70–77.

170. Lefkowitch JH, Falkow S, Whitlock RT. Hepatic Hodgkin's disease simulating cholestatic hepatitis with liver failure. *Arch Pathol Lab Med* 1985; **109**: 424–426.

170a. Man KM, Drejet A. Keefe EB et al. Primary sclerosing cholangitis and Hodgkins' disease. *Hepatology* 1993; **18**: 1127–1131.

171. Trudel M, Aramendi T, Caplan S. Large-cell lymphoma presenting with hepatic sinusoidal infiltration. *Arch Pathol Lab Med* 1991; **115**: 821–824.

172. Dubois A, Dauzat M, Pignodel C et al. Portal hypertension in lymphoproliferative and myeloproliferative disorders: hemodynamic and histological correlations. *Hepatology* 1993; **17**: 246–250.

173. Saló J, Nomdedeu B, Bruguera M et al. Acute liver failure due to non-Hodgkin's lymphoma. *Am J Gastroenterol* 1993; **88**: 774–776.

174. Verdi CJ, Grogan TM, Protell R, Richter L, Rangel C. Liver biopsy immunotyping to characterize lymphoid malignancies. *Hepatology* 1986; **6**: 6–13.

175. Freeman C, Berg JW, Cutler SJ. Occurrence and prognosis of extranodal lymphomas. *Cancer* 1972; **29**: 252–260.

176. Zafrani ES, Gaulard P. Primary lymphoma of the liver. *Liver* 1993; **13**: 57–61.

177. Stemmer S, Geffen DB, Goldstein J, Cohen Y. Primary small noncleaved cell lymphoma of the liver. *J Clin Gastroenterol* 1993; **16**: 65–69.

178. Scoazec J-Y, Degott C, Brousse N et al. Non-Hodgkin's lymphoma presenting as a primary tumor of the liver: presentation, diagnosis and outcome in eight patients. *Hepatology* 1991; **13**: 870–875.

179. Gaulard P, Zafrani ES, Mavier P et al. Peripheral T-cell lymphoma presenting as predominant liver disease: a report of three cases. *Hepatology* 1986; **6**: 864–868.

180. Farcet J-P, Gaulard P, Marolleau J-P et al. Hepatosplenic T-cell lymphoma: sinusal/sinusoidal localization of malignant cells expressing the T-cell receptor γδ. *Blood* 1990; **75**: 2213–2219.

181. Thomas FB, Clausen KP, Greenberger NJ. Liver disease in multiple myeloma. *Arch Intern Med* 1973; **132**: 195–202.

182. Brooks AP. Portal hypertension in Waldenstrom's macroglobulinaemia. *Br Med J* 1976; **1**: 689–690.

183. Yam LT, Chan CH, Li CY. Hepatic involvement in systemic mast cell disease. *Am J Med* 1986; **80**: 819–826.

184. Schwartz JB, Shamsuddin AM. The effects of leukemic infiltrates in various organs in chronic lymphocytic leukemia. *Hum Pathol* 1981; **12**: 432–440.

185. Roquet ML, Zafrani ES, Farcet JP, Reyes F, Pinaudeau Y. Histopathological lesions of the liver in hairy cell leukemia: a report of 14 cases. *Hepatology* 1985; **5**: 496–500.

186. Yam LT, Janckila AJ, Chan CH, Li C-Y. Hepatic involvement in hairy cell leukemia. *Cancer* 1983; **51**: 1497–1504.

187. Zafrani ES, Degos F, Guigui B et al. The hepatic sinusoid in hairy cell leukemia: an ultrastructural study of 12 cases. *Hum Pathol* 1987; **18**: 801–807.

188. Grouls V, Stiens R. Hepatic involvement in hairy cell leukemia: diagnosis by tartrate-resistant acid phosphatase enzyme histochemistry on formalin fixed and paraffin-embedded liver biopsy specimens. *Pathol Res Prac* 1984; **178**: 332–334.

189. Wheeler DA, Edmondson HA, Reynolds TB. Spontaneous liver cell adenoma in children. *Am J Clin Pathol* 1986; **85**: 6–12.

190. Janes CH, McGill DB, Ludwig J, Krom RAF. Liver cell adenoma at the age of 3 years and transplantation 19 years later after development of carcinoma: a case report. *Hepatology* 1993; **17**: 583–585.

191. Moran CA, Mullick FG, Ishak KG. Nodular regenerative hyperplasia of the liver in children. *Am J Surg Pathol* 1991; **15**: 449–454.

192. Srouji MN, Chatten J, Schulman WM, Ziegler MM, Koop CE. Mesenchymal hamartoma of the liver in infants. *Cancer* 1978; **42**: 2483–2489.

193. Stocker JT, Ishak KG. Mesenchymal hamartoma of the liver: report of 30 cases and review of the literature. *Ped Pathol* 1983; **1**: 245–267.

194. Dehner LP, Ishak KG. Vascular tumors of the liver in infants and children. A study of 30 cases and review of the literature. *Arch Pathol* 1971; **92**: 101–111.

195. Dachman AH, Lichtenstein JE, Friedman AC, Hartman DS. Infantile hemangioendothelioma of the liver: a radiologic–pathologic–clinical correlation. *AJR* 1983; **140**: 1091–1096.

196. Stocker JT, Ishak KG. Hepatoblastoma. In Okuda K, Ishak KG (eds): Neoplasms of the Liver. Tokyo: Springer-Verlag, 1987, pp 127–136.

197. Ishak KG, Glunz PR. Hepatoblastoma and hepatocarcinoma in infancy and childhood. Report of 47 cases. *Cancer* 1967; **20**: 396–422.

198. Lack EE, Neave C, Vawter GF. Hepatoblastoma. A clinical and pathologic study of 54 cases. *Am J Surg Pathol* 1982; **6**: 693–705.

199. Kasai M, Watanabe I. Histologic classification of liver cell carcinoma in infancy and childhood and its clinical evaluation. *Cancer* 1970; **25**: 551–563.

200. Weinberg AG, Finegold MJ. Primary hepatic tumors of childhood. *Hum Pathol* 1983; **14**: 512–537.

201. Gonzalez-Crussi F, Upton MP, Maurer HS. Hepatoblastoma. Attempt at characterization of histologic subtypes. *Am J Surg Pathol* 1982; **6**: 599–612.

202. Abenoza P, Manivel JC, Wick MR, Hagen K, Dehner LP. Hepatoblastoma: an immunohistochemical and ultrastructural study. *Hum Pathol* 1987; **18**: 1025–1035.

203. Stocker JT, Ishak KG. Undifferentiated (embryonal) sarcoma of the liver: report of 31 cases. *Cancer* 1978; **42**: 336–348.

204. Keating S, Taylor GP. Undifferentiated (embryonal) sarcoma of the liver: ultrastructural and immunohistochemical similarities with malignant fibrous histiocytoma. *Hum Pathol* 1985; **16**: 693–699.

205. Aoyama C, Hachitanda Y, Sato JK, Said JW, Shimada H. Undifferentiated (embryonal) sarcoma of the

liver. A tumor of uncertian histogenesis showing divergent differentiation. *Am J Surg Pathol* 1991; **15**: 615–624.

206. Lack EE, Schloo BL, Azumi N, Travis WD, Grier HE, Kozakewich HPW. Undifferentiated (embryonal) sarcoma of the liver. Clinical and pathologic study of 16 cases with emphasis on immunohistochemical features. *Am J Surg Pathol* 1991; **15**: 1–16.

207. Mills AE. Undifferentiated primary hepatic non-Hodgkin's lymphoma in childhood. *Am J Surg Pathol* 1988; **12**: 721–726.

GENERAL READING

Anthony PP. Tumours and tumour-like lesions of the liver and biliary tract. In MacSween RNM, Anthony PP, Scheuer PJ, Portmann B, Burt AD (eds): Pathology of the Liver, 3rd edn. Edinburgh: Churchill Livingstone, 1994.

Anthony PP. Liver tumours: an update. In Anthony PP, MacSween RNM (eds): Recent Advances in Histopathology, Vol. 14. Edinburgh: Churchill Livingstone, 1989.

Okuda K, Ishak KG, (eds). Neoplasms of the Liver. Tokyo: Springer-Verlag, 1987.

VASCULAR DISORDERS

12

THE HEPATIC ARTERIES

The branches of the hepatic artery are subject to the same diseases as other systemic arteries. **Polyarteritis nodosa** may affect the hepatic arterial tree[1] but is rarely seen in needle liver biopsy material. The disease is sometimes found in carriers of the hepatitis B virus. The liver is occasionally involved in the arteritis of **systemic lupus erythematosus**[2] and **giant cell arteritis.**[3] Hepatic fibrin-ring granulomas have been reported in association with the latter.[4] In some older subjects, especially those with systemic hypertension, small arteries and arterioles in portal tracts appear thickened and hyaline. **Amyloidosis** (p. 251) can give rise to thickening of arterial walls in the absence of sinusoidal deposits.

The vascular lesions of **hereditary haemorrhagic telangiectasia** are sometimes found in the liver, with or without surrounding fibrosis.[5–7] The parenchyma may undergo nodular hyperplasia.[8]

Infarcts of the liver result from arteritis, aneurysms, thrombosis, embolism or surgical ligation. They may complicate pregnancy or liver transplantation. Infarction can also follow occlusion of portal-vein branches,[8a] and may even be found in the absence of demonstrable vascular obstruction.[9,10] The pathological features are as in other organs: well-defined zones of coagulative necrosis have a congested and inflamed border (Fig. 12.1). Portal tracts sometimes survive within the infarcted areas. Coagulative necrosis of the centres of cirrhotic nodules following hypoperfusion is sometimes called nodular infarction. An alternative term is ischaemic hepatitis (see below).[11]

Shock and Heart Failure

Severe hypoperfusion of the hepatic parenchyma leads to necrosis, usually in acinar zone 3 but sometimes, additionally or alternatively, in zone 2.[12] Portal tracts and the periportal parenchyma typically remain normal (Fig. 12.2). In contrast to the necrosis of acute hepatitis there is usually little or no inflammation, but in some patients neutrophils and mononuclear cells accumulate in limited numbers.[13] Affected areas may be congested and contain large, ceroid-laden macrophages. There may be cholestasis and evidence of regenerative hyperplasia in the surviving parenchyma. The reticulin network shows regular condensation in the necrotic areas. Similar, usually mild changes are seen in patients with **heat-stroke**.[14,15]

One of the most important causes of this type of necrosis is heart failure with consequent hypoperfusion of the liver. The term ischaemic hepatitis is commonly used for

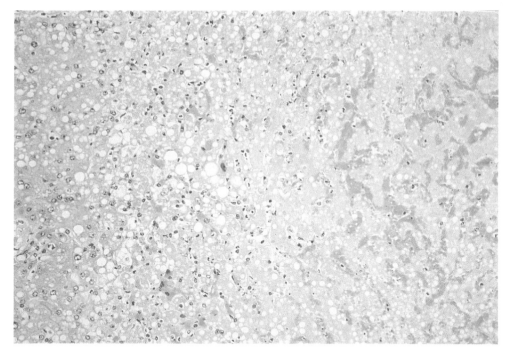

Figure 12.1. *Infarct.* The dead parenchyma to the right is intensely congested. Surviving liver tissue (left) is fatty. Post-mortem liver, H & E.

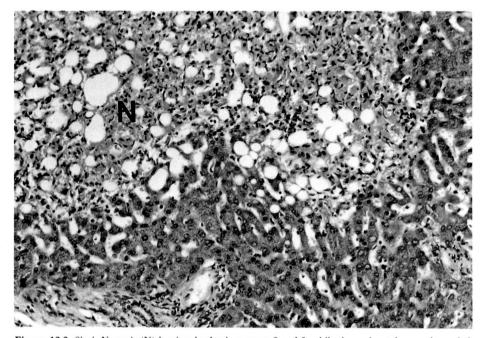

Figure 12.2. *Shock.* Necrosis (N) has involved acinar zones 2 and 3, while the periportal parenchyma below and to the right is intact. There are fat vacuoles in the necrotic areas. Post-mortem liver, H & E.

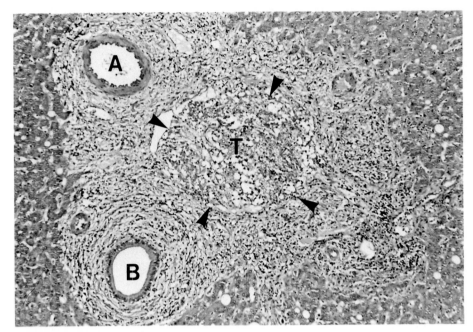

Figure 12.3. *Pylephlebitis.* Thrombus (T), outlined by arrowheads, fills a portal-vein branch. A = artery, B = bile duct. Thrombus and portal tract contain inflammatory cells. Wedge biopsy, H & E.

the viral hepatitis-like clinical picture which may ensue.[16–18] Congestive heart failure leads to sinusoidal dilatation (see "Venous congestion and outflow obstruction", p. 188).

THE PORTAL VEINS

Thrombosis of the main portal veins may result from infection, local or in the portal venous drainage area, cirrhosis, liver transplantation and disorders of coagulation. Invasion by hepatocellular carcinoma is a common cause. In some patients no reason for the thrombosis can be discovered. In the acute phase of pylephlebitis, septic thrombi may be seen in portal-vein branches in portal tracts (Fig. 12.3).

Possible results of portal thrombosis include diffuse or focal parenchymal atrophy, parenchymal nodularity (see "Nodular regenerative hyperplasia", p. 155), and a mild degree of portal fibrosis. Focal atrophy is also known as Zahn's infarction and is often found at the margins of tumour nodules. Occasionally portal venous obstruction leads to true infarction of the hepatic parenchyma.[8a] In many patients with thrombosis of the main portal veins the liver remains histologically normal.

Portal Hypertension

Portal hypertension is most often the result of cirrhosis. Other causes include schistosomiasis, alcohol-related liver disease,[19] congenital hepatic fibrosis, the tropical splenomegaly syndrome, hepatic venous outflow obstruction and portal venous thrombosis. The latter probably contributes to portal hypertension in polycythaemia and other haematological diseases.[20] In lymphoproliferative and myeloproliferative disorders, the portal infiltration may be a further pathogenetic factor.[21]

There remains a group of patients with **non-cirrhotic portal hypertension (idio-**

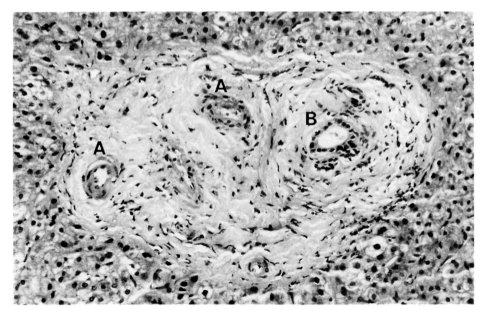

Figure 12.4. *Non-cirrhotic portal hypertension.* An enlarged, sclerotic portal tract contains arteries (A) and bile ducts (B). Portal vein branches are inconspicuous. Wedge biopsy, H & E.

pathic portal hypertension, hepatoportal sclerosis, non-cirrhotic portal fibrosis, obliterative portal venopathy), with or without demonstrable thrombosis or narrowing of portal-vein branches.[22,23] In many patients the disease is of unknown cause. In a minority there is a defined cause such as a toxin (e.g. arsenic,[24] vinyl chloride,[25,26] cytotoxic drugs[27]). Needle liver biopsies from patients with non-cirrhotic portal hypertension are often normal or show only non-specific changes. Abnormalities are more likely to be seen in operative wedge biopsies. Portal-vein branches are sometimes thickened and narrowed, unusually inconspicuous or replaced by multiple small, thin-walled channels. Dilated veins appear to herniate into the adjacent parenchyma.[28] There may be portal fibrosis and enlargement, with or without inflammatory-cell infiltration (Fig. 12.4). Slender fibrous septa extending from the portal tracts give an appearance indistinguishable from incomplete septal cirrhosis.[29] In some instances these septa connect with bridge-like zones of necrosis.[28] There may be randomly distributed thin-walled vessels in the acini ("megasinusoids"), and sclerosis or dilatation of efferent veins.[28] Diffuse or localized nodular hyperplasia of the parenchyma is commonly seen, so that there is overlap with the condition of nodular regenerative hyperplasia (p. 155). In patients exposed to vinyl chloride monomer and other carcinogens, there may be, in addition to the above features, perisinusoidal fibrosis and an increase in the number and size of sinusoidal cells.[25,26] Perisinusoidal fibrosis may also contribute to the portal hypertension which develops in some patients after renal transplantation.[30] Prolonged drug therapy has been suggested as a possible mechanism.

THE HEPATIC SINUSOIDS

The width of the sinusoids in liver biopsy specimens is very variable. It is influenced not only by the state of the patient's circulation at the time of biopsy, but also by fixation and tissue processing. Slight variations in width are therefore of doubtful significance.

The amount of connective tissue in sinusoidal walls should also be assessed critically,

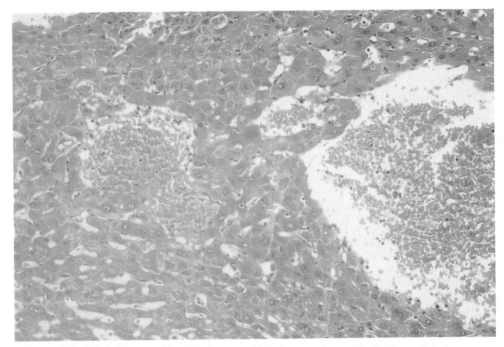

Figure 12.5. *Peliosis.* There are blood-filled spaces within the parenchyma. Needle biopsy, H & E.

since its appearance varies with section thickness. A definite increase in fibres is characteristic of steatohepatitis (p. 86). Other causes and associations, some of them already mentioned above, include congenital syphilis, vinyl chloride toxicity, heroin addiction,[31] hypervitaminosis A, renal transplantation, myeloid metaplasia[32] and thrombocytopenic purpura.[33]

Definite and regular dilatation of the sinusoidal network is associated with several conditions, the most important being venous outflow obstruction (p. 188). It has been reported in patients with tumours or granulomas even when these did not involve the liver,[34] and in Crohn's disease.[35] Dilatation of periportal sinusoids has been described in a small number of patients taking oral contraceptives.[36] In some patients with renal cell carcinoma there is focal dilatation of midzonal sinusoids.[37]

The borderline between regular diffuse dilatation and the focal dilatation known as **peliosis hepatis** is not always sharp.[37,38] In peliosis blood-filled cysts are found in the parenchyma (Fig. 12.5), ranging in size from less than one to several millimetres in diameter. The endothelial lining is usually incomplete.[39] Peliosis is found in association with many different conditions and circumstances including wasting diseases, malignant tumours, thorotrast liver disease,[40] liver or renal transplantation[41,42] and treatment with steroid hormones[43-45] or anti-tumour therapy.[46] The lesion is often discovered incidentally but rupture leading to fatal haemoperitoneum has been reported.[47,48] and peliosis may cause cholestasis[46] or contribute to liver failure.[40] **Bacillary peliosis hepatis** (see also p. 236) is attributed to the bacteria which cause cutaneous bacillary angiomatosis in patients with AIDS.[49,50] Their presence in silver preparations distinguishes the condition from simple peliosis.

Disseminated intravascular coagulation commonly involves the liver.[51] Sinusoids and small portal vessels contain fibrin thrombi (Fig. 12.6). The fibrin is often difficult to identify with certainty in conventional sections. Similar changes are seen in eclampsia, in association with periportal necrosis and acute inflammation.

In most patients with **sickle-cell disease** clumps of sickled erythrocytes are found in

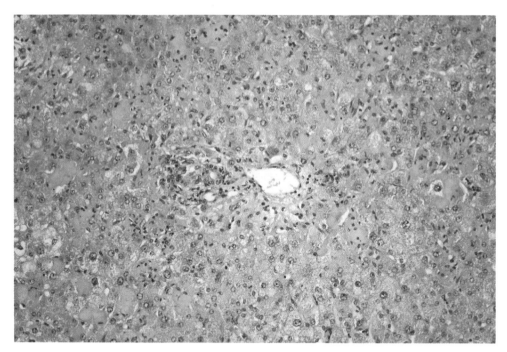

Figure 12.6. *Disseminated intravascular coagulation.* Periportal sinusoids are filled with fibrin and neutrophils. Needle biopsy, H & E.

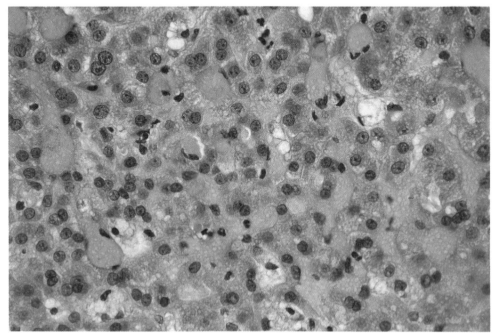

Figure 12.7. *Sickle-cell disease.* Clumped erythrocytes are seen in distended sinusoids and there is mild cholestasis. Needle biopsy, H & E.

sinusoids (Fig. 12.7) and there is erythrophagocytosis. Hypertrophied Kupffer cells and hepatocytes contain iron. Hepatocytes may show regenerative hyperplasia. The commonly seen sinusoidal dilatation is distinguishable from simple venous congestion by the presence of sickled erythrocytes and fibrin. The degree of sickling seen does not correlate with biochemical or clinical evidence of liver damage, and many hepatic manifestations in patients with sickle-cell disease are thought to be the result of complications.[52–54] These include transfusion-related hepatitis and siderosis, cholelithiasis and venous outflow obstruction. Cirrhosis is occasionally found, and may be a consequence of viral hepatitis or siderosis.

VENOUS CONGESTION AND OUTFLOW OBSTRUCTION

Interference with the venous outflow of the liver results from a multitude of causes ranging from congestive cardiac failure to occlusion of the smallest tributaries of the hepatic veins within the liver. Space-occupying lesions such as tumours may cause localized obstruction affecting only parts of the liver. The term **Budd–Chiari syndrome** is often used to describe the clinical findings when the inferior vena cava or main hepatic veins are obstructed, and is sometimes extended to obstruction at the level of the heart. Ludwig and colleagues[55] argue convincingly that classification should be based on the nature and location of the obstruction, and that the label Budd–Chiari syndrome should be used sparingly and only until the cause of the obstruction is known. Indeed, the pathologist faced with a severely congested liver biopsy is often unsure about the level and nature of the block. Use of the term **venous outflow obstruction** is then appropriate.

In **congestive cardiac failure** the terminal hepatic venules and adjacent sinusoids are dilated.[56] As already noted, this congestion may be accompanied by hepatocellular necrosis if there is also a significant element of hypoperfusion (Fig. 12.8), as in the

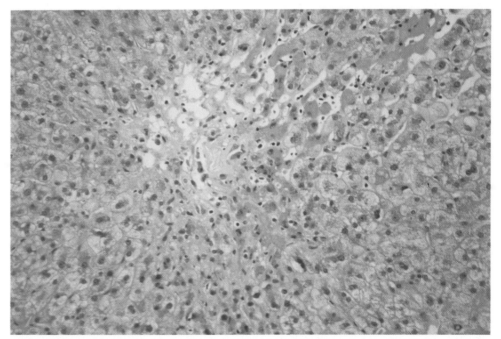

Figure 12.8. *Venous congestion.* Perivenular sinusoids are dilated. The pale zone of necrosis indicates an element of hypoperfusion. Kupffer cells in and around this area are loaded with brown ceroid pigment. Needle biopsy, H & E.

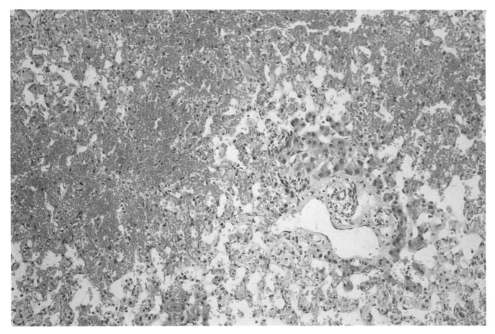

Figure 12.9. *Acute venous outflow obstruction.* In this example, due to obstruction of major veins (Budd–Chiari syndrome), much of the parenchyma has been replaced by blood. A few hepatocytes have survived around the portal tract (below right). Wedge biopsy, H & E.

combination of congestive and left-sided heart failure. Blood may infiltrate the liver-cell plates.[57] Cholestasis is sometimes present but must be distinguished from the commonly found ceroid pigment in Kupffer cells. Inflammation is typically mild or absent, and portal tracts usually remain normal. There may be regenerative hyperplasia of hepatocytes, and chronic venous congestion is one cause of nodular regenerative hyperplasia (p. 155) and, very rarely, cirrhosis. In some patients hepatocytes contain PAS-positive globules which probably represent phagosomes containing imbibed plasma proteins.[58] The globules are usually located in or near the congested areas. They can be distinguished from the globules of α_1-antitrypsin deficiency by their location and if necessary by immunochemical staining.

Obstruction to large veins typically causes more severe congestion. There are many causes, including thrombosis related to myeloproliferative disorders[59] and other haematological diseases. An association with the use of oral contraceptives lacks conclusive proof.[60] Fibrous webs may represent a late consequence of thrombosis.[61–63] Occasionally the obstruction results from administration of anti-tumour drugs,[64] primary vascular disease[65,66] or infection.[67] In some patients no cause can be discovered.

In the acute stages much of the parenchyma may be replaced by blood. Sinusoids at the border between the haemorrhagic zones and the surviving parenchyma are dilated and empty (Fig. 12.9). Small efferent veins may be narrowed or blocked, depending on the cause of the obstruction (see discussion of veno-occlusive disease, below). Eventually the haemorrhage and congestion lead to fibrosis or even cirrhosis (Fig. 12.10). Fibrosis is often difficult to distinguish from simple acute condensation of pre-existing reticulin and collagen. Stains for elastic fibres are then sometimes helpful, as in the distinction between bridging necrosis and fibrosis discussed on p. 70. Two further diagnostic problems should be noted. First, blocked veins may be missed in haematoxylin and eosin-stained sections so that a collagen stain should be examined if venous outflow obstruction is suspected. Thin-walled bypass channels should not be mistaken for patent veins. Secondly the obstruction

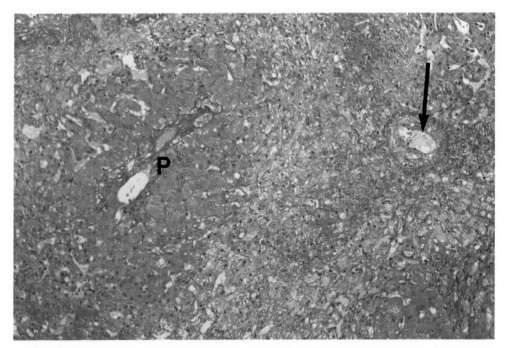

Figure 12.10. *Chronic venous outflow obstruction.* Late in the disease fibrous tissue, stained blue, has been laid down in the congested areas. Surviving parenchyma shows reversed lobulation around a portal tract (P). An efferent vein (arrow) is partly occluded by fibrous tissue. Needle biopsy, chromotrope aniline blue.

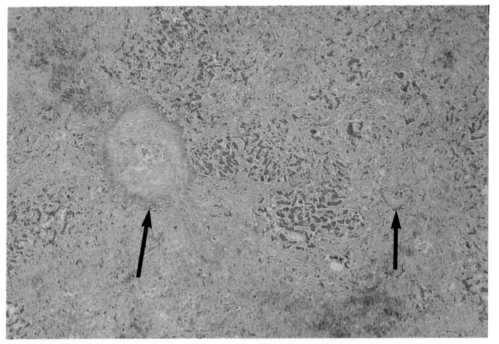

Figure 12.11. *Veno-occlusive disease.* Efferent veins (arrows) are greatly narrowed by fibrosis. Post-mortem liver, MSB stain.

may not affect all the hepatic veins, so that parts of the liver escape serious congestion. This can lead to diagnostic confusion. It follows that a near-normal liver biopsy does not necessarily exclude a diagnosis of venous outflow obstruction.

Veno-occlusive disease refers to conditions in which the smallest tributaries of the hepatic veins, the terminal hepatic venules and sublobular veins, are occluded by fibrous tissue (Fig. 12.11). The venous lesions can thus be detected in needle biopsies. Apart from these lesions the changes are as for obstruction of large veins. As already noted, the borderline between obstruction to large and small veins is not sharp, since both may be affected by thrombosis, for example, in patients with coagulation disorders. Furthermore, thrombosis of large or medium-sized hepatic veins may lead to fibrous intimal thickening of smaller vessels. As in the case of obstruction to larger veins, there are many causes of veno-occlusive disease. The classical cause, ingestion of pyrrolizidine alkaloids, remains a hazard.[68,69] Venous occlusion is increasingly seen following bone-marrow, renal or liver transplantation.[70-72] Other associations and causes are irradiation of the liver,[73] primary vascular disease,[74] tumour therapy,[75] arsenic poisoning[76] and heroin addiction.[31] Finally, careful examination of connective tissue stains may reveal occluded veins in the livers of patients with alcohol-related liver disease[77,78] and in cirrhosis from any cause.[79]

REFERENCES

1. Parangi S, Oz MC, Blume RS et al. Hepatobiliary complications of polyarteritis nodosa. *Arch Surg* 1991; **126**: 909–912.
2. Matsumoto T, Yoshimine T, Shimouchi K et al. The liver in systemic lupus erythematosus: pathologic analysis of 52 cases and review of Japanese Autopsy Registry Data. *Hum Pathol* 1992; **23**: 1151–1158.
3. Rousselet M-Ch, Kettani S, Rohmer V, Saint-Andre J-P. A case of temporal arteritis with intrahepatic arterial involvement. *Pathol Res Pract* 1989; **185**: 329–331.
4. De Bayser L, Roblot P, Ramassamy A, Silvain C, Levillain P, Becq-Giraudon B. Hepatic fibrin-ring granulomas in giant cell arteritis. *Gastroenterology* 1993; **105**: 272–273.
5. Daly JJ, Schiller AL. The liver in hereditary hemorrhagic telangiectasia (Osler–Weber–Rendu disease). *Am J Med* 1976; **60**: 723–726.
6. Martini GA. The liver in hereditary haemorrhagic telangiectasia: an inborn error of vascular structure with multiple manifestations: a reappraisal. *Gut* 1978; **19**: 531–537.
7. Deviere J, Brohee D, Hiden M, Bourgeois N. Hepatic telangiectasia and cirrhosis. *J Clin Gastroenterol* 1988; **10**: 111–114.
8. Wanless IR, Gryfe A. Nodular transformation of the liver in hereditary hemorrhagic telangiectasia. *Arch Pathol Lab Med* 1986; **110**: 331–335.
8a. Saegusa, M, Takano Y, Okudaira M. Human hepatic infarction: histopathological and postmortem angiological studies. *Liver* 1993; **13**: 239–245.
9. Seeley TT, Blumenfeld CM, Ikeda R, Knapp W, Ruebner BH. Hepatic infarction. *Hum Pathol* 1972; **3**: 265–276.
10. Chen V, Hamilton J, Qizilbash A. Hepatic infarction. A clinicopathologic study of seven cases. *Arch Pathol Lab Med* 1976; **100**: 32–36.
11. Henrion J, Colin L, Schmitz A, Schapira M, Heller FR. Ischemic hepatitis in cirrhosis. Rare but lethal. *J Clin Gastroenterol* 1993; **16**: 35–39.
12. de la Monte SM, Arcidi JM, Moore GW, Hutchins GM. Midzonal necrosis as a pattern of hepatocellular injury after shock. *Gastroenterology* 1984; **86**: 627–631.
13. Lefkowitch JH, Mendez L. Morphologic features of hepatic injury in cardiac disease and shock. *J Hepatol* 1986; **2**: 313–327.
14. Kew M, Bersohn I, Seftel H, Kent G. Liver damage in heatstroke. *Am J Med* 1970; **49**: 192–202.
15. Bianchi L, Ohnacker H, Beck K, Zimmerli-Ning M. Liver damage in heatstroke and its regression. A biopsy study. *Hum Pathol* 1972; **3**: 237–248.
16. Cohen JA, Kaplan MM. Left-sided heart failure presenting as hepatitis. *Gastroenterology* 1978; **74**: 583–587.
17. Bynum TE, Boitnott JK, Maddrey WC. Ischemic hepatitis. *Dig Dis Sci* 1979; **24**: 129–135.
18. Gitlin N, Serio KM. Ischemic hepatitis: widening horizons. *Am J Gastroenterol* 1992; **87**: 831–836.
19. Vidins EI, Britton RS, Medline A, Blendis LM, Israel Y, Orrego H. Sinusoidal caliber in alcoholic and nonalcoholic liver disease: diagnostic and pathogenic implications. *Hepatology* 1985; **5**: 408–414.
20. Wanless IR, Peterson P, Das A, Boitnott JK, Moore GW, Bernier V. Hepatic vascular disease and portal hypertension in polycythemia vera and agnogenic myeloid metaplasia: a clinicopathological study of 145 patients examined at autopsy. *Hepatology* 1990; **12**: 1166–1174.

21. Dubois A, Dauzat M, Pignodel C et al. Portal hypertension in lymphoproliferative and myeloproliferative disorders: hemodynamic and histological correlations. *Hepatology* 1993; **17**: 246–250.

22. Okuda K, Nakashima T, Okudaira M et al. Liver pathology of idiopathic portal hypertension. Comparison with non-cirrhotic portal fibrosis of India. The Japan idiopathic portal hypertension study. *Liver* 1982; **2**: 176–192.

23. Okuda K, Kono K, Ohnishi K et al. Clinical study of eighty-six cases of idiopathic portal hypertension and comparison with cirrhosis with splenomegaly. *Gastroenterology* 1984; **86**: 600–610.

24. Nevens F, Fevery J, Van Steenbergen W, Sciot R, Desmet V, De Groote J. Arsenic and non-cirrhotic portal hypertension. A report of eight cases. *J Hepatol* 1990; **11**: 80–85.

25. Thomas LB, Popper H, Berk PD, Selikoff I, Falk H. Vinyl-chloride-induced liver disease. From idiopathic portal hypertension (Banti's syndrome) to angiosarcomas. *N Engl J Med* 1975; **292**: 17–22.

26. Popper H, Thomas LB, Telles NC, Falk H, Selikoff IJ. Development of hepatic angiosarcoma in man induced by vinyl chloride, thorotrast, and arsenic. Comparison with cases of unknown etiology. *Am J Pathol* 1978; **92**: 349–369.

27. Shepherd P, Harrison DJ. Idiopathic portal hypertension associated with cytotoxic drugs. *J Clin Pathol* 1990; **43**: 206–210.

28. Ludwig J, Hashimoto E, Obata H, Baldus WP. Idiopathic portal hypertension; a histopathological study of 26 Japanese cases. *Histopathology* 1993; **22**: 227–234.

29. Levison DA, Kingham JG, Dawson AM, Stansfeld AG. Slow cirrhosis – or no cirrhosis? A lesion causing benign intrahepatic portal hypertension. *J Pathol* 1982; **137**: 253–272.

30. Nataf C, Feldmann G, Lebrec D et al. Idiopathic portal hypertension (perisinusoidal fibrosis) after renal transplantation. *Gut* 1979; **20**: 531–537.

31. Trigueiro de Araújo MS, Gerard F, Chossegros P, Porto LC, Barlet P, Grimaud J-A. Vascular hepatotoxicity related to heroin addiction. *Virchows Arch (A)* 1990; **417**: 497–503.

32. Degott C, Capron J-P, Bettan L et al. Myeloid metaplasia, perisinusoidal fibrosis, and nodular regenerative hyperplasia of the liver. *Liver* 1985; **5**: 276–281.

33. Lafon ME, Bioulac-Sage P, Grimaud JA et al. Perisinusoidal fibrosis of the liver in patients with thrombocytopenic purpura. *Virchows Arch (A)* 1987; **411**: 553–559.

34. Bruguera M, Aranguibel F, Ros E, Rodes J. Incidence and clinical significance of sinusoidal dilatation in liver biopsies. *Gastroenterology* 1978; **75**: 474–478.

35. Capron JP, Lemay JL, Gontier MF, Dupas JL, Capron-Chivrac D, Lorriaux A. Hepatic sinusoidal dilatation in Crohn's disease. *Scand J Gastroenterol* 1979; **14**: 987–992.

36. Winkler K, Christoffersen P. A reappraisal of Poulsen's disease (hepatic zone 1 sinusoidal dilatation). *APMIS* 1991; Suppl. **23**: 86–90.

37. Aoyagi T, Mori I, Ueyama Y, Tamaoki N. Sinusoidal dilatation of the liver as a paraneoplastic manifestation of renal cell carcinoma. *Hum Pathol* 1989; **20**: 1193–1197.

38. Oligny LL, Lough J. Hepatic sinusoidal ectasia. *Hum Pathol* 1992; **23**: 953–956.

39. Wold LE, Ludwig J. Peliosis hepatis: two morphologic variants? *Hum Pathol* 1981; **12**: 388–389.

40. Okuda K, Omata M, Itoh Y, Ikezaki H, Nakashima T. Peliosis hepatis as a late and fatal complication of thorotrast liver disease. Report of five cases. *Liver* 1981; **1**: 110–122.

41. Degott C, Rueff B, Kreis H, Duboust A, Potet F, Benhamou JP. Peliosis hepatis in recipients of renal transplants. *Gut* 1978; **19**: 748–753.

42. Scheuer PJ, Schachter LA, Mathur S, Burroughs AK, Rolles K. Peliosis hepatitis after liver transplantation. *J Clin Pathol* 1990; **43**: 1036–1037.

43. Nadell J, Kosek J. Peliosis hepatis. Twelve cases associated with oral androgen therapy. *Arch Pathol Lab Med* 1977; **101**: 405–410.

44. Karasawa T, Shikata T, Smith RD. Peliosis hepatis. Report of nine cases. *Acta Pathol Jpn* 1979; **29**: 457–469.

45. Soe KL, Soe M, Gluud C. Liver pathology associated with the use of anabolic-androgenic steroids. *Liver* 1992; **12**: 73–79.

46. Larrey D, Fréneaux E, Berson A et al. Peliosis hepatis induced by 6-thioguanine administration. *Gut* 1988; **29**: 1265–1269.

47. Bagheri SA, Boyer JL. Peliosis hepatis associated with androgenic-anabolic steroid therapy. A severe form of hepatic injury. *Ann Intern Med* 1974; **81**: 610–618.

48. Takiff H, Brems JJ, Pockros PJ, Elliott ML. Focal hemorrhagic necrosis of the liver. A rare cause of hemoperitoneum. *Dig Dis Sci* 1992; **37**: 1910–1914.

49. Perkocha LA, Geaghan SM, Yen TS et al. Clinical and pathological features of bacillary peliosis hepatis in association with human immunodeficiency virus infection. *N Engl J Med* 1990; **323**: 1581–1586.

50. Garcia-Tsao G, Panzini L, Yoselevitz M, West AB. Bacillary peliosis hepatis as a cause of acute anemia in a patient with the acquired immunodeficiency syndrome. *Gastroenterology* 1992; **102**: 1065–1070.

51. Shimamura K, Oka K, Nakazawa M, Kojima M. Distribution patterns of microthrombi in disseminated intravascular coagulation. *Arch Pathol Lab Med* 1983; **107**: 543–547.

52. Omata M, Johnson CS, Tong M, Tatter D. Pathological spectrum of liver diseases in sickle cell disease. *Dig Dis Sci* 1986; **31**: 247–256.

53. Mills LR, Mwakyusa D, Milner PF. Histopathologic features of liver biopsy specimens in sickle cell disease. *Arch Pathol Lab Med* 1988; **112**: 290–294.

54. Comer GM, Ozick LA, Sachdev RK et al. Transfusion-related chronic liver disease in sickle cell anemia. *Am J Gastroenterol* 1991; **86**: 1232–1234.

55. Ludwig J, Hashimoto E, McGill DB, van Heerden JA. Classification of hepatic venous outflow obstruction: ambiguous terminology of the Budd–Chiari syndrome. *Mayo Clin Proc* 1990; **65**: 51–55.

56. Arcidi JMJ, Moore GW, Hutchins GM. Hepatic morphology in cardiac dysfunction: a clinicopathologic study of 1000 subjects at autopsy. *Am J Pathol* 1981; **104**: 159–166.
57. Kanel GC, Ucci AA, Kaplan MM, Wolfe HJ. A distinctive perivenular hepatic lesion associated with heart failure. *Am J Clin Pathol* 1980; **73**: 235–239.
58. Klatt EC, Koss MN, Young TS, Macauley L, Martin SE. Hepatic hyaline globules associated with passive congestion. *Arch Pathol Lab Med* 1988; **112**: 510–513.
59. Boughton BJ. Hepatic and portal vein thrombosis. Closely associated with chronic myeloproliferative disorders. *Br Med J* 1991; **302**: 192–193.
60. Maddrey WC. Hepatic vein thrombosis (Budd Chiari syndrome): possible association with the use of oral contraceptives. *Semin Liver Dis* 1987; **7**: 32–39.
61. Okuda K. Membranous obstruction of the inferior vena cava: etiology and relation to hepatocellular carcinoma. *Gastroenterology* 1982; **82**: 376–379.
62. Sevenet F, Deramond H, Hadengue A, Casadevall N, Delamarre J, Capron J-P. Membranous obstruction of the inferior vena cava associated with a myeloproliferative disorder: a clue to membrane formation? *Gastroenterology* 1989; **97**: 1019–1021.
63. Vickers CR, West RJ, Hubscher SG, Elias E. Hepatic vein webs and resistant ascites. Diagnosis, management and implications. *J Hepatol* 1989; **8**: 287–293.
64. Greenstone MA, Dowd PM, Mikhailidis DP, Scheuer PJ. Hepatic vascular lesions associated with dacarbazine treatment. *Br Med J Clin Res* 1981; **282**: 1744–1745.
65. Young ID, Clark RN, Manley PN, Groll A, Simon JB. Response to steroids in Budd–Chiari syndrome caused by idiopathic granulomatous venulitis. *Gastroenterology* 1988; **94**: 503–507.
66. Bismuth E, Hadengue A, Hammel P, Benhamou J-P. Hepatic vein thrombosis in Behçet's disease. *Hepatology* 1990; **11**: 969–974.
67. Vallaeys JH, Praet MM, Roels HJ, Van Marck E, Kaufman L. The Budd–Chiari syndrome caused by a zygomycete. A new pathogenesis of hepatic vein thrombosis. *Arch Pathol Lab Med* 1989; **113**: 1171–1174.
68. Weston CFM, Cooper BT, Davies JD, Levine DF. Veno-occlusive disease of the liver secondary to ingestion of comfrey. *Br Med J* 1987; **295**: 183.
69. Ridker PM, McDermott WV. Comfrey herb tea and hepatic veno-occlusive disease. *Lancet* 1989; **i**: 657–658.
70. Katzka DA, Saul SH, Jorkasky D, Sigal H, Reynolds JC, Soloway RD. Azathioprine and hepatic venocclusive disease in renal transplant patients. *Gastroenterology* 1986; **90**: 446–454.
71. Shulman HM, Gown AM, Nugent DJ. Hepatic veno-occlusive disease after bone marrow transplantation. Immunohistochemical identification of the material within occluded central venules. *Am J Pathol* 1987; **127**: 549–558.
72. McDonald GB, Hinds MS, Fisher LD et al. Veno-occlusive disease of the liver and multiorgan failure after bone marrow transplantation: a cohort study of 355 patients. *Ann Intern Med* 1993; **118**: 255–267.
73. Fajardo LF, Colby TV. Pathogenesis of veno-occlusive liver disease after radiation. *Arch Pathol Lab Med* 1980; **104**: 584–588.
74. Ito N, Kimura A, Nishikawa M et al. Veno-occlusive disease of the liver in a patient with allergic granulomatous angiitis. *Am J Gastroenterol* 1988; **83**: 316–319.
75. Nakhleh RE, Wesen C, Snover DC, Grage T. Venooclusive lesions of the central veins and portal vein radicles secondary to intraarterial 5-fluoro-2'-deoxyuridine infusion. *Hum Pathol* 1989; **20**: 1218–1220.
76. Labadie H, Stoessel P, Callard P, Beaugrand M. Hepatic venoocclusive disease and perisinusoidal fibrosis secondary to arsenic poisoning. *Gastroenterology* 1990; **99**: 1140–1143.
77. Goodman ZD, Ishak KG. Occlusive venous lesions in alcoholic liver disease. A study of 200 cases. *Gastroenterology* 1982; **83**: 786–796.
78. Burt AD, MacSween RN. Hepatic vein lesions in alcoholic liver disease: retrospective biopsy and necropsy study. *J Clin Pathol* 1986; **39**: 63–67.
79. Nakanuma Y, Ohta G, Doishita K. Quantitation and serial section observations of focal venoocclusive lesions of hepatic veins in liver cirrhosis. *Virchows Arch (A)* 1985; **405**: 429–438.

GENERAL READING

Sarin SK. Non-cirrhotic portal fibrosis. *Gut* 1989; **30**: 406–415.

Wanless IR. Vascular disorders. In MacSween RNM, Anthony PP, Scheuer PJ, Portmann B, Burt AD (eds): Pathology of the Liver, 3rd edn. Edinburgh: Churchill Livingstone, 1994.

Zafrani ES, von Pinaudeau Y, Dhumeaux D. Drug-induced vascular lesions of the liver. *Arch Intern Med* 1983; **143**: 495–502.

13
CHILDHOOD LIVER DISEASE AND METABOLIC DISORDERS

Paediatric liver biopsies present a unique set of diagnostic problems for the pathologist, many of which become clinically apparent in the first few months of life as **neonatal cholestasis**.[1] Among the important disorders one must consider in evaluating neonatal liver biopsies are **extrahepatic biliary atresia**, **paucity of intrahepatic bile ducts** (syndromatic and non-syndromatic types), **metabolic diseases**, **viral hepatitis** and the hepatic effects of **parenteral nutrition** (Table 13.1). Common to many of these conditions are the histological features of **cholestasis** and **giant-cell hepatitis** (formation of multinucleated hepatocytes). Because these features are not specifically diagnostic of any one neonatal liver disease, the pathologist must be acquainted with other biopsy changes by which to establish or suggest the diagnosis. In many instances, assays of metabolic enzymes and products in serum and liver tissue take diagnostic precedence to routine histopathological interpretation. Electron microscopy may be required to assess the structure of organelles or storage material in hepatocytes or Kupffer cells, particularly when lysosomal storage disorders are being considered. In older children, the biopsy diagnosis of **chronic viral hepatitis**, **primary sclerosing cholangitis**, and liver involvement in **acquired immune deficiency syndrome** (**AIDS**) is essentially that seen in adults, as described elsewhere in this book. Childhood liver tumours are discussed in Chapter 11.

DIAGNOSTIC APPROACH TO THE NEONATAL LIVER BIOPSY

Histopathological examination of neonatal liver biopsies may benefit from a systematic checklist of questions by which the major diagnostic concerns in neonatal liver disease can be evaluated. A simplified, stepwise set of seven questions can be asked:

1. *Is the acinar structure normal for age?* As described in Chapter 3, the hepatic plates are two cells thick until 5 or 6 years of age, and should not be misconstrued as a pathological change. As with adult biopsies, the presence of fibrosis, nodularity or cirrhosis should be noted early in the biopsy evaluation and correlated with other histological features which may define the aetiology.

2. *Are cholestasis and giant cells present?* As indicated above, neither of these is diagnostically specific. If present, the next interpretive steps should be examination of portal tracts for evidence of biliary tract obstruction (atresia, etc.) and of portal tracts and parenchyma for evidence of hepatitis.

Table 13.1. Liver Biopsy Interpretation in Neonatal Cholestasis*

Aetiology	Histological Features
Extrahepatic biliary atresia	Proliferation of bile ductules in portal tracts; portal fibrosis; ductular cholestasis
Paucity of intrahepatic bile ducts	Loss of interlobular bile ducts (bile duct:hepatic artery ratio < 1)
Neonatal hepatitis	Portal and acinar mononuclear cell inflammation; acidophil bodies
Metabolic disorders	Fat; fibrosis or cirrhosis; storage product in liver cells or Kupffer cells (see specific disorder)
Parenteral nutrition	Proliferation of bile ductules, portal fibrosis or cirrhosis

* Many of the conditions shown in this table are associated with cholestasis and formation of giant multinucleated hepatocytes, in addition to the diagnostic features listed.

3. *Are histological changes of hepatitis present?* Mononuclear cell infiltrates within acini and portal tracts associated with liver-cell degeneration should be sought when considering cytomegalovirus, Epstein–Barr virus, rubella or hepatitis virus infections.

4. *Are the interlobular bile ducts normal?* This question has three major ramifications. **Proliferation of bile ductules** usually signifies some form of biliary obstruction, such as extrahepatic atresia or choledochal cyst. **Paucity of bile ducts** may be due to developmental, metabolic, or infectious causes. Last, **malformations of bile ducts** comprise a spectrum of problems related to abnormal remodelling of the embryonic bile duct plate (fibropolycystic diseases).

5. *Does the biopsy specimen contain iron or copper?* Although rare, neonatal haemochromatosis and Indian childhood cirrhosis (copper toxicosis in young children) are serious liver diseases with high mortality rates that must be excluded. In the older child and adolescent, Wilson's disease (Chapter 14) must not be overlooked. It should be noted, however, that fetal and neonatal liver contains much higher copper levels compared to adults, with an irregular tissue distribution.[2]

6. *Has the biopsy specimen been studied by diastase-PAS or immunoperoxidase staining to exclude* α_1-*antitrypsin deficiency?* The expression of α_1-antitrypsin deficiency is variable and biopsies may not show diagnostic staining of retained enzyme within liver cells prior to 13–15 weeks of age. This condition should be histologically excluded whenever possible.

7. *Are storage cells present?* Abnormal storage products in liver cells or Kupffer cells may be seen in various metabolic diseases which cause hepatomegaly and failure to thrive. These should be sought on routine haematoxylin and eosin as well as special stains.

NEONATAL HEPATITIS

Inflammation and hepatocellular damage in the neonatal period may result from infections and from inborn errors of metabolism. The former include type B hepatitis, cytomegalovirus infection and rubella among others, the latter α_1-antitrypsin deficiency and galactosaemia. A diagnosis of neonatal hepatitis is therefore a signal for further investigation. The histological picture is broadly similar whatever the cause. There is a variable degree of hepatocellular swelling and multinucleation, cholestasis and portal inflammation. Intra-acinar inflammation may be mild. Liver-cell necrosis and swelling result in collapse and distortion of the reticulin framework (Fig. 13.1). Fibrosis is sometimes already well developed, as in neonatal haemochromatosis (Chapter 14, p. 226) or the severe perinatal liver disease which may rarely be seen in Down syndrome.[3] Giant multinucleated hepatocytes are commonly seen, whatever the cause of the hepatitis (Fig. 13.2). The outcome of neonatal giant-cell hepatitis is resolution, liver failure, cirrhosis or a chronic cholestatic course. The variety of different outcomes is well illustrated in α_1-antitrypsin deficiency.[4]

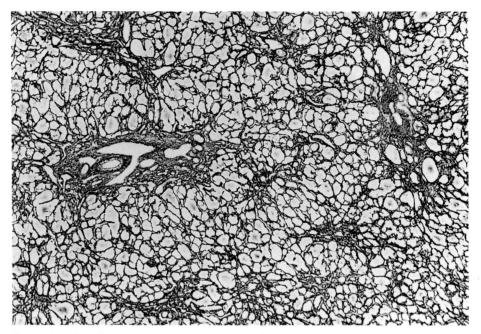

Figure 13.1. *Neonatal (giant-cell) hepatitis.* Fibrosis extends from portal tracts into the acini and architecture is distorted. Wedge biopsy, reticulin.

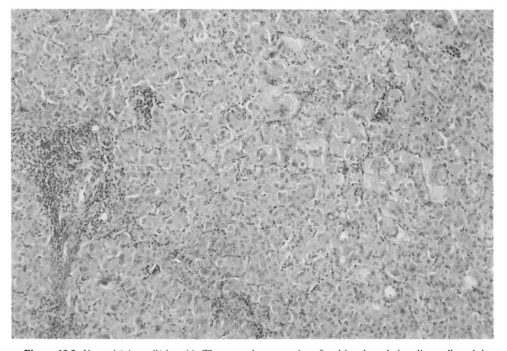

Figure 13.2. *Neonatal (giant-cell) hepatitis.* The parenchyma consists of multinucleated giant liver cells and the portal tract shown is infiltrated by lymphocytes. Wedge biopsy, H & E.

From a histological point of view, the main differential diagnosis of neonatal hepatitis is extrahepatic biliary obstruction which may require surgical treatment. Giant multinucleated hepatocytes and an altered reticulin structure are more prominent in hepatitis than in biliary obstruction, while cholestasis is usually more severe in atresia and there is typically proliferation of bile ductules.

EXTRAHEPATIC BILIARY ATRESIA

This condition results from inflammation and destruction of all or part of the extrahepatic bile duct system *in utero* or in the perinatal period. Pathological studies of atretic bile duct segments[5-7] show chronic inflammation and obliterative fibrosis, sometimes with a few remaining bile-duct cells.[8] Satisfactory bile drainage and an improved outcome after the Kasai portoenterostomy[9] have been associated with identification of bile ducts with lumens of 150 μm or greater at the proximal resection margin.[6] Frozen section of this margin may therefore be requested at the time of surgery to assess bile duct lumenal size. Optimal surgical results are obtained if the Kasai procedure is performed within the first 8 weeks of life.[10]

The trigger for the destructive process in extrahepatic atresia is unknown, although animal models have suggested roles for Reovirus type 3 infection,[11] and expression of histocompatibility antigens type I and II on biliary epithelium.[12] There may be associated congenital abnormalities, including polysplenia[13] and intrahepatic biliary cysts.[14] The process of biliary atresia is a dynamic one which may also involve the intrahepatic bile ducts,[15,16] even after Kasai surgery.[17]

Liver biopsy shows cholestasis and portal tract changes resembling those of large bile-duct obstruction in the adult (p. 40). Portal tracts are enlarged by oedema, a striking proliferation of bile ductules and infiltrating neutrophils with fewer numbers of chronic inflammatory cells (Fig. 13.3). Proliferating ductules may contain inspissated bile ("ductular cholestasis"). The profiles of proliferating ductules occasionally resemble the embryonic bile duct plate described by Jørgensen[18] (Figs 13.4 and 13.5). Proliferation of bile ductules is a major histological point of distinction from neonatal hepatitis.[19] There is panacinar cholestasis with accentuation in zone 3. Giant cells are common, but not as numerous or as striking as in neonatal hepatitis. The degree of portal fibrosis depends on the duration of the obstruction and the age at diagnosis. The overall acinar architecture remains intact except in patients diagnosed late in the disease who may then show secondary biliary cirrhosis (Fig. 13.6). The differential diagnosis includes biliary obstruction by a choledochal cyst, chronic injury associated with parenteral nutrition (p. 211) and various inborn errors of metabolism.

PAUCITY OF INTRAHEPATIC BILE DUCTS IN CHILDHOOD

Two varieties of intrahepatic bile duct paucity (formerly called intrahepatic biliary atresia) are recognized in childhood: **syndromatic** and **non-syndromatic**.[20] In syndromatic paucity[21,22] (Alagille's syndrome, arteriohepatic dysplasia), loss of small intrahepatic bile ducts is associated with abnormal facies, vertebral anomalies and various other malformations. In non-syndromatic paucity, duct loss is not associated with facial or other anomalies. In some patients it may be related to a definable cause such as α_1-antitrypsin deficiency or cytomegalovirus infection,[23] while in others there is no detectable aetiological factor. The exact time of onset of bile duct injury is difficult to establish

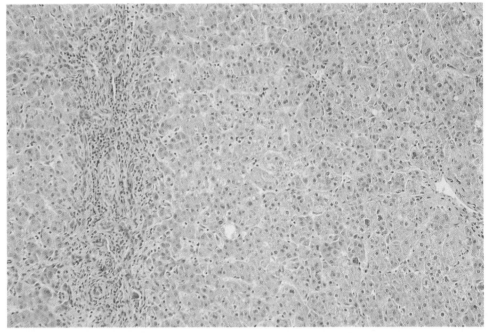

Figure 13.3. *Extrahepatic biliary atresia.* An expanded, inflamed portal tract at left contains many proliferated bile ducts, some of which are filled with inspissated bile. There is also panacinar cholestasis. Wedge biopsy, H & E.

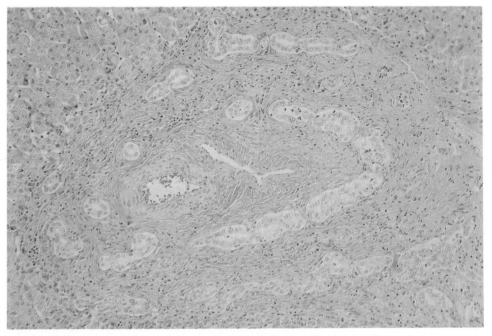

Figure 13.4. *Extrahepatic biliary atresia with bile duct plate-like structures.* The proliferating bile duct structures in this case resemble the embryonic bile duct plate. Wedge biopsy, H & E.

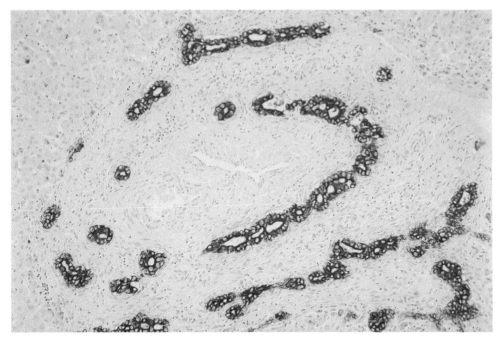

Figure 13.5. *Extrahepatic biliary atresia with bile duct plate-like structures.* The field shown in Figure 13.4 stained with antibodies to cytokeratin highlights the circumferential portal bile duct structures resembling the embryonic bile duct plate. Wedge biopsy, specific immunoperoxidase.

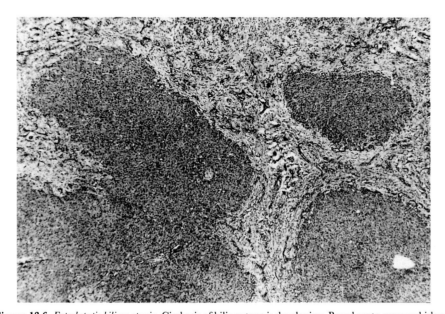

Figure 13.6. *Extrahepatic biliary atresia.* Cirrhosis of biliary type is developing. Broad septa surround islands of parenchyma in which there is little evidence of regeneration. Wedge biopsy, H & E.

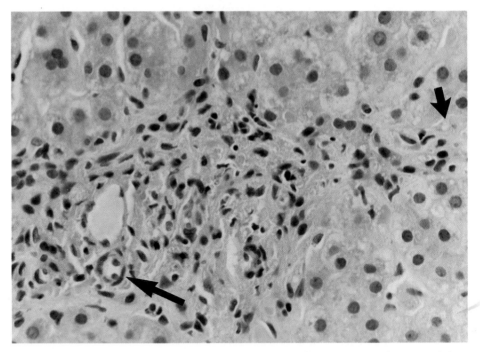

Figure 13.7. *Paucity of bile ducts in childhood.* The portal tract shows an artery (large arrow) but no corresponding bile duct of similar calibre. There is periportal cholestasis (small arrow). Needle biopsy, H & E.

accurately and probably varies from case to case. Some patients have active destruction of ducts in the first few weeks of life[22] and later stabilize, potentially with few symptoms or only mild chronic cholestasis into young adulthood. In others, cirrhosis and liver failure may develop within months or many years later.[24] It has been speculated that there may be a small subgroup of patients with non-syndromatic paucity in which cholestatic disease first presents in adulthood[24] (**"idiopathic adulthood ductopenia"**[25]).

Histologically, in both forms of intrahepatic duct paucity there is canalicular cholestasis and chronic periportal cholestasis. Portal tracts show a variable degree of fibrosis, and small bile ducts are scanty or absent[26] (Fig. 13.7). Step sections may be needed for thorough assessment of duct numbers which, as in primary biliary cirrhosis, should approximately correspond to the number of arteries of similar size. Inflammation is often slight or even absent but lymphoid aggregates may be seen in the place of bile ducts. Secondary biliary cirrhosis develops in some patients.[24,27] α_1-Antitrypsin deficiency should be looked for in all patients with paucity of ducts. Duct paucity has also been described in association with histiocytosis X.[28] As primary sclerosing cholangitis can also present in childhood,[29-31] it should be considered in the differential diagnosis.

FIBROPOLYCYSTIC DISEASES

This term covers a number of congenital abnormalities involving bile ducts, many of them related to an abnormal remodelling of the embryonic "bile duct plate".[32-34] They include congenital hepatic fibrosis, Caroli's disease (congenital dilatation of the intrahepatic bile ducts), microhamartoma (von Meyenburg complex), choledochal cyst, and both infantile and adult forms of polycystic disease. The first four of these carry an increased risk of carcinoma of the biliary tree.[35-38] The bile duct plate, first seen at

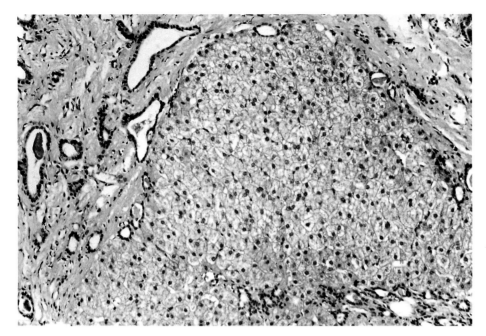

Figure 13.8. *Congenital hepatic fibrosis.* Normal parenchyma is surrounded by fibrous septa containing many epithelium-lined structures of biliary origin. Needle biopsy, H & E.

approximately 8 weeks of gestation, is a layer of primitive small cells encircling the portal tract mesenchyme (Figs 13.4 and 13.5). Progressive involution of most of these cells, with acquisition of strong cytokeratin 7 and 19 positivity in those remaining, is the process by which mature interlobular bile ducts of the portal tracts are formed.[33] Persistence of portions of the ductal plate and abnormal remodelling (the "ductal plate malformation" described by Jørgensen[18]) lead to ectatic and irregularly shaped bile ducts set in fibrous stroma, the basic histopathological features common to all fibropolycystic diseases.

Congenital Hepatic Fibrosis

This recessively inherited condition presents as hepatomegaly or the effects of portal hypertension, usually in childhood but occasionally in adults.[39] The liver is enlarged and very hard. Islands of normal liver parenchyma with unaltered vascular relationships are separated by broad and narrow septa of dense, mature fibrous tissue containing elongated or cystic spaces lined by regular biliary epithelium (Fig. 13.8). These represent cross-sections of the hollow structures comprising the ductal plate malformation. Two separate sets of duct-like structures can often be identified, one lying centrally in the septa, the other near the parenchyma. The lumens may contain inspissated bile. Portal vein branches are small and inconspicuous in some cases. There is usually no necrosis, inflammation or hepatocellular regeneration.

Congenital hepatic fibrosis must be differentiated from cirrhosis, in which there is nodular regeneration and often inflammation and necrosis, and in which the abnormal biliary channels are not seen. The shape of the parenchymal islands in congenital hepatic fibrosis is very similar to that seen in secondary biliary cirrhosis (Fig. 5.11, p. 46). In this condition the septa contain irregular, newly proliferated bile ducts rather than congenitally abnormal plates, the connective tissue of the septa is loose and inflamed, and there may be cholestatic features. Histological cholangitis, other types of inflammation or

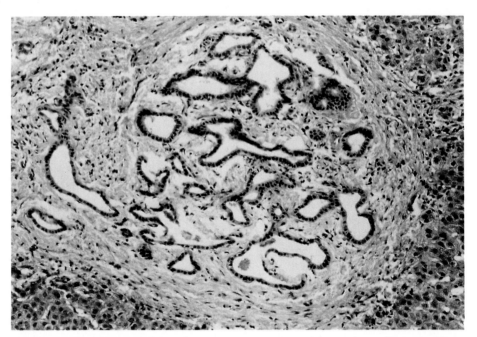

Figure 13.9. *Microhamartoma.* A cluster of duct-like structures is seen in a portal tract. Note resemblance to congenital hepatic fibrosis, shown in Figure 13.8. Wedge biopsy, H & E.

cholestasis in a liver with the characteristic features of congenital hepatic fibrosis should raise the possibility of co-existing Caroli's disease.

Caroli's Disease (Congenital Dilatation of the Intrahepatic Bile Ducts)

This cystic malformation can affect different parts of the intrahepatic biliary tree, and is seen alone or in combination with other congenital abnormalities, notably congenital hepatic fibrosis.[40] Because the cysts communicate with the rest of the biliary tree, there is a risk of ascending bacterial infection. Liver biopsy then shows the changes of cholangitis, with or without associated congenital hepatic fibrosis. The lesion of Caroli's disease must be distinguished from the acquired cholangiectases sometimes found in primary sclerosing cholangitis.[41]

Microhamartoma

Microhamartomas (von Meyenburg complexes) are rounded nodules closely related to portal tracts, containing multiple biliary channels lined by regular epithelium and set in a stroma of dense fibrous tissue (Fig. 13.9). They may be grossly visible on the liver surface as 1–2 mm white nodules. The lumens of the biliary structures sometimes contain inspissated bile. Serial sectioning shows that they are interconnected.[42] Microhamartomas are usually found incidentally and do not normally give rise to symptoms or abnormalities of liver function. They are often multiple, in which case they may very occasionally be associated with portal hypertension; distinction from congenital hepatic fibrosis is then difficult. If a small nodule on the liver surface is seen during surgery, frozen section may occasionally be requested in order to exclude metastatic carcinoma. The irregularly

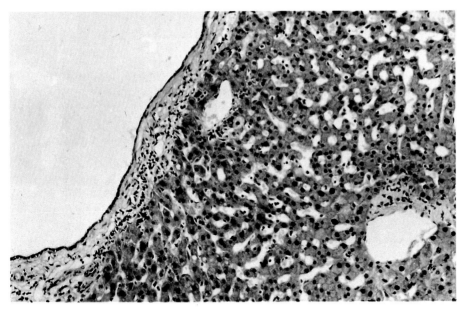

Figure 13.10. *Cystic liver.* A cyst (top left) is lined by a single layer of low cuboidal epithelium. Wedge biopsy, H & E.

dilated duct structures, inspissated bile and circumscription seen in microhamartomas are helpful in making this distinction.

Polycystic Disease

The infantile type of polycystic disease is regularly associated with renal involvement.[33,43] Portal tracts contain multiple cystic channels set in a fibrous stroma. In the adult type the cysts are lined by epithelium of biliary type (Fig. 13.10) but are not connected with the rest of the biliary tree. Solitary congenital cysts are histologically similar. The presence of microhamartomas and features of Caroli's disease in individuals with polycystic disease favours a continuum in the expression of fibropolycystic disease.[44-46]

INHERITED METABOLIC DISORDERS

Cystic Fibrosis

In this inherited disease in which abnormally viscous exocrine secretions are present in the pancreas, salivary glands, alimentary tract and lungs, the prevalence of liver disease is variable and in part age-dependent.[47-49] Subclinical liver disease may be significant.[48] Jaundice in the neonatal period has been attributed to bile-duct obstruction by abnormally viscous bile and to gastrointestinal obstruction by meconium. Intercurrent hepatitis may also be responsible. Fatty change is common, although not always related to malnutrition.[50] Paucity of intrahepatic bile ducts in cystic fibrosis has also been reported.[51] In a proportion of older children a characteristic lesion of intrahepatic bile ducts is found.[52] Dense plugs of PAS-positive material are seen within dilated, proliferated ducts (Fig. 13.11). Bile-duct cells may undergo degeneration and necrosis.[50] There is surrounding fibrosis and a variable degree of inflammatory infiltration which may be associated

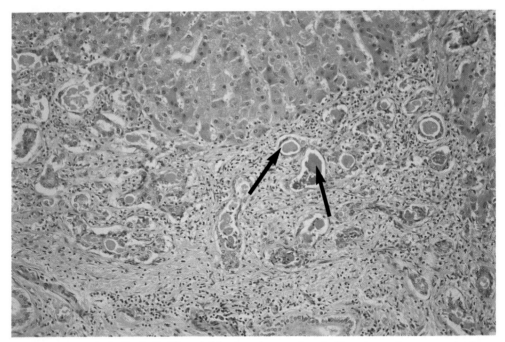

Figure 13.11. *Cystic fibrosis.* Proliferated bile ducts in an enlarged, fibrosed portal tract contain dense inspissated material (arrows). Post-mortem liver, H & E.

with abnormal intrahepatic ducts on cholangiography.[48] Eventually the fibrous areas may join, separating parenchymal islands. The term **focal biliary fibrosis** expresses the uneven involvement of the intrahepatic bile ducts in this process, with parts of the liver remaining unaffected. In some patients the disease evolves to secondary biliary cirrhosis.[52]

Storage Disorders: General Remarks

Inherited metabolic defects leading to the abnormal accumulation of lipids, proteins and carbohydrates in the liver are many and varied; for a full description of the morphological changes, recent reviews should be consulted.[53-55] Ishak[53] helpfully discusses the differential diagnosis of individual histological features. Liver biopsy is sometimes useful in diagnosis, though by no means always decisive. The following points are offered as practical suggestions for occasions when biopsy is contemplated in children suspected of having storage disorders.

1. Storage disorders can involve hepatocytes (e.g. glycogenoses, α_1-antitrypsin deficiency), macrophages (e.g. Gaucher's disease), or both (e.g. Niemann–Pick disease, cholesterol ester storage disease). When Kupffer cells are involved, they may swell to the size of hepatocytes and their involvement may not at first be apparent; the use of stains other than haematoxylin and eosin, especially PAS and trichrome stains, then usually makes the Kupffer cell involvement obvious.

2. Suspicion of a possible storage disorder is one of the few indications for electron microscopy of part of the biopsy specimen as a diagnostic procedure, because characteristic ultrastructural appearances sometimes enable a correct diagnosis to be established quickly.[56] Even when the changes are not diagnostic they can direct attention to a particular group of diseases, and suggest the next line of investigation. Arrangements for electron microscopy should be made beforehand, so that part of the specimen can be put into the correct fixative without delay (p. 298). In centres without

facilities for electron microscopy, part of the specimen should still be correctly fixed and/or embedded, and sent to a referral centre later if light microscopic findings warrant this.

3. Arrangements should also be made to freeze part of the specimen and to store it in liquid nitrogen for possible biochemical analysis and histochemical staining of frozen sections. Speed is essential to avoid loss of enzyme activity. Again, a specialist centre may need to be consulted, because few centres or pathologists have the necessary expertise to investigate the rarer metabolic diseases.

Many inherited metabolic diseases affect the liver and several may lead to **cirrhosis**[53] (glycogenosis type IV, galactosaemia, tyrosinaemia type I, α_1-antitrypsin deficiency, Wilson's disease, genetic haemochromatosis). Liver transplantation may be indicated in some patients.[57–59] The discussion in this chapter will be limited primarily to the disorders mentioned under point 1 above. Wilson's disease, to which the above remarks about electron microscopy apply equally, and haemochromatosis are described in the next chapter.

Glycogen Storage Diseases (Glycogenoses)

Most forms of glycogen storage disease involve the liver.[60] In type I glycogenosis (von Gierke's disease) fat and glycogen accumulate in the cytoplasm of hepatocytes. These appear swollen, pale-staining and sometimes vacuolated with haematoxylin and eosin, and have centrally placed nuclei (Fig. 13.12). Mallory bodies may be found in the cytoplasm.[61] The abundant glycogen displaces the organelles of affected cells to the periphery, giving them a plant cell-like appearance. Some liver-cell nuclei also contain glycogen. Sinusoids are compressed. The overall appearance has been described as a uniform mosaic pattern.[60] Liver-cell adenomas[62,63] or even, rarely, carcinomas[64] may

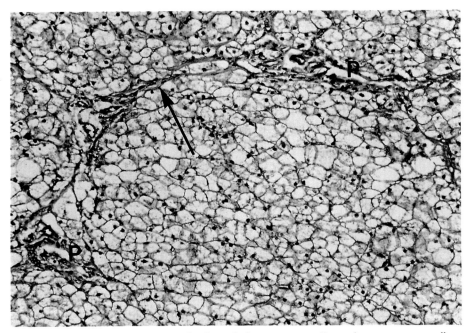

Figure 13.12. *Glycogenosis.* In this example of type I glycogen storage disease, hepatocytes are swollen and resemble plant cells. A slender septum (arrow) extends between two portal tracts (P). Wedge biopsy, H & E.

develop. Rapid fixation in buffered formal saline usually enables abundant glycogen to be demonstrated in hepatocytes in paraffin sections, but it should be noted that the diagnosis does not rest only on the demonstration of glycogen, which is plentiful in normal liver.

In type II glycogenosis (Pompe's disease), the highly soluble storage material is contained in enlarged lysosomes, visible as vacuoles in hepatocytes and Kupffer cells by light microscopy. Many other tissues are involved. Type III glycogenosis has been subdivided into several biochemical subtypes. Histological appearances are like those of type I, but fat is less abundant and there may be fibrosis or cirrhosis.[64a] Type IV (amylopectinosis) is characterized by abnormal glycogen in the form of well-defined cytoplasmic inclusions in hepatocytes.[65] The glycogen is only incompletely removed by diastase digestion. In other types of glycogenosis there is often much variation in the degree of hepatocellular swelling in different areas, in contrast to the regular distribution of the changes in type I.[60]

α_1-Antitrypsin Deficiency

Individuals with decreased levels of the serum protease inhibitor α_1-antitrypsin (α_1-antitrypsin deficiency) may present with liver disease as neonates (neonatal cholestasis), in adolescence or in adulthood, even beyond 60 years of age.[66,67] There are at least 75 different alleles of the α_1-antitrypsin (AAT) gene, two of which determine an individual's phenotype. The most common phenotype, PiMM, is associated with normal serum levels of AAT. Individuals with heterozygous (PiMZ) and homozygous deficiency (PiZZ) have moderately and profoundly reduced serum levels of AAT, respectively. The accumulation of characteristic PAS-positive, diastase-resistant globules in the hepatocytes of AAT-deficient individuals (Fig. 13.13) is based on a structural change in the glycoprotein which is encoded by the mutant Z gene.[68] An amino-acid substitution (lysine for glutamic acid at position 342) results in abnormal folding of the protein and failure of secretion from the

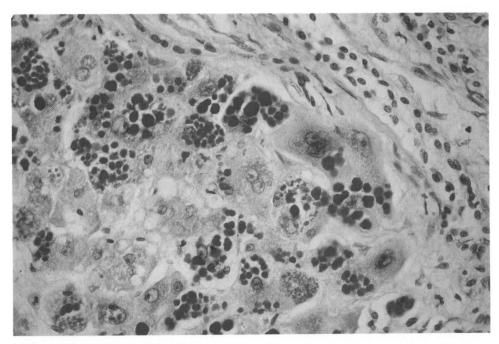

Figure 13.13. α_1-Antitrypsin deficiency. Hepatocytes near a fibrous septum contain many magenta globules of different sizes. Post-mortem liver, diastase-PAS.

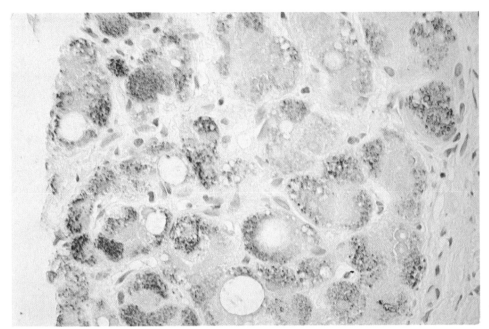

Figure 13.14. α_1-*Antitrypsin deficiency*. Periportal hepatocytes contain numerous globules of α_1-antitrypsin, stained brown by the immunoperoxidase method. Each globule typically is stained around the perimeter, with a central unstained region. Needle biopsy, specific immunoperoxidase.

endoplasmic reticulum.[68] The globules of AAT which accumulate range from less than 1 μm to 10 μm or more in diameter. They are mainly found in periportal hepatocytes, a similar distribution to the much smaller granules of copper-associated protein and haemosiderin, from which they need to be distinguished. In doubtful cases, immunohistochemical staining enables AAT to be identified with certainty (Fig. 13.14). Moreover, immunohistochemical staining is more sensitive than diastase-PAS positivity, and is helpful when diastase-PAS positive globules are scanty or unevenly distributed. Conversely, immunohistochemically positive material is found in some patients without the genetic deficiency, usually with a panacinar or perivenular rather than a periportal distribution,[69,70] and particularly in livers with sinusoidal congestion and hypoxia.[71] From a practical point of view it is wise to regard the presence of diastase-resistant PAS-positive globules in periportal liver cells as evidence for α_1-antitrypsin deficiency until proved otherwise.[72] Intracellular AAT globules have been vividly demonstrated in a transgenic mouse model of the disease.[73,73a]

A minority of children with homozygous AAT deficiency develop neonatal cholestasis. Histological changes include bile ductular proliferation and fibrosis, but the typical globules may not be seen until the age of 3 or 4 months.[74] The subsequent course varies; many children improve, while others develop a chronic cholestatic syndrome with paucity of bile ducts (p. 200) or cirrhosis.[4,75] Cirrhosis in children with AAT deficiency often has "biliary" features, such as ductular proliferation and partial preservation of acinar architecture.

Adults carrying two Z alleles present with pulmonary emphysema or liver disease, but may also be symptom-free and healthy. Liver biopsy may show little apart from the PAS-positive globules, or varying degrees of fibrosis. Cirrhosis may have developed, and is either inactive or shows features of chronic hepatitis. An increased prevalence of hepatitis B and C viral infections in AAT deficiency may contribute to this picture.[76] The characteristic globules are found predominantly in periportal or periseptal hepatocytes.

They are seen most easily in sections stained with diastase-PAS, phosphotungstic acid haematoxylin or specific immunoperoxidase, but are also seen in trichrome preparations and, when large and abundant, are faintly visible with haematoxylin and eosin. Similar globules are seen in some hepatocellular carcinomas in patients with or without the Z allele.[77,78] Furthermore, an increased risk of hepatocellular carcinoma has been reported in male patients with AAT deficiency.[79] Chronic hepatitis, cirrhosis, liver-cell dysplasia and hepatocellular carcinoma may also be seen in heterozygous (PiMZ) AAT deficiency, and in individuals with other allelic variants such as Mmalton.[80–82]

Brief mention should be made of several other endoplasmic reticulum inclusions found in hepatocytes in patients who may have chronic hepatitis or cirrhosis. Diastase-PAS-negative periportal granules of α_1-antichymotrypsin can be identified by specific immunohistochemical staining in **partial α_1-antichymotrypsin deficiency**.[83,84] In **fibrinogen storage disease** there are diastase-PAS-negative intracellular pale inclusions resembling ground-glass hepatocytes.[83]

Gaucher's Disease (Glycosyl Ceramide Lipidosis)

Cerebrosides accumulate in Kupffer cells and portal macrophages, which are enlarged, moderately diastase-PAS positive and have a finely striated appearance (Fig. 13.15). The affected cells compress hepatocytes and sinusoids, and may give rise to portal hypertension. Pericellular fibrosis is a common finding.[85]

Niemann–Pick Disease (Sphingomyelin Lipidosis)

There are several variants of this disorder, and the clinical features range from severe and fatal neurological disease in infancy to symptomless hepatosplenomegaly in adults.

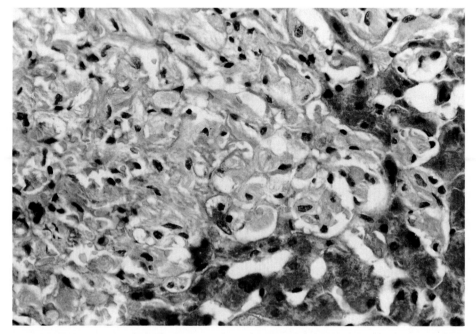

Figure 13.15. *Gaucher's disease.* Pale-staining, striated cells containing stored lipid have caused hepatocellular atrophy. Surviving hepatocytes are seen below and to the right. Wedge biopsy, H & E.

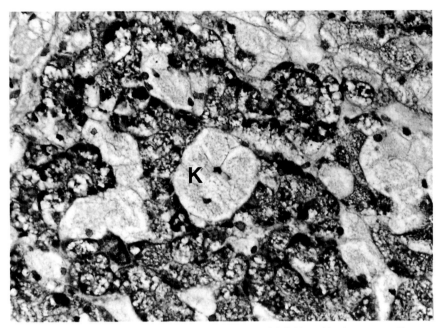

Figure 13.16. *Niemann–Pick disease.* The dark cells are glycogen-rich PAS-positive hepatocytes. Between them are large, pale-staining Kupffer cells (K) filled with lipid. Wedge biopsy, PAS.

The typical morphological feature of Niemann–Pick disease is the accumulation of sphingomyelin in both hepatocytes and macrophages. The latter are greatly swollen, foamy and diastase-PAS positive to a variable extent. They can readily be distinguished from glycogen-rich liver cells in sections stained by the PAS method (Fig. 13.16). In addition to sphingomyelin, portal phagocytes, especially in the adult form, may also contain a brown lipofuscin-like pigment; these, as well as similar cells in bone marrow, stain a sea-blue colour by the Giemsa method. Niemann–Pick disease is thus one cause of the so-called sea-blue histiocyte syndrome.[86] Type B Niemann–Pick disease may progress to cirrhosis.[59,87]

Wolman's Disease and Cholesterol Ester Storage Disease

In these apparently related conditions, the first a severe and usually fatal disease of infants, the second a milder disease of older children, cholesterol esters accumulate in hepatocytes and macrophages.[88,89] Hepatocytes also contain much triglyceride. The diagnosis may be suspected from the bright orange colour of the liver biopsy core. By light microscopy hepatocytes appear fat-laden, and macrophages are enlarged and foamy. Crystalline deposits may be seen within affected cells, particularly in frozen sections. The excess lipid is birefringent. Other features which may be found include ductular proliferation, pericellular fibrosis and even cirrhosis.[89]

Galactosaemia

Severe fatty change appears early in children with an inherited deficiency of galactose-1-phosphate uridyl transferase. Bile ductular proliferation and cholestasis may also be present. Within a few weeks, liver-cell plates become transformed into tubular, duct-like structures which dominate the histological picture, and there is siderosis and extramedullary haemopoiesis. Fibrosis and cirrhosis then develop. Institution of a galactose-free diet may result in substantial histological improvement.[90]

Histologically, the differential diagnosis includes **hereditary fructose intolerance**, in which the changes are somewhat similar but less severe. Also similar but more severe are the histological changes of **tyrosinaemia**. In this condition adenoma-like nodules are often seen, containing much fat.[53,54] Siderosis is also prominent. Hepatocellular carcinoma can develop, particularly in children over the age of 2 years, and liver transplantation is an important therapeutic option to forestall this event.[91]

REYE'S SYNDROME

This is a serious and often fatal condition of encephalopathy and fatty change in the viscera of children under the age of 18. Viral infections (influenza B or A, varicella), salicylate ingestion and endotoxaemia have been implicated in the pathogenesis.[92-94] The incidence of Reye's syndrome declined throughout the 1980s in parallel with a decrease in the use of salicylates for childhood viral illnesses. Liver biopsy is an important part of the investigation. The specimen is abnormally pale or yellow on naked-eye examination, and on light microscopy there is fine-droplet fatty change. This is panacinar in distribution and may be difficult to see without specific staining for fat because of the small size of the vacuoles (Fig. 13.17). Droplets are smaller at the periphery of acini than near portal tracts. Necrosis and inflammation are usually slight or absent, but in a few patients there is periportal ballooning or necrosis of hepatocytes.[95,96] Electron microscopy shows characteristic degenerative changes in liver-cell mitochondria; these are swollen and

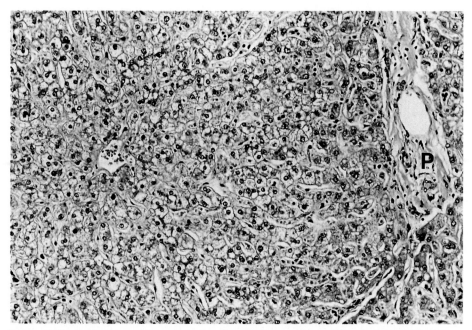

Figure 13.17. *Reye's syndrome.* Hepatocytes near the terminal hepatic venule to the left are pale because of abundant fat but vacuoles are inconspicuous. More normal hepatocytes are seen near a portal tract (P) to the right. Compare with Figure 15.27 (p. 255), showing fatty liver of pregnancy. Post-mortem liver, H & E.

irregular in shape, with flocculent, electron-lucent matrix and reduced numbers of granules.[97] Succinic dehydrogenase activity is reduced.

PARENTERAL NUTRITION

The effects of parenteral nutrition have already been discussed in Chapter 8 (p. 104— 105, 113). It is pertinent to note here that in infants **cholestasis** is the major lesion associated with parenteral nutrition;[98,99] this may occasion diagnostic difficulties when other causes of cholestasis, such as sepsis or biliary obstruction, are also under clinical consideration. These difficulties are compounded by the fact that, with prolonged administration of parenteral nutrition, the portal tracts show progressive changes which are very similar to those of bile-duct obstruction. Cohen and Olsen[100] have described bile ductular proliferation in infants who received parenteral nutrition for over 3 weeks. After 90 days several infants developed portal fibrosis, and, in one case, micronodular cirrhosis after 5 months. Correlation of biopsy features with detailed clinical information regarding the duration of parenteral nutrition is clearly paramount in establishing the cause of jaundice in this population.

CHRONIC GRANULOMATOUS DISEASE

Chronic granulomatous disease of childhood (see also p. 232) is an inherited disorder of leucocytes, which are unable to kill ingested organisms.[54] Patients are therefore susceptible to infections of different kinds. A variety of types of granulomas and microabscesses is found in the liver parenchyma. Pigmented, PAS-positive macrophages are seen in portal tracts and acini.[101] Patients may die in childhood, but the disease is occasionally found in young adults.

HYPERBILIRUBINAEMIAS

In **Gilbert's syndrome**, a common form of familial unconjugated hyperbilirubinae- mia, the liver is histologically normal by light microscopy except that small amounts of stainable iron are often seen in hepatocytes. In the **Dubin–Johnson syndrome**, in which the serum bilirubin is mainly conjugated, canalicular excretion of bilirubin and some other organic substances is defective.[102] Other constituents of bile are excreted normally and there is no cholestasis. A complex dark brown pigment accumulates in hepatocytes, especially in perivenular areas, giving the liver a dark, speckled appearance to the naked eye. The pigment granules somewhat resemble normal lipofuscin pigment and occupy a similar pericanalicular site in hepatocytes, but are darker, more abundant, larger and more variable in size (Fig. 13.18). When the pigment is very abundant, its pericanalicular location is no longer evident. Simple histochemical characteristics such as PAS-positivity and acid-fastness do not reliably distinguish between Dubin–Johnson pigment and lipofuscin because both stain variably (Table 3.1, p. 22), but the distinction is usually clear on the basis of the above morphological features. When there is doubt, this may be resolved by electron microscopy which shows the Dubin–Johnson pigment granules to be composed of characteristic strands of electron-dense material in an electron-lucent background, together with scanty lipid droplets (Fig. 17.2, p. 283).

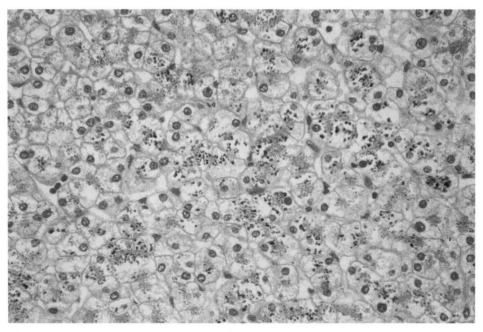

Figure 13.18. *Dubin–Johnson syndrome*. Hepatocytes contain abundant coarse, dark-brown pigment granules. Needle biopsy, H & E.

OTHER CAUSES OF CHOLESTASIS IN CHILDHOOD

In addition to the causes of neonatal and childhood cholestasis discussed earlier in this chapter, there are several congenital or familial cholestatic syndromes such as Norwegian cholestasis, North American Indian cholestasis and Byler disease.[20,103] In **Byler disease**, named after an affected Amish family, cholestasis and ductular proliferation are followed by cirrhosis, and hepatocellular carcinoma sometimes develops.[104] **Benign recurrent cholestasis** is characterized by multiple attacks of jaundice and itching, often starting in childhood or early adult life.[105] The condition is sometimes familial. Histologically, canalicular cholestasis is seen in attacks, usually unaccompanied by any substantial degree of inflammation. Between attacks the liver returns to normal and there is no fibrosis or progression to cirrhosis.

CIRRHOSIS IN CHILDHOOD

Children are susceptible to many of the causal agents affecting adults, including hepatitis virus infections. As already noted, several inherited metabolic disorders lead to cirrhosis and the possibility of Wilson's disease (p. 218) should always be considered in a child with chronic liver disease. Cirrhosis in young women should raise the question of autoimmune hepatitis, either type I (with anti-actin antibodies) or type II (anti-liver–kidney microsomal antibodies)[106] (see Chapter 9, p. 130). Rarely, familial forms of cirrhosis have been described.[107] Not infrequently, the aetiology of some forms of childhood cirrhosis is obscure as, for example, in the cerebral degenerative disorder Alpers disease.[108]

Indian childhood cirrhosis is a disease of young Indian children, with a high

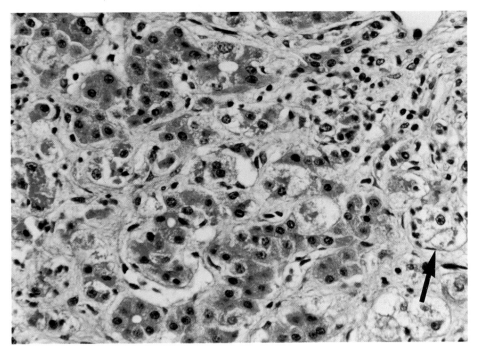

Figure 13.19. *Indian childhood cirrhosis.* Many liver cells are swollen (centre), and surrounded by fibrosis and mononuclear cells. Mallory bodies are present within some hepatocytes (arrow). Regenerating hepatocytes are organized into small clusters. Post-mortem liver, H & E.

mortality and sometimes a familial incidence.[109] Scattered cases outside the Indian subcontinent have been reported.[110–113] Genetic factors and increased dietary copper ingestion through tap water or cooking utensils appear to play an important role in the pathogenesis.[113,114] Hepatocellular swelling in early stages is followed by ballooning, Mallory body formation and necrosis. Focal accumulations of neutrophils and pericellular fibrosis are seen as in alcoholic hepatitis, but there is little or no fatty change (Fig. 13.19). Large amounts of copper and copper-associated protein accumulate in affected hepatocytes.[115,116] In some patients, tissue copper decreases after d-penicillamine therapy[114]. The small clusters of damaged hepatocytes surrounded by fibrosis eventually evolve to a cirrhosis characterized by very small nodules ("micro-micronodular cirrhosis").

REFERENCES

1. Balistreri WF. Neonatal cholestasis. *J Pediatrics* 1985; **106**: 171–184.
2. Faa G, Liguori C, Columbano A, Diaz G. Uneven copper distribution in the human newborn liver. *Hepatology* 1987; **7**: 838–842.
3. Ruchelli ED, Uri A, Dimmick JE et al. Severe perinatal liver disease and Down syndrome: an apparent relationship. *Hum Pathol* 1991; **22**: 1274–1280.
4. Hadchouel M, Gautier M. Histopathologic study of the liver in the early cholestatic phase of alpha-1-antitrypsin deficiency. *J Pediatrics* 1976; **89**: 211–215.
5. Gautier M, Eliot N. Extrahepatic biliary atresia. Morphological study of 98 biliary remnants. *Arch Pathol Lab Med* 1981; **105**: 397–402.
6. Chandra RS, Altman RP. Ductal remnants in extrahepatic biliary atresia: a histopathologic study with clinical correlation. *J Pediatrics* 1978; **93**: 196–200.
7. Gautier M, Jehan P, Odièvre M. Histologic study of biliary fibrous remnants in 48 cases of extrahepatic biliary atresia: correlation with postoperative bile flow restoration. *J Pediatrics* 1976; **89**: 704–709.
8. Haas JE. Bile duct and liver pathology in biliary atresia. *World J Surg* 1978; **2**: 561–569.

9. Kasai M, Suzuki S. A new operation for "non-correctable" biliary atresia. *Shujitsu* 1959; **13**: 173–179.
10. Logan S, Stanton A. Screening for biliary atresia. *Lancet* 1993; **342**: 256.
11. Cornelius CE, Rosenberg DP. Neonatal biliary atresia. *Am J Pathol* 1985; **118**: 168–171.
12. Schreiber RA, Kleinman RE, Barksdale EM, Maganaro TF, Donahoe PK. Rejection of murine congenic bile ducts: a model for immune-mediated bile duct disease. *Gastroenterology* 1992; **102**: 924–930.
13. Silveira TR, Salzano FM, Howard ER, Mowat AP. Congenital structural abnormalities in biliary atresia: evidence for etiopathogenic heterogeneity and therapeutic implications. *Acta Paediatr Scand* 1991; **80**: 1192–1199.
14. Fain JS, Lewin KJ. Intrahepatic biliary cysts in congenital biliary atresia. *Arch Pathol Lab Med* 1989; **113**: 1383–1386.
15. Raweily EA, Gibson AAM, Burt AD. Abnormalities of intrahepatic bile ducts in extrahepatic biliary atresia. *Histopathology* 1990; **17**: 521–527.
16. Nietgen GW, Vacanti JP, Perez-Atayde AR. Intrahepatic bile duct loss in biliary atresia despite portoenterostomy: a consequence of ongoing obstruction? *Gastroenterology* 1992; **102**: 2126–2133.
17. Alagille D. Extrahepatic biliary atresia. *Hepatology* 1984; **4**: 7S–10S.
18. Jørgensen MJ. The ductal plate malformation: a study of the intrahepatic bile-duct lesion in infantile polycystic disease and congenital hepatic fibrosis. *Acta Pathol Microbiol Scand (Suppl)* 1977; **257**: 1–88.
19. Brough AJ, Bernstein J. Conjugated hyperbilirubinemia in early infancy. A reassessment of liver biopsy. *Hum Pathol* 1974; **5**: 507–516.
20. Riely CA. Familial intrahepatic cholestatic syndromes. *Semin Liver Dis* 1987; **7**: 119–133.
21. Dahms BB, Petrelli M, Wyllie R et al. Arteriohepatic dysplasia in infancy and childhood: a longitudinal study of six patients. *Hepatology* 1982; **2**: 350–358.
22. Kahn EI, Daum F, Markowitz J et al. Arteriohepatic dysplasia. II. Hepatobiliary morphology. *Hepatology* 1983; **3**: 77–84.
23. Finegold MJ, Carpenter RJ. Obliterative cholangitis due to cytomegalovirus: a possible precursor of paucity of intrahepatic bile ducts. *Hum Pathol* 1982; **13**: 662–665.
24. Bruguera M, Llach J, Rodés J. Nonsyndromic paucity of intrahepatic bile ducts in infancy and idiopathic ductopenia in adulthood: the same syndrome? *Hepatology* 1992; **15**: 830–834.
25. Ludwig J, Wiesner RH, La Russo NF. Idiopathic adulthood ductopenia: a cause of chronic cholestatic liver disease and biliary cirrhosis. *J Hepatol* 1988; **7**: 193–199.
26. Kahn E, Daum F, Markowitz J et al. Nonsyndromatic paucity of interlobular bile ducts: light and electron microscopic evaluation of sequential liver biopsies in early childhood. *Hepatology* 1986; **6**: 890–901.
27. Heathcote J, Deodhar KP, Scheuer PJ, Sherlock S. Intrahepatic cholestasis in childhood. *N Engl J Med* 1976; **295**: 801–805.
28. Leblanc A, Hadchouel M, Jehan P, Odièvre M, Alagille D. Obstructive jaundice in children with histiocytosis X. *Gastroenterology* 1981; **80**: 134–139.
29. Johnson DA, Cattau EL, Hancock JE. Pediatric primary sclerosing cholangitis. *Dig Dis Sci* 1986; **31**: 773–777.
30. DiPalma JA, Strobel CT, Farrow JG. Primary sclerosing cholangitis associated with hyperimmunoglobulin M immunodeficiency (dysgammaglobulinemia). *Gastroenterology* 1986; **91**: 464–468.
31. el-Shabrawi M, Wilkinson ML, Portmann B, Mieli-Vergani G, Chong SK, Mowat AP. Primary sclerosing cholangitis in childhood. *Gastroenterology* 1987; **92**: 1226–1235.
32. Summerfield JA, Nagafuchi Y, Sherlock S, Cadafalch J, Scheuer PJ. Hepatobiliary fibropolycystic diseases. A clinical and histological review of 51 patients. *J Hepatol* 1986; **2**: 141–156.
33. Desmet VJ. Congenital diseases of intrahepatic bile ducts: variations on the theme "ductal plate malformation". *Hepatology* 1992; **16**: 1069–1083.
34. Desmet VJ. What is congenital hepatic fibrosis? *Histopathology* 1992; **20**: 465–477.
35. Scott J, Shousha S, Thomas HC, Sherlock S. Bile duct carcinoma: a late complication of congenital hepatic fibrosis. Case report and review of literature. *Am J Gastroenterol* 1980; **73**: 113–119.
36. Chaudhuri PK, Chaudhuri B, Schuler JJ, Nyhus LM. Carcinoma associated with congenital cystic dilation of bile ducts. *Arch Surg* 1982; **117**: 1349–1351.
37. Honda N, Cobb C, Lechago J. Bile duct carcinoma associated with multiple von Meyenburg complexes in the liver. *Hum Pathol* 1986; **17**: 1287–1290.
38. Case records of the Massachusetts General Hospital. Case 48-1988. *N Engl J Med* 1988; **319**: 1465–1474.
39. Hodgson HJF, Davies DR, Thompson RPH. Congenital hepatic fibrosis. *J Clin Pathol* 1976; **29**: 11–16.
40. Nakanuma Y, Terada T, Ohta G, Kurachi M, Matsubara F. Caroli's disease in congenital hepatic fibrosis and infantile polycystic disease. *Liver* 1982; **2**: 346–354.
41. Ludwig J, MacCarty RL, LaRusso NF, Krom RA, Wiesner RH. Intrahepatic cholangiectases and large-duct obliteration in primary sclerosing cholangitis. *Hepatology* 1986; **6**: 560–568.
42. Thommesen N. Biliary hamartomas (von Meyenburg complexes) in liver needle biopsies. *Acta Pathol Microbiol Scand A* 1978; **86**: 93–99.
43. Landing BH, Wells TR, Claireaux AE. Morphometric analysis of liver lesions in cystic diseases of childhood. *Hum Pathol* 1980; **11**: 549–560.
44. Forbes A, Murray-Lyon IM. Cystic disease of the liver and biliary tract. *Gut* 1991; Suppl: S116–S122.
45. Terada T, Nakanuma Y. Congenital biliary dilatation in autosomal dominant adult polycystic disease of the liver and kidneys. *Arch Pathol Lab Med* 1988; **112**: 1113–1116.
46. Ramos A, Torres VE, Holley KE, Offord KP, Rakela J, Ludwig J. The liver in autosomal dominant polycystic kidney disease. Implications for pathogenesis. *Arch Pathol Lab Med* 1990; **114**: 180–184.

47. Scott-Jupp R, Lama M, Tanner MS. Prevalence of liver disease in cystic fibrosis. *Arch Dis Child* 1991; **66**: 698–701.
48. Nagel RA, Westaby D, Javaid A et al. Liver disease and bileduct abnormalities in adults with cystic fibrosis. *Lancet* 1989; **ii**: 1422–1425.
49. Marino CR, Gorelick FS. Scientific advances in cystic fibrosis. *Gastroenterology* 1992; **103**: 681–693.
50. Lindblad A, Hultcrantz R, Strandvik B. Bile-duct destruction and collagen deposition: a prominent ultrastructural feature of the liver in cystic fibrosis. *Hepatology* 1992; **16**: 372–381.
51. Furuya KN, Roberts EA, Canny GJ, Phillips MJ. Neonatal hepatitis syndrome with paucity of interlobular bile ducts in cystic fibrosis. *J Ped Gastroenterol Nutr* 1991; **12**: 127–130.
52. Isenberg JI. Cystic fibrosis: its influence on the liver, biliary tree, and bile salt metabolism. *Semin Liver Dis* 1982; **4**: 302–313.
53. Ishak KG. Hepatic morphology in the inherited metabolic diseases. *Semin Liver Dis* 1986; **6**: 246–258.
54. Ishak KG, Sharp HL. Metabolic errors and liver disease. In MacSween RNM, Anthony PP, Scheuer PJ, Portmann BC, Burt AD (eds): Pathology of the Liver, 3rd edn. Edinburgh: Churchill Livingstone, 1994.
55. Portmann BC. Liver biopsy in the diagnosis of inherited metabolic disorders. In Anthony PP, MacSween RNM (eds): Recent Advances in Histopathology, Vol. 14. Edinburgh: Churchill Livingstone, 1989, pp. 139–159.
56. Phillips MJ, Poucell S, Patterson J, Valencia P. The Liver. An Atlas and Text of Ultrastructural Pathology. New York: Raven Press, 1987.
57. Whitington PF, Balistreri WF. Liver transplantation in pediatrics: indications, contraindications, and pretransplant management. *J Pediatrics* 1991; **118**: 169–177.
58. Resnick JM, Krivit W, Snover DC et al. Pathology of the liver in mucopolysaccharidosis: light and electron microscopic assessment before and after bone marrow transplantation. *Bone Marrow Transplant* 1992; **10**: 273–280.
59. Smanik EJ, Tavill AS, Jacobs GH et al. Orthotopic liver transplantation in two adults with Niemann–Pick and Gaucher's diseases: implications for the treatment of inherited metabolic disease. *Hepatology* 1993; **17**: 42–49.
60. McAdams AJ, Hug G, Bove KE. Glycogen storage disease, types I to X: criteria for morphologic diagnosis. *Hum Pathol* 1974; **5**: 463–487.
61. Itoh S, Ishida Y, Matsuo S. Mallory bodies in a patient with type Ia glycogen storage disease. *Gastroenterology* 1987; **92**: 520–523.
62. Howell RR, Stevenson RE, Ben-Menachem Y, Phyliky RL, Berry DH. Hepatic adenomata with type 1 glycogen storage disease. *JAMA* 1976; **236**: 1481–1484.
63. Coire CI, Qizilbash AH, Castelli MF. Hepatic adenomata in type Ia glycogen storage disease. *Arch Pathol Lab Med* 1987; **111**: 166–169.
64. Limmer J, Fleig WE, Leupold D, Bittner R, Ditschuneit H, Beger H-G. Hepatocellular carcinoma in type I glycogen storage disease. *Hepatology* 1988; **8**: 531–537.
64a. Markowitz AJ, Chen Y-T, Muenzer J, Del Buono EA, Lucey MR. A man with type III glycogenosis associated with cirrhosis and portal hypertension. *Gastroenterology* 1993; **105**: 1882–1885.
65. Bannayan GA, Dean WJ, Howell RR. Type IV glycogen-storage disease. Light-microscopic, electron-microscopic, and enzymatic study. *Am J Clin Pathol* 1976; **66**: 702–709.
66. Jack CIA, Evans CC. Three cases of alpha-1-antitrypsin deficiency in the elderly. *Postgrad Med J* 1991; **67**: 840–842.
67. Rakela J, Goldschmiedt M, Ludwig J. Late manifestation of chronic liver disease in adults with alpha-1-antitrypsin deficiency. *Dig Dis Sci* 1987; **32**: 1358–1362.
68. Perlmutter DH. The cellular basis for liver injury in α1-antitrypsin deficiency. *Hepatology* 1991; **13**: 172–185.
69. Callea F, Fevery J, De Groote J, Desmet VJ. Detection of Pi Z phenotype individuals by alpha-1-antitrypsin (AAT) immunohistochemistry in paraffin-embedded liver tissue specimens. *J Hepatol* 1986; **2**: 389–401.
70. Theaker JM, Fleming KA. Alpha-1-antitrypsin and the liver: a routine immunohistological screen. *J Clin Pathol* 1986; **39**: 58–62.
71. Qizilbash A, Young-Pong O. Alpha 1 antitrypsin liver disease differential diagnosis of PAS-positive, diastase-resistant globules in liver cells. *Am J Clin Pathol* 1983; **79**: 697–702.
72. Hay CR, Preston FE, Triger DR, Underwood JC. Progressive liver disease in haemophilia: an understated problem? *Lancet* 1985; **1**: 1495–1498.
73. Geller SA, Nichols WS, Dycaico MJ, Felts KA, Sorge JA. Histopathology of α1-antitrypsin liver disease in a transgenic mouse model. *Hepatology* 1990; **12**: 40–47.
73a. Geller SA, Nichols WS, Kim S et al. Hepatocarcinogenesis is the equal to hepatitis in Z 2α₁-antitrypsin transgenic mice: histopathological and DNA ploidy studies. *Hepatology* 1994; **19**: 389–397.
74. Talbot IC, Mowat AP. Liver disease in infancy: histological features and relationship to alpha-antitrypsin phenotype. *J Clin Pathol* 1975; **28**: 559–563.
75. Odièvre M, Martin JP, Hadchouel M, Alagille D. Alpha1-antitrypsin deficiency and liver disease in children: phenotypes, manifestations, and prognosis. *Pediatrics* 1976; **57**: 226–231.
76. Propst T, Propst A, Dietze O, Judmaier G, Braunsteiner H, Vogel W. High prevalence of viral infection in adults with homozygous and heterozygous alpha-1-antitrypsin deficiency and chronic liver disease. *Ann Intern Med* 1992; **117**: 641–645.

77. Palmer PE, Wolfe HJ. Alpha-antitrypsin deposition in primary hepatic carcinomas. *Arch Pathol Lab Med* 1976; **100**: 232–236.
78. Reintoft I, Hagerstrand I. Demonstration of alpha 1-antitrypsin in hepatomas. *Arch Pathol Lab Med* 1979; **103**: 495–498.
79. Eriksson S, Carlson J, Velez R. Risk of cirrhosis and primary liver cancer in alpha 1-antitrypsin deficiency. *N Engl J Med* 1986; **314**: 736–739.
80. Pittschieler K. Liver disease and heterozygous alpha-1-antitrypsin deficiency. *Acta Paediatr Scand* 1991; **80**: 323–327.
81. Marwick TH, Cooney PT, Kerlin P. Cirrhosis and hepatocellular carcinoma in a patient with heterozygous (MZ) alpha-1-antitrypsin deficiency. *Pathol* 1985; **17**: 649–652.
82. Reid CL, Wiener GJ, Cox DW, Richter JE, Geisinger KR. Diffuse hepatocellular dysplasia and carcinoma associated with the Mmalton variant of α1-antitrypsin. *Gastroenterology* 1987; **93**: 181–187.
83. Callea F, Brisigotti M, Fabbretti G, Bonino F, Desmet VJ. Hepatic endoplasmic reticulum storage diseases. *Liver* 1992; **12**: 357–362.
84. Lindmark B, Eriksson S. Partial deficiency of α1-antichymotrypsin is associated with chronic cryptogenic liver disease. *Scand J Gastroenterol* 1991; **26**: 508–512.
85. James SP, Stromeyer FW, Chang C, Barranger JA. Liver abnormalities in patients with Gaucher's disease. *Gastroenterology* 1981; **80**: 126–133.
86. Long RG, Lake BD, Pettit JE, Scheuer PJ, Sherlock S. Adult Niemann–Pick disease: its relationship to the syndrome of the sea-blue histiocyte. *Am J Med* 1977; **62**: 627–635.
87. Tassoni JP, Fawaz KA, Johnston DE. Cirrhosis and portal hypertension in a patient with adult Niemann–Pick disease. *Gastroenterology* 1991; **100**: 567–569.
88. Lake BD, Patrick AD. Wolman's disease: deficiency of E600-resistant acid esterase activity with storage of lipids in lysosomes. *J Pediatrics* 1970; **76**: 262–266.
89. Beaudet AL, Ferry GD, Nichols BL Jr, Rosenberg HS. Cholesterol ester storage disease: clinical, biochemical, and pathological studies. *J Pediatrics* 1977; **90**: 910–914.
90. Applebaum MN, Thaler MM. Reversibility of extensive liver damage in galactosemia. *Gastroenterology* 1975; **69**: 496–502.
91. Mieles LA, Esquivel COO, Van Thiel DH et al. Liver transplantation for tyrosinemia: a review of 10 cases from the University of Pittsburgh. *Dig Dis Sci* 1990; **35**: 153–157.
92. Kilpatrick-Smith L, Hale DE, Douglas SD. Progress in Reye syndrome: epidemiology, biochemical mechanisms and animal models. *Dig Dis* 1989; **7**: 135–146.
93. Lichtenstein PK, Heubi JE, Daugherty CC et al. Grade I Reye's syndrome. A frequent cause of vomiting and liver dysfunction after varicella and upper-respiratory-tract infection. *N Engl J Med* 1983; **309**: 133–139.
94. Mowat AP. Reye's syndrome: 20 years on (editorial). *Br Med J Clin Res* 1983; **286**: 1999–2001.
95. Brown RE, Ishak KG. Hepatic zonal degeneration and necrosis in Reye's syndrome. *Arch Pathol Lab Med* 1976; **100**: 123–126.
96. Kimura S, Kobayashi T, Tanaka Y, Sasaki Y. Liver histopathology in clinical Reye syndrome. *Brain Dev* 1991; **13**: 95–100.
97. Tonsgard JH. Effect of Reye's syndrome serum on the ultrastructure of isolated liver mitochondria. *Lab Invest* 1989; **60**: 568–573.
98. Balistreri WF, Bove KE. Hepatobiliary consequences of parenteral alimentation. In Popper H, Schaffner F (eds): Progress in Liver Diseases, Vol. IX. Philadelphia: WB Saunders Co., 1990, pp 567-602.
99. Quigley EMM, Marsh MN, Shaffer JL, Markin RS. Hepatobiliary complications of total parenteral nutrition. *Gastroenterology* 1993; **104**: 286–301.
100. Cohen C, Olsen MM. Pediatric total parenteral nutrition. Liver histopathology. *Arch Pathol Lab Med* 1981; **105**: 152–156.
101. Nakhleh RE, Glock M, Snover DC. Hepatic pathology of chronic granulomatous disease of childhood. *Arch Pathol Lab Med* 1992; **116**: 71–75.
102. Berthelot P, Dhumeaux D. New insights into the classification and mechanisms of hereditary, chronic, non-haemolytic hyperbilirubinaemias. *Gut* 1978; **19**: 474–480.
103. Desmet VJ. Cholestasis: extrahepatic obstruction and secondary biliary cirrhosis. In MacSween RNM, Anthony PP, Scheuer PJ, Portmann BC, Burt AD (eds): Pathology of the Liver, 3rd edn. Edinburgh: Churchill Livingstone, 1994.
104. Ugarte N, Gonzalez-Crussi F. Hepatoma in siblings with progressive familial cholestatic cirrhosis of childhood. *Am J Clin Pathol* 1981; **76**: 172–177.
105. Beaudoin M, Feldmann G, Erlinger S, Benhamou JP. Benign recurrent cholestasis. *Digestion* 1973; **9**: 49–65.
106. Johnson PJ, McFarlane IG, Eddleston ALWF. The natural course and heterogeneity of autoimmune-type chronic active hepatitis. *Semin Liver Dis* 1991; **11**: 187–196.
107. Barnett JL, Appelman HD, Moseley RH. A familial form of incomplete septal cirrhosis. *Gastroenterology* 1992; **102**: 674–678.
108. Narkewicz MR, Sokol RJ, Beckwith B, Sondheimer J, Silverman A. Liver involvement in Alpers disease. *J Pediatrics* 1991; **119**: 260–267.
109. Millward-Sadler GH. Cirrhosis. In MacSween RNM, Anthony PP, Scheuer PJ, Portmann BC, Burt AD (eds): Pathology of the Liver, 3rd edn. Edinburgh: Churchill Livingstone, 1994.
110. Klass HJ, Kelly JK, Warnes TW. Indian childhood cirrhosis in the United Kingdom. *Gut* 1980; **21**: 344–350.

111. Lefkowitch JH, Honig CL, King ME, Hagstrom JW. Hepatic copper overload and features of Indian childhood cirrhosis in an American sibship. *N Engl J Med* 1982; **307**: 271–277.
112. Müller-Höcker J, Meyer U, Wiebecke B et al. Copper storage disease of the liver and chronic dietary copper intoxication in two further German infants mimicking Indian childhood cirrhosis. *Path Res Pract* 1988; **183**: 39–45.
113. Adamson M, Reiner B, Olson JL et al. Indian childhood cirrhosis in an American child. *Gastroenterology* 1992; **102**: 1771–1777.
114. Bhusnurmath SR, Walia BNS, Singh S, Parkash D, Radotra BD, Nath R. Sequential histopathologic alterations in Indian childhood cirrhosis treated with d-penicillamine. *Hum Pathol* 1991; **22**: 653–658.
115. Popper H, Goldfischer S, Sternlieb I, Nayak NC, Madhavan TV. Cytoplasmic copper and its toxic effects. Studies in Indian childhood cirrhosis. *Lancet* 1979; **1**: 1205–1208.
116. Tanner MS, Portmann B, Mowat AP, Williams R, Pandit AN, Mills CF. Increased hepatic copper concentration in Indian childhood cirrhosis. *Lancet* 1979; **1**: 1203–1205.

GENERAL READING

Chandra RS, Stocker JT. The liver, gallbladder, and biliary tract. In Stocker JT, Dehner LP (eds): Pediatric Pathology. Philadelphia: JB Lippincott Company, 1992, pp 703–790.

Ishak KG. Hepatic morphology in the inherited metabolic diseases. *Semin Liver Dis* 1986; **6**: 246–258.

Ishak KG, Sharp HL. Developmental abnormality and liver disease in childhood. In MacSween RNM, Anthony PP, Scheuer PJ, Portmann BC, Burt AD (eds): Pathology of the Liver, 3rd edn. Edinburgh: Churchill Livingstone, 1994.

Ishak KG, Sharp HL. Metabolic errors and liver disease. In MacSween RNM, Anthony PP, Scheuer PJ, Portmann BC, Burt AD (eds): Pathology of the Liver, 3rd edn. Edinburgh: Churchill Livingstone, 1994.

Portmann BC. Liver biopsy in the diagnosis of inherited metabolic disorders. In Anthony PP, MacSween RNM (eds): Recent Advances in Histopathology, Vol. 14. Edinburgh: Churchill Livingstone, 1989, pp 139-159.

DISTURBANCES OF COPPER AND IRON METABOLISM

14

WILSON'S DISEASE (HEPATOLENTICULAR DEGENERATION)

Wilson's disease is an uncommon but important and treatable condition, inherited in an autosomal recessive manner. Liver disease develops as a result of the accumulation of copper in hepatocytes. Liver biopsy is important for histological diagnosis and monitoring.

Estimation of copper concentration in the biopsy sample helps to establish the diagnosis and is sometimes used for determination of the genetic status of a patient's siblings.[1,2] For chemical estimation the biopsy sample should be taken with a copper-free or specially washed needle. Homozygous subjects have increased liver copper levels from an early age but do not develop symptoms of liver disease in the first few years of life. Increased liver copper levels precede the development of histological abnormalities.

Histological lesions develop before the disease is clinically apparent. In the early, pre-cirrhotic phase there is fatty change,[2] sometimes with the formation of fat granulomas.[1] Slender fibrous septa extend from portal tracts (Fig. 14.1). There may be unusually abundant lipofuscin pigment in hepatocytes and glycogen vacuolation of hepatocyte nuclei, but neither feature is easy to evaluate; both are found in normal subjects, and nuclear vacuolation is particularly common in the young. Lipofuscin granules may be larger and less regular in outline than normal.[3] Inflammation is absent or mild in the early stages. Kupffer cells are sometimes enlarged and may stain for iron as a result of haemolysis. Electron microscopy helps in the diagnosis of both early and late disease because of characteristic changes in mitochondria and lysosomes (p. 286).

In some patients a phase of chronic hepatitis next develops, difficult to distinguish histologically from chronic viral hepatitis. Stains for copper and copper-associated protein may be helpful, as discussed below. Cirrhosis develops in untreated patients, with or without a recognizable preceding phase of chronic hepatitis. A common though not invariable pattern is of an active cirrhosis with fatty change, ballooned hepatocytes, focally dense eosinophilic cytoplasm and glycogen vacuolation of nuclei (Fig. 14.2). Cholestasis may be present. Hepatocytes often contain Mallory bodies and these are sometimes very abundant. They are associated with an infiltrate rich in neutrophils, as in alcoholic hepatitis (Fig. 14.3). Partial fibrous occlusion of efferent veins has been reported.[3] Hepatocellular carcinoma is a rare sequel of cirrhosis in Wilson's disease.[4,5]

Fulminant hepatic failure may be the first manifestation of Wilson's disease. In one group of 11 patients studied the livers were cirrhotic and showed evidence of recent collapse. Nodules were mostly small and separated by septa in which there were

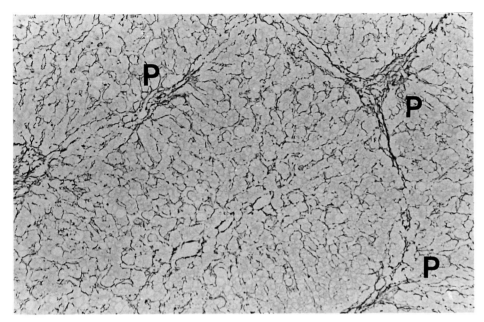

Figure 14.1. *Wilson's disease.* At this early stage slender septa extend from portal tracts (P) but acinar architecture is intact. There is steatosis, just visible in this reticulin preparation. Wedge biopsy, reticulin.

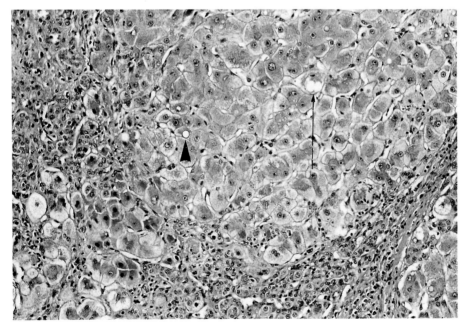

Figure 14.2. *Wilson's disease.* Active cirrhosis with liver-cell swelling, steatosis (thin arrow) and nuclear vacuolation (arrowhead). Wedge biopsy, H & E.

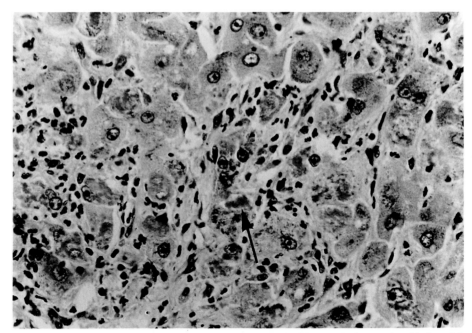

Figure 14.3. *Wilson's disease.* Mallory bodies (arrow) are seen in this severely damaged and inflamed liver. Post-mortem liver, H & E.

proliferated ductules but relatively few inflammatory cells.[6] In an earlier study, all nine patients with fulminant hepatic failure were reported to have massive hepatic necrosis, eight of them with nodular regeneration.[7] It is not clear whether the pathological findings in these two studies were similar or fundamentally different, but in either case the presence of much stainable copper and/or copper-associated protein distinguishes Wilson's disease from other causes of fulminant hepatic failure.

Staining for copper and copper-associated protein (p. 13) plays a part in the diagnosis of Wilson's disease. However, failure to stain either is common at some stages of the disease and does not therefore exclude the diagnosis. Conversely, both copper and copper-associated protein are found in other liver diseases, usually as a result of failure to secrete copper into the bile. Thus in a child with liver disease strong staining for copper might reflect loss of bile ducts rather than Wilson's disease. Other copper storage disorders have been described, including Indian childhood cirrhosis (p. 212) which is also occasionally seen in the Western world. Furthermore, neonatal liver is normally rich in copper.

In the early phases of Wilson's disease, liver copper levels are high but the copper is difficult to demonstrate histochemically. This is because it is diffusely distributed in hepatocytes and not concentrated in lysosomes. Sensitive histochemical methods (e.g. Timm's silver method or rhodanine) may show faint cytoplasmic staining. Later in the course of the disease copper begins to accumulate in liver-cell lysosomes and is then more easily stained. Once cirrhosis has developed, the distribution of copper is typically uneven, some nodules staining strongly while others are negative (Fig. 14.4). Staining for copper and copper-protein may be dissociated, although in most cases both are positive.[8,9]

Because of the great variety of histological lesions in the liver, Wilson's disease can easily be mistaken for other liver disorders. Clinicians and pathologists should consider Wilson's disease in the differential diagnosis of hepatocellular disease at all ages and especially in the young. The disease can be arrested by treatment and its development prevented in siblings. The penalties for missing the diagnosis are therefore very great.

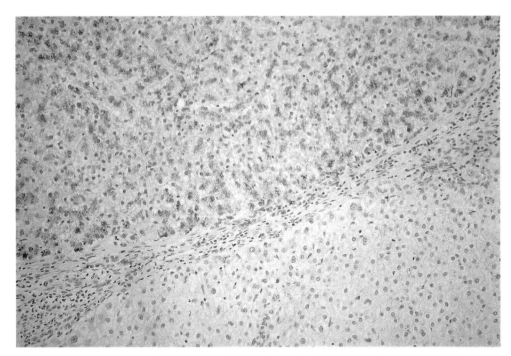

Figure 14.4. *Wilson's disease.* The upper nodule is strongly positive for copper, stained orange-red. The lower nodule is completely negative. Wedge biopsy, rhodanine.

IRON OVERLOAD

Siderosis

Siderosis (or haemosiderosis) means the presence of demonstrable iron in tissues, irrespective of cause. Its many causes include genetic haemochromatosis, haemochromatosis secondary to blood diseases such as thalassaemia, neonatal haemochromatosis, blood transfusion, haemolysis, renal transplantation and porphyria cutanea tarda. Macroregenerative nodules in cirrhotic livers may contain much iron in the absence of iron storage disease.[10] In viral hepatitis and alcoholic liver disease small amounts of stainable iron are commonly found. The reason for hepatic siderosis is not always obvious but the possibility of genetic haemochromatosis must always be considered, as discussed below.

The distribution of stainable iron among the various cell types varies according to cause.[11] In genetic and neonatal haemochromatosis the excess iron is mainly hepatocellular. In thalassaemia both hepatocytes and macrophages are positive, while exogenous iron overload leads to Kupffer cell storage in the first instance. Dense iron-positive granules are common in endothelial cells in a variety of conditions including acute hepatitis[12] and alcoholic liver disease, but their significance is not known.

The main forms of iron in hepatocytes are ferritin, haemosiderin and heme.[11] Stainable iron is mainly haemosiderin which is principally located in lysosomes and is seen as granules concentrated towards the biliary poles of the cells. Ferritin gives rise to more diffuse staining. Hepatocellular siderosis is almost always most severe in acinar zones 1, near small portal tracts, and least in zones 3.

Numerical Assessment of Tissue Iron

Many different systems have been devised for the quantification of iron in tissue sections.[13] Hepatocellular iron can be simply graded on a scale from 1 to 4, grade 1 representing minimal deposition, grade 4 massive deposits with obliteration of the usual acinar gradient, and grades 2 and 3 intermediate amounts. Examples are shown in various illustrations to this chapter. Other systems measure iron not only in hepatocytes but also in mesenchymal cells, bile duct epithelium, blood vessels and connective tissue. The comprehensive grading system of Deugnier and colleagues[14] generates a score between 0 and 60, and has proved helpful in the assessment of patients with genetic haemochromatosis. Bassett and colleagues[15] have emphasized the value of a hepatic iron index, derived by dividing the chemically measured liver iron concentration (μmol/g dry weight) by the subject's age in years; because of the progressive accumulation of iron in genetic haemochromatosis, this enables patients with the disease (who have an iron index of 1.9 or more) to be distinguished from heterozygous subjects and those with siderosis from other causes.[16] Tissue for iron measurement can be taken separately from the specimen for histology or the block deparaffinized after histological examination is complete. This has the advantage that the nature of the sample is known.[17] The chemically measured hepatic iron index has been found to correlate well with a similar index derived from histological assessment and age.[18] This avoids destruction of the blocked tissue and can be performed when chemical iron estimation is not available. Measurement of iron deposition by computerized image analysis provides a further approach to the problem, again correlating well with biochemical assay.[13]

Genetic Haemochromatosis

In this disorder iron accumulates progressively in the liver, heart, pancreas and other organs. The rate of accumulation varies even among homozygous subjects within the same family,[19] which may help to explain why the clinical disease is not seen more often; in some populations about one person in 200 is thought to be homozygous for haemochromatosis, whereas overt disease is only seen in one in 5000.[11] The disease is inherited in an autosomal recessive manner. The gene is located near the histocompatibility antigen HLA-A3 locus on the short arm of chromosome 6, and about three-quarters of homozygotes have this haplotype. Whether the fundamental biochemical defect leading to the iron overload is located in the gut or the liver has long been a matter for debate; the question has not been conclusively answered in spite of evidence from liver transplantation.[20,21]

Diagnosis rests on a combination of clinical, biochemical, genetic and histological information. The first histological abnormality is the appearance of stainable iron in periportal hepatocytes. This may be found incidentally in the course of investigation for other diseases. The unexplained presence of more than very small amounts of iron in hepatocytes should always raise the possibility of early genetic haemochromatosis. The diagnosis can then be confirmed or refuted by means of the hepatic iron index. Measurement of serum iron, iron-binding capacity and ferritin may also be helpful. Early diagnosis is most important, because cirrhosis can be prevented by appropriate treatment both in patients and in their homozygous relatives, and life expectancy returned to normal.[22] In heterozygotes, stainable liver iron is either absent or very scanty.[18]

As iron stores increase in the homozygous patient with genetic haemochromatosis, fibrosis begins to expand the portal tracts and slender septa extend from these to give a pattern of fibrosis resembling holly leaves (Fig. 14.5). The enlarged tracts contain iron-

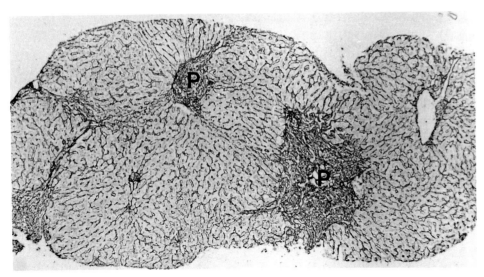

Figure 14.5. *Genetic haemochromatosis.* At this early stage of fibrosis acinar architecture is still intact and vascular relationships are maintained. The portal tracts (P) are expanded by fibrous tissue. Needle biopsy, reticulin.

rich macrophages and proliferated bile ductules, but usually show little or no inflammatory infiltration. Iron may be seen in the new ductules and in the epithelium of interlobular ducts in small amounts; larger quantities are not found until a later stage, when parenchymal siderosis is severe. It is a challenging paradox that in early haemochromatosis most of the iron is in hepatocytes but there is little or no evidence of liver-cell damage, liver-cell function remains virtually unimpaired, and the progressive lesion is portal in location. However, with increasing iron overload foci of sideronecrosis[14] are found, comprising eosinophilic or lytic necrosis of iron-laden hepatocytes, often in close association with clusters of macrophages. The ratio of non-hepatocytic to hepatocytic iron, as assessed histologically, rises progressively.

In fully developed genetic haemochromatosis the acinar gradient of iron staining is obliterated; iron in hepatocytes is now seen throughout the acini whereas earlier it is more abundant in zones 1 and 2.[14] Within individual hepatocytes the iron is seen to be deposited in pericanalicular granules, outlining the bile canalicular system (Fig. 14.6). Cirrhosis slowly develops as fibrosis and hepatocellular hyperplasia alter the normal architectural relationships. True nodule formation is, however, a late event and for a long period there is fibrosis rather than cirrhosis, with irregular islands of parenchyma demarcated by fibrous septa (Fig. 14.7). The pattern is somewhat like that of chronic biliary tract disease. At this stage some regression of fibrosis as a result of treatment remains possible. Once cirrhosis has developed, biopsy assessment of the effect of treatment on structural changes becomes more difficult because of a tendency for increasing nodule size and compression or remodelling of septa. The onset of cirrhosis marks a fall in life expectancy and an increased risk of hepatocellular carcinoma.[22] The presence of iron-free foci may represent an early stage of malignant transformation.[23] Carcinoma has been recorded in non-cirrhotic patients with genetic haemochromatosis, but is very rare.[23,24]

Effective treatment leads to a steady reduction in stainable iron. Iron encrusted onto portal collagen is usually the most resistant to removal and may be the only stainable iron remaining in the liver. Removal of iron unmasks a brown lipofuscin-like pigment in hepatocytes and connective tissue.

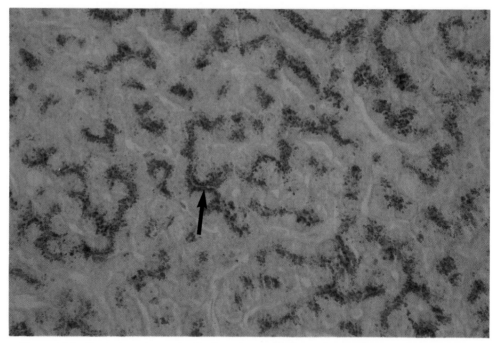

Figure 14.6. *Genetic haemochromatosis.* Grade 4 (maximal) liver-cell siderosis. Iron-rich granules in a pericanalicular location outline bile canaliculi (arrow). Needle biopsy, Perls' stain.

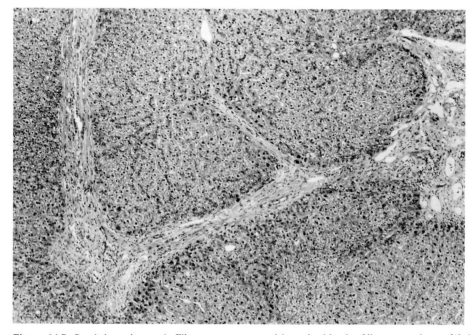

Figure 14.7. *Genetic haemochromatosis.* Fibrous septa surround irregular islands of liver parenchyma. Wedge biopsy, H & E.

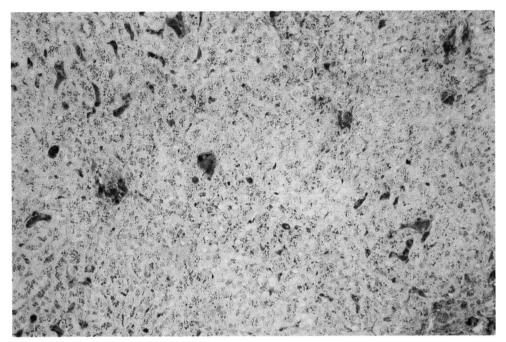

Figure 14.8. *Thalassaemia*. In this example of secondary haemochromatosis hepatocytes show grade 3 siderosis. The darker clumps are iron-laden macrophages. Needle biopsy, Perls' stain.

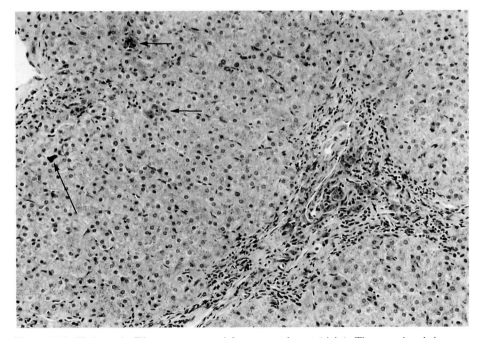

Figure 14.9. *Thalassaemia*. Fibrous septa extend from a portal tract (right). There are iron-laden macrophages in portal tract and acini (short arrows). The long arrow marks a megakaryocyte in a sinusoid. The portal inflammation is probably due to transfusion-transmitted hepatitis C. Needle biopsy, H & E.

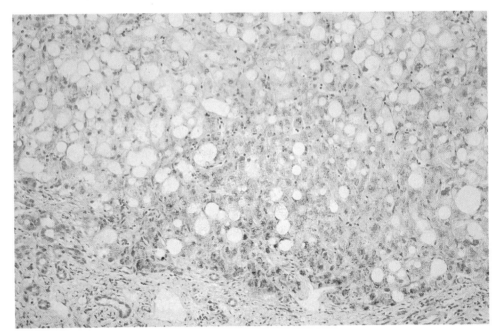

Figure 14.10. *Cirrhosis with siderosis.* In this fatty cirrhosis in an alcohol abuser there is grade 2 hepatocellular siderosis, the cause of which needs investigation. Needle biopsy, Perls' stain.

Neonatal (Perinatal) Haemochromatosis

This is characterized by extensive hepatocellular necrosis, giant-cell formation, siderosis, fibrosis and nodule formation in fetal life and the perinatal period.[25–27] Whether the disease is an aetiological entity or represents a reaction to a variety of agents remains uncertain.[28] Intrauterine infection has been suggested as a possible cause,[29] but an inherited defect has not been excluded. Siderosis is a common finding in pathological livers of neonates and may not itself be responsible for the liver damage in neonatal haemochromatosis.[29a]

Secondary Haemochromatosis

Secondary haemochromatosis is found in patients with thalassaemia and, less commonly, other haematological disorders. The iron overload is partly the result of blood transfusion. In addition to the hepatocytic siderosis, portal fibrosis and septum formation seen in genetic haemochromatosis, there is iron in macrophages from an early stage (Fig. 14.8) and haemopoietic cells may be present. There is often more infiltration of portal tracts, septa and sinusoids by lymphocytes than in genetic haemochromatosis (Fig. 14.9). This, together with focal hepatocellular damage, is attributable to transfusion-related hepatitis, now most commonly type C.[30,31] The pattern of fibrosis and degree of inflammation in a liver biopsy often help to determine the relative roles of iron overload and hepatitis C in the progression of the disease.

Siderosis and Liver Disease of Varied Aetiology

As already stated, unexpected iron overload may be an indication that the patient has genetic haemochromatosis. The presence of disease of other aetiology does not exclude this diagnosis. In chronic hepatitis, serum iron and ferritin are sometimes increased as a result of release of iron from damaged hepatocytes, and iron may be seen on liver biopsy; calculation of the hepatic iron index is then helpful for the distinction between simple siderosis and concomitant genetic haemochromatosis.[32] In alcoholic liver disease, histological siderosis presents a similar problem (Fig. 14.10). In patients with genetic haemochromatosis together with another cause for liver disease such as alcohol abuse[33] or chronic viral hepatitis,[34] progression of liver disease is accelerated.

REFERENCES

1. Scheinberg IH, Sternlieb I. Wilson's disease. Major Problems in Internal Medicine XXIII. Philadelphia: WB Saunders, 1984.
2. Walshe JM. Diagnosis and treatment of presymptomatic Wilson's disease. *Lancet* 1988; **ii**: 435–437.
3. Stromeyer FW, Ishak KG. Histology of the liver in Wilson's disease: a study of 34 cases. *Am J Clin Pathol* 1980; **73**: 12–24.
4. Polio J, Enriquez RE, Chow A, Wood WM, Atterbury CE. Hepatocellular carcinoma in Wilson's disease. Case report and review of the literature. *J Clin Gastroenterol* 1989; **11**: 220–224.
5. Cheng WSC, Govindarajan S, Redeker AG. Hepatocellular carcinoma in a case of Wilson's disease. *Liver* 1992; **12**: 42–45.
6. Davies SE, Williams R, Portmann B. Hepatic morphology and histochemistry of Wilson's disease presenting as fulminant hepatic failure: a study of 11 cases. *Histopathology* 1989; **15**: 385–394.
7. McCullough AJ, Fleming CR, Thistle JL et al. Diagnosis of Wilson's disease presenting as fulminant hepatic failure. *Gastroenterology* 1983; **84**: 161–167.
8. Elmes ME, Clarkson JP, Mahy NJ, Jasani B. Metallothionein and copper in liver disease with copper retention – a histopathological study. *J Pathol* 1989; **158**: 131–137.
9. Mulder TPJ, Janssens AR, Verspaget HW, van Hattum J, Lamers CBHW. Metallothionein concentration in the liver of patients with Wilson's disease, primary biliary cirrhosis, and liver metastasis of colorectal cancer. *J Hepatol* 1992; **16**: 346–350.
10. Terada T, Nakanuma Y. Survey of iron-accumulative macroregenerative nodules in cirrhotic livers. *Hepatology* 1989; **10**: 851–854.
11. Tavill AS, Sharma BK, Bacon BR. Iron and the liver: genetic hemochromatosis and other hepatic iron overload disorders. In Popper H, Schaffner F (eds): Progress in Liver Diseases, Vol. IX. Philadelphia: WB Saunders, 1990, pp 281–305.
12. Bardadin KA, Scheuer PJ. Endothelial cell changes in acute hepatitis. A light and electron microscopic study. *J Pathol* 1984; **144**: 213–220.
13. Olynyk J, Hall P, Sallie R, Reed W, Shilkin K, Mackinnon M. Computerized measurement of iron in liver biopsies: a comparison with biochemical iron measurement. *Hepatology* 1990; **12**: 26–30.
14. Deugnier YM, Loréal O, Turlin B et al. Liver pathology in genetic hemochromatosis: a review of 135 homozygous cases and their bioclinical correlations. *Gastroenterology* 1992; **102**: 2050–2059.
15. Bassett ML, Halliday JW, Powell LW. Value of hepatic iron measurements in early hemochromatosis and determination of the critical iron level associated with fibrosis. *Hepatology* 1986; **6**: 24–29.
16. Sallie RW, Reed WD, Shilkin KB. Confirmation of the efficacy of hepatic tissue iron index in differentiating genetic haemochromatosis from alcoholic liver disease complicated by alcoholic haemosiderosis. *Gut* 1991; **32**: 207–210.
17. Ludwig J, Batts KP, Moyer TP, Baldus WP, Fairbanks VF. Liver biopsy diagnosis of homozygous hemochromatosis: a diagnostic algorithm. *Mayo Clin Proc* 1993; **68**: 263–267.
18. Deugnier YM, Turlin B, Powell LW et al. Differentiation between heterozygotes and homozygotes in genetic hemochromatosis by means of a histological hepatic iron index: a study of 192 cases. *Hepatology* 1993; **17**: 30–34.
19. Adams PC. Intrafamilial variation in hereditary hemochromatosis. *Dig Dis Sci* 1992; **37**: 361–363.
20. Powell LW. Does transplantation of the liver cure genetic hemochromatosis? *J Hepatol* 1992; **16**: 259–261.
21. Dabkowski PL, Angus PW, Smallwood RA, Ireton J, Jones RM. Site of principal metabolic defect in idiopathic haemochromatosis: insights from transplantation of an affected organ. *Br Med J* 1993; **306**: 1726.
22. Niederau C, Fischer R, Sonnenberg A, Stremmel W, Trampisch HJ, Strohmeyer G. Survival and causes of death in cirrhotic and in noncirrhotic patients with primary hemochromatosis. *N Engl J Med* 1985; **313**: 1256–1262.
23. Deugnier YM, Guyader D, Crantock L et al. Primary liver cancer in genetic hemochromatosis: a clinical, pathological, and pathogenetic study of 54 cases. *Gastroenterology* 1993; **104**: 228–234.
24. Fellows IW, Stewart M, Jeffcoate WJ, Smith PG, Toghill PJ. Hepatocellular carcinoma in primary haemochromatosis in the absence of cirrhosis. *Gut* 1988; **29**: 1603–1606.
25. Goldfischer S, Grotsky HW, Chang CH. Idiopathic neonatal iron storage involving the liver, pancreas, heart and endocrine and exocrine glands. *Hepatology* 1981; **1**: 58–64.
26. Blisard KS, Bartow SA. Neonatal hemochromatosis. *Hum Pathol* 1986; **17**: 376–383.

27. Moerman P, Pauwels P, Vandenberghe K et al. Neonatal haemochromatosis. *Histopathology* 1990; **17**: 345–351.

28. Witzleben CL, Uri A. Perinatal hemochromatosis: entity or end result? *Hum Pathol* 1989; **20**: 335–340.

29. Kershisnik MM, Knisely AS, Sun C-CJ, Andrews JM, Wittwer CT. Cytomegalovirus infection, fetal liver disease, and neonatal hemochromatosis. *Hum Pathol* 1992; **23**: 1075–1080.

29a. Silver MM, Valberg LS, Cutz E, Lines LD, Phillips MJ. Hepatic morphology and iron quantitation in perinatal hemochromatosis. Comparison with a large perinatal control population including cases with chronic liver disease. *Am J Pathol* 1993; **143**: 1312–1325.

30. Wonke B, Hoffbrand AV, Brown D, Dusheiko G. Antibody to hepatitis C virus in multiply transfused patients with thalassaemia major. *J Clin Pathol* 1990; **43**: 638–640.

31. Donohue SM, Wonke B, Hoffbrand AV et al. Alpha interferon in the treatment of chronic hepatitis C infection in thalassaemia major. *Br J Haematol* 1993; **83**: 491–497.

32. Di Bisceglie AM, Axiotis CA, Hoofnagle JH, Bacon BR. Measurements of iron status in patients with chronic hepatitis. *Gastroenterology* 1992; **102**: 2108–2113.

33. Loréal O, Deugnier Y, Moirand R et al. Liver fibrosis in genetic hemochromatosis. Respective roles of iron and non-iron-related factors in 127 homozygous patients. *J Hepatol* 1992; **16**: 122–127.

34. Piperno A, Fargion S, D'Alba R et al. Liver damage in Italian patients with hereditary hemochromatosis is highly influenced by hepatitis B and C virus infection. *J Hepatol* 1992; **16**: 364–368.

GENERAL READING

Copper

Brewer GJ, Yuzbasiyan-Gurkan V. Wilson disease. *Medicine* 1992; **71**: 139–164.

Sternlieb I. Perspectives on Wilson's disease. *Hepatology* 1990; **12**: 1234–1239.

Sternlieb I. The outlook for the diagnosis of Wilson's disease. *J Hepatol* 1993; **17**: 263–264.

Yarze JC, Martin P, Muñoz SJ, Friedman LS. Wilson's disease: current status. *Am J Med* 1992; **92**: 643–654.

Iron

Iancu TC. Ultrastructural pathology of iron overload. *Baillières Clin Haematol* 1989; **2**: 475-495.

Powell LW. Does transplantation of the liver cure genetic hemochromatosis? *J Hepatol* 1992; **16**: 259–261.

Searle J, Kerr JFR, Halliday JW, Powell LW. Iron storage disease. In MacSween RNM, Anthony PP, Scheuer PJ, Portmann B, Burt AD (eds): Pathology of the Liver, 3rd edn. Edinburgh: Churchill Livingstone, 1994.

Stål P, Glaumann H, Hultcrantz R. Liver cell damage and lysosomal iron storage in patients with idiopathic hemochromatosis. A light and electron microscopic study. *J Hepatol* 1990; **11**: 172–180.

Tavill AS, Sharma BK, Bacon BR. Iron and the liver: genetic hemochromatosis and other hepatic iron overload disorders. In Popper H, Schaffner F (eds): Progress in Liver Diseases, Vol. IX. Philadelphia: WB Saunders, 1990, pp 281–305.

15

THE LIVER IN SYSTEMIC DISEASE AND PREGNANCY

Liver biopsies are often obtained to evaluate abnormalities of liver function tests in patients with known or suspected systemic disease and in the investigation of pyrexia of unknown origin. In the latter, liver biopsy provides diagnostic information in approximately 15–30% of cases.[1] The hepatic changes associated with systemic diseases vary from obvious granulomas or steatosis (discussed in Chapter 7) to more subtle findings such as an increase in liver-cell mitoses. The pathologist will want to know, whenever possible, whether or not the biopsy changes are specific for a systemic disease. For example, when granulomas are present, their aetiology usually has important therapeutic implications. Liver biopsy in patients with acquired immune deficiency syndrome may demonstrate hepatic involvement by a microorganism already identified elsewhere in the patient, or may disclose a new diagnosis such as lymphoma. Liver biopsy also provides tissue for culture and special stains. This chapter examines the pathology of hepatic granulomas, hepatic changes in a variety of infectious diseases, and liver involvement in gastrointestinal and haemopoietic diseases and the porphyrias.

In the unusual situation where liver dysfunction is found in pregnancy, the histopathologist may be called upon to differentiate intercurrent conditions such as viral hepatitis from several varieties of liver disease unique to pregnancy. This differential diagnosis is discussed in the latter portion of this chapter.

GRANULOMAS

There are many causes of hepatic granulomas, including local irritants, infections, infestations and hypersensitivity to drugs. The constituents of these lesions, depending on the aetiology, include large epithelioid cells, multinucleated giant cells, varied numbers of mononuclear cells and eosinophils. The causes, which vary in frequency from one country to another, greatly outnumber morphological points of distinction, so that it is often impossible to reach an aetiological diagnosis on histological criteria alone. Sometimes culture of part of the biopsy specimen yields a causal organism. The cause of hepatic granulomas may remain unknown in 15–36% of cases.[2] From a practical point of view biopsies containing granulomas fall into one of four groups:

1. The cause of the granuloma is seen under the microscope. Examples are the granulomas around schistosome ova, and the mineral oil lipogranulomas found in portal tracts or near terminal hepatic venules (p. 82).

Table 15.1. Histological Features of Hepatic Granulomas

Aetiology	Favoured site(s)	Special Features
Sarcoidosis	Portal/periportal	Clustering Hyalinization Inclusions in giant cells May destroy bile ducts
Tuberculosis	None	Necrosis
PBC	Portal	Near damaged bile duct Acinar granulomas uncommon
Drug	None	Eosinophils Other lesions often present (hepatitis, fat, cholestasis)
Mineral oil	Portal, perivenous	Oil vacuoles
Q fever, CMV, Allopurinol, etc.	None	Fibrin-ring granuloma
CGDC*	None	Brown pigment in macrophages; may be necrotizing

* Chronic granulomatous disease of childhood.

2. The cause is not seen, but other histological features and clinical circumstances make the diagnosis clear. For example, granulomas near damaged bile ducts in a patient with clinically and immunologically typical primary biliary cirrhosis are almost certainly due to this disease.

3. The cause is uncertain but appearances favour one particular line of further investigation rather than another. For instance, sarcoidosis should be suspected when clusters of large granulomas with prominent epithelioid cells, large multinucleated giant cells and dense fibrosis are found in portal tracts.

4. The cause of the granulomas cannot be determined from the histological appearances. This is unfortunately common, and the help that the pathologist can then give to the clinician is limited.

These four circumstances can be summarized as **see the cause**, **know the cause**, **suspect the cause** and **don't know the cause**. Some of the histological guidelines for evaluating granulomas are shown in Table 15.1.

Granulomas are found in up to 10% of liver biopsies.[3,4] They may be sparse and suspicion of granulomatous disease is an indication for examining step sections from different levels of a paraffin block, if no lesions are seen initially. Because identifiable granulomas are generally more than 50 μm in diameter, serial sections 5 μm thick are unnecessary unless a single granuloma is to be further investigated.

Granulomas are commonly found in the liver in **sarcoidosis**. The liver is usually one of several organs involved, but occasionally extrahepatic lesions are difficult to demonstrate and chest X-ray may be normal.[5] Liver biopsy is helpful for diagnosis, especially in patients with fever and arthralgia.[6] The lesions may be found both in portal tracts and in acini, and consist of well-defined rounded granulomas with variable infiltration by inflammatory cells including plasma cells and eosinophils (Figs. 15.1 and 15.2). The granulomas contain reticulin fibres (Fig. 15.3). Multinucleated giant cells may contain inclusions of different types. Central necrosis is quite common but never as extensive as in tuberculosis. The granulomas often cluster in portal and periportal regions[7] (Fig. 15.1) and older lesions show dense hyalinized collagen. The fibrosis may extend to interfere with normal acinar structure. A surprising degree of reactive portal and acinar inflammation may occasionally be seen in association with sarcoid granulomas, raising the question of concomitant hepatitis.[7a] The acinar component consists predominantly of hyperplastic Kupffer cells; acidophil bodies are rare. The portal tracts show considerable variability in the amount of lymphocytic inflammation and the most active portal inflammation is usually near granulomas. Serological tests for viral hepatitis should be obtained if there is

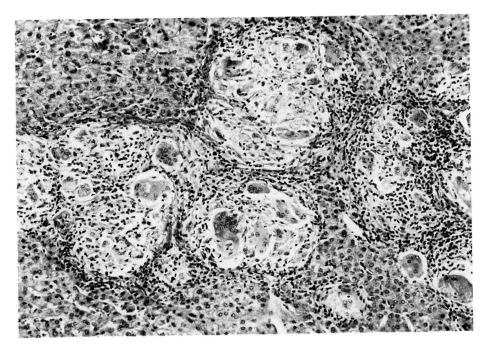

Figure 15.1. *Sarcoidosis*. A cluster of epithelioid-cell granulomas with giant cells has expanded a portal tract. Wedge biopsy, H & E.

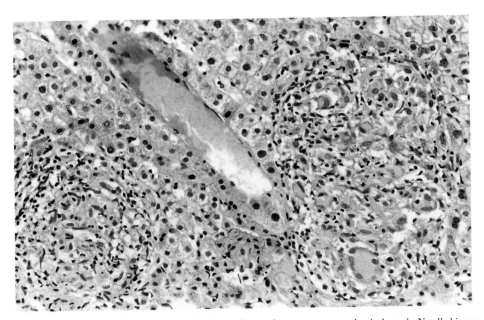

Figure 15.2. *Sarcoidosis*. There are two epithelioid-cell granulomas near a portal-vein branch. Needle biopsy, H & E.

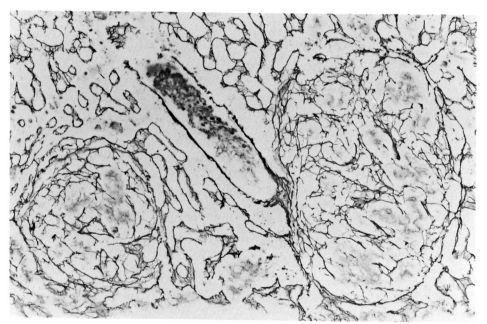

Figure 15.3. *Sarcoidosis.* The same field as in Figure 15.2. The granulomas contain strands of reticulin. Needle biopsy, reticulin.

serious diagnostic concern. A few patients with sarcoidosis develop portal hypertension with or without cirrhosis.[8,9] Another rare complication of sarcoidosis is a primary biliary cirrhosis-like lesion, with destruction of bile ducts and a clinical picture of chronic cholestasis.[10] It should be noted that a diagnosis of sarcoidosis cannot be proved by histological examination of the liver alone because very similar lesions are found in other granulomatous diseases.

In **chronic granulomatous disease of childhood** defective neutrophil leucocyte function leads to the development of infective granulomas of different sizes, containing homogeneous eosinophilic material, necrotic debris or pus. Portal tracts are inflamed and there may be fibrosis. A brown pigment of ceroid type accumulates in portal macrophages and to a lesser extent in Kupffer cells.[11–13] The disease is sometimes first diagnosed in adult life.[14]

Drugs and toxins should be considered in the evaluation of hepatic granulomas (see Chapter 8), particularly if eosinophils are prominent.[15] A diverse array of particulate materials may cause granulomas, including aluminium[16] and silicone.[17] Biopsies with granulomas should therefore be examined under polarized light for evidence of particulate material. Dense reactive fibrosis may develop in the form of **sclerohyaline nodules** in individuals exposed in the workplace or by intravenous drug abuse to silica, chromium, cobalt and magnesium.[18]

The **fibrin-ring granuloma** is a distinctive, though non-specific, form described in Q fever,[19–23] Hodgkin's disease,[24] allopurinol hypersensitivity,[25] cytomegalovirus[26] and Epstein–Barr virus infections,[27] leishmaniasis,[28] toxoplasmosis,[24] hepatitis A,[29,30] giant-cell arteritis,[30a] and systemic lupus erythematosis.[31] This granuloma is composed of a fat vacuole surrounded by a ring of fibrin, epithelioid cells, giant cells and neutrophils (Fig. 15.4). Serial sections may be needed to demonstrate the typical fibrin-ring or "doughnut" lesion.[20]

Simon and Wolff[32] have described a syndrome characterized by fever, constitutional symptoms and hepatic granulomas, not responding to anti-tuberculous drugs but

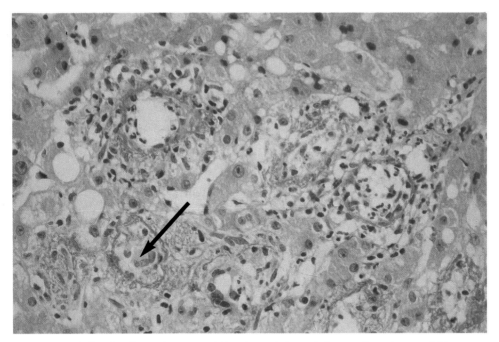

Figure 15.4. *Q fever*. Small granulomas containing giant cells (arrow), fat vacuoles and neutrophil leucocytes are surrounded by rings of fibrin, stained red. Needle biopsy, MSB.

improving on corticosteroid therapy. In some patients the syndrome resolves spontaneously without treatment.[33] The cause has not been established.

VIRAL DISEASES

The pathological changes in the liver resulting from virus infections other than hepatitis viruses have been reviewed by Lucas.[34] The viral haemorrhagic fevers, such as mosquito-borne **Flavivirus** infection (**Dengue fever**[35]) and rodent-borne **Hantavirus** infections,[36] are characterized by midzonal or more extensive hepatic necrosis. In **yellow fever**, acidophil bodies are typically abundant; they were first described in this disease by Councilman in the last century.[37]

Several viruses not normally associated with liver disease can occasionally cause liver damage. Examples include **herpes simplex virus** infection leading to irregular and randomly distributed areas of coagulative necrosis[38,39] and **adenovirus** infection.[40,41] In both infections, virus particles or antigens can be identified in hepatocytes. **Paramyxovirus**-like particles have been associated with **syncytial giant-cell hepatitis** in adults,[42] a lesion that may also be seen in autoimmune hepatitis and other liver diseases.[43,44]

Cytomegalovirus Infection

Cytomegalovirus (CMV) has been implicated in some children with neonatal hepatitis (p. 195). Histological features include giant-cell formation as in other forms of neonatal liver damage, inflammation and cholestasis. Bile ducts are damaged and may be destroyed.[45] CMV genome can be identified by polymerase chain reaction in many cases.[46]

In later life CMV infection can present as a mononucleosis-like illness but also as a

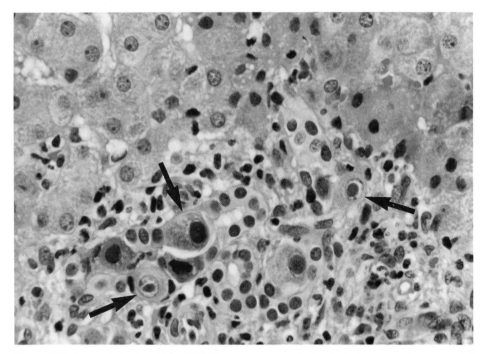

Figure 15.5. *Cytomegalovirus hepatitis in AIDS.* Numerous cytomegalovirus inclusions (arrows) are seen within bile duct epithelial cells. Needle biopsy, H & E.

hepatitis. Asymptomatic infection is common in immunocompromised patients. In these, the histological changes are often mild but typical CMV inclusions are found in hepatocytes, bile duct epithelium and endothelial cells (Fig. 15.5). Specific immunocyto-chemical staining reveals CMV antigens even in cells without inclusions,[47] but sometimes with an abnormal granular basophilic cytoplasm.[48] Patients with CMV infection may also show aggregation of neutrophils in sinusoids, with or without evidence of CMV in neighbouring cells,[48] an important diagnostic consideration in immunocompromised patients or individuals who have received organ transplants. Larger accumulations of macrophages and lymphocytes can be seen and epithelioid-cell granulomas have been reported.[49] In immunocompetent patients, there are varying degrees of focal liver-cell and bile-duct damage, portal inflammation, infiltration of sinusoids with lymphoid cells and increased mitoses in hepatocytes.[50] In such patients, it may not be possible to demonstrate CMV inclusions or antigen, a situation possibly analogous to hepatitis B virus infection where inclusions and antigen may be scanty or absent during the acute attack while characteristic of the carrier state.[50]

Infectious Mononucleosis

The liver is histologically abnormal in infectious mononucleosis even when there is no clinical jaundice.[51] Dense accumulations of atypical lymphocytes are found in portal tracts and sinusoids (Fig. 15.6). Sinusoidal aggregates must be distinguished from the more heterogeneous collections of cells found in extramedullary haemopoiesis. The infiltration also mimics that of leukaemia. Kupffer cells are enlarged. Epithelioid-cell granulomas are occasionally present.[4] Small foci of hepatocellular necrosis and acidophil bodies may be seen, but the diffuse hepatocellular damage characteristic of viral hepatitis is usually absent and extensive necrosis[52] is rare. Cholestasis is absent or mild.

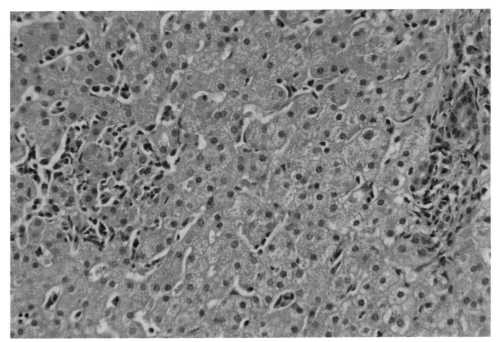

Figure 15.6. *Infectious mononucleosis.* At left, a prominent sinusoidal "beads-on-a-string" pattern is seen, consisting of atypical lymphocytes and hyperplastic Kupffer cells. Atypical lymphocytes are also present in the portal tract at right. Needle biopsy, H & E.

Acquired Immune Deficiency Syndrome (AIDS)

Liver involvement in AIDS is chiefly by opportunistic infections, lymphoma and Kaposi's sarcoma which develop as a consequence of the immune deficiency.[53-60] The most likely hepatic targets for direct infection by human immunodeficiency virus type 1 (HIV-1) are Kupffer cells and sinusoidal endothelial cells.[61-63,63a] There are no specific hepatic lesions due to HIV-1, however, and identification of the virus rests with immunohistochemistry, *in situ* hybridization, or polymerase chain reaction.

Liver biopsy is an important diagnostic tool in patients with HIV infection or AIDS who have abnormal liver function tests. Specimens should routinely be studied with acid-fast and silver stains for detection of high-incidence pathogens such as mycobacteria and fungi. Other methods such as Gram stain or Warthin–Starry stain can be applied, depending on the clinical and histological indications. A portion of the biopsy should be sent for culture.

Opportunistic infections and infestations involving the liver and bile ducts in AIDS include *Mycobacterium avium-intracellulare* and *Mycobacterium tuberculosis* infection, cytomegalovirus infection, cryptococcosis, candidiasis, histoplasmosis, malaria, crypto-sporidiosis,[64] and microsporidiosis.[65-67] *Pneumocystis carinii* may disseminate to the liver, producing acellular exudative masses which closely resemble the pulmonary alveolar exudates.[68] **Lymphomas** involve the liver as nodular masses or portal tract infiltrates (see Chapter 7, Fig. 7.3) and are high-grade large-cell, immunoblastic and Burkitt types.[69,70]

There are several distinctive histopathological presentations of liver involvement, including infiltration by **granulomas**, a **sclerosing cholangitis-like syndrome (AIDS cholangiopathy)** due to several microorganisms which infect the biliary tree, and **peliosis hepatis. Fatty change** is common and is frequently periportal (see Chapter 7, Fig. 7.3). **Siderosis** of Kupffer cells is related to transfusion or viraemia-associated erythrophagocytosis. In some cases, **non-specific changes** consisting of sparse portal or

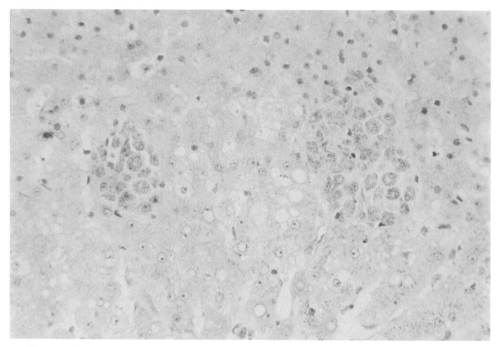

Figure 15.7. *Mycobacterium avium-intracellulare in AIDS.* Several granulomas are filled with abundant red-staining mycobacteria. Needle biopsy, Ziehl–Neelsen.

acinar lymphocytic inflammation with scattered acidophil bodies are seen, with no apparent aetiology.

One of the most frequently encountered hepatic lesions in AIDS is the presence of numerous granulomas containing *Mycobacterium avium-intracellulare* (MAI), readily demonstrated by staining with diastase-PAS or the Ziehl–Neelsen method[71–74] (Fig. 15.7). Each granuloma consists of foamy histiocytes with few lymphocytes. The histiocytes often show a striated appearance on haematoxylin and eosin stain due to the abundant packing of organisms in each cell. MAI organisms are also well stained with Gomori methenamine silver. For screening of liver biopsies, particularly for *Mycobacterium tuberculosis* which may be present in fewer numbers than MAI, the auramine-rhodamine fluorescent method[75,76] gives excellent results (Fig. 15.8). Careful examination of special stains is of particular importance as some AIDS patients have mycobacterial infection without typical granuloma formation; scant, single mycobacteria may be present within sinusoids or portal tracts.

AIDS cholangiopathy resembles sclerosing cholangitis clinically and radiographically and is due to infections of the large bile ducts by several possible pathogens, including CMV, cryptosporidia and microsporidia.[65–67,77–79] Liver biopsy changes are those of large duct obstruction. Cryptosporidia and microsporidia are best identified in aspirates obtained at endoscopy, duodenal biopsies, or post-mortem tissue samples of the major bile ducts.[65–67]

Peliosis hepatis[73,80,81] in AIDS has been postulated to be due to endothelial damage by HIV-1 infection.[63] Alternatively, **bacillary peliosis hepatis** may develop as a consequence of hepatic infection by rickettsial organisms *Rochalimaea henselae* and *Rochalimaea quintana*.[82–84] Smudge-like or granular pink-to-purple material associated with a myxoid stroma is seen within dilated vascular spaces (Fig. 15.9) and Warthin–Starry stain shows clumped bacilli in these areas.

AIDS patients have many of the same risk factors for infection by hepatitis viruses, and

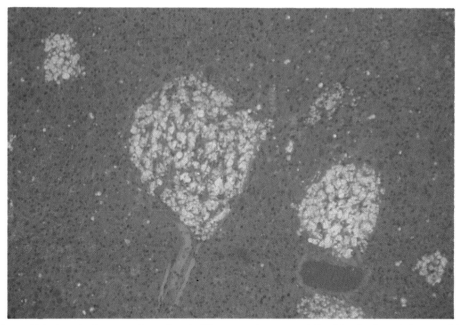

Figure 15.8. *Auramine fluorescence for mycobacteria*. Three granulomas containing *M. avium-intracellulare* as well as discrete mycobacteria are readily observed on fluorescence microscopy. A terminal hepatic venule is at lower right. Post-mortem liver, auramine fluorescence. Illustration kindly provided by Dr Stephen Chin, New York.

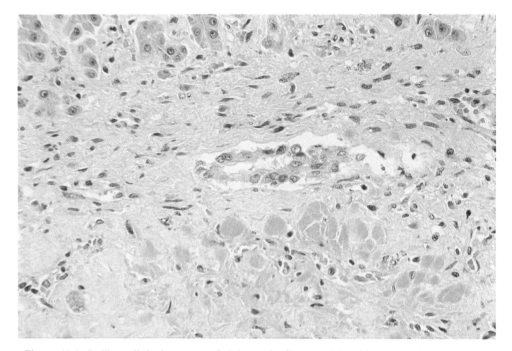

Figure 15.9. *Bacillary peliosis*. Aggregates of pink, smudge-like material within periportal sinusoids in the lower half of this field represent clusters of rickettsia in a patient with AIDS. Post-mortem liver, H & E.

serum markers of prior infection or active viral hepatitis are often present. The course of hepatitis B, C or delta is variable in persons infected with HIV. Fulminant hepatitis may occur[85] and in drug addicts a propensity for more severe chronic hepatitis with progression to cirrhosis has been noted.[86]

Other lesions reported include **nodular regenerative hyperplasia**[87] and **hypertrophied perisinusoidal Ito cells** containing numerous lipid droplets.[88] In children, **giant-cell hepatitis**,[89,90] **chronic hepatitis** of uncertain cause[91] and **primary leiomyosarcoma**[92] are described.

RICKETTSIAL, BACTERIAL AND FUNGAL INFECTIONS

Q Fever

In Q fever, due to infection with *Coxiella burnetii*, liver involvement is common although only a few patients present clinically with liver disease. Histological changes include focal necrosis, non-specific inflammation and fatty change. The most characteristic lesion is the **fibrin-ring granuloma**[19-24] (Fig. 15.4), a granulomatous lesion also seen in several other infections and in some patients taking allopurinol[25] (see p. 232). Atypical lesions without annular arrangement or a central clear area but containing irregular fibrin strands are also found, as are non-specific granulomas without fibrin. In chronic Q fever progressive fibrosis and cirrhosis have been reported.[93]

Brucellosis

In most patients with brucellosis, liver biopsy shows non-specific reactive changes comprising sinusoidal-cell hypertrophy, portal inflammation and focal necrosis. Non-necrotizing granulomas, often small and located within the acini, are more commonly found in the acute phase of the infection.[94]

Typhoid Fever

Liver involvement is uncommon, but most patients with "typhoid hepatitis" are jaundiced.[95] Liver biopsy shows a mild hepatitis with marked hyperplasia of mononuclear phagocytes and lymphocytoid cells in sinusoids.[96] Characteristic granuloma-like collections of mononuclear cells, the typhoid nodules, are described.[97] Other features include fatty change and portal inflammation.[95,98]

Tuberculosis

Tuberculous lesions are present in the liver either as part of a generalized infection[99] or, less often, in the hepatobiliary form of the disease.[100] A normal chest X-ray does not exclude the diagnosis.[101] Granulomas are found randomly scattered in the parenchyma and also in the portal tracts. They range from small accumulations of macrophage-like cells to well-developed, large epithelioid-cell nodules with Langhans giant cells (Fig. 15.10). Central necrosis may or may not be present, and its absence does not exclude the diagnosis. Mycobacteria are seen in a minority of biopsies. Acute lesions contain little reticulin, while chronic ones undergo scarring. Remaining liver tissue shows non-specific reactive features and fatty change. Patients with AIDS sometimes have mycobacterial

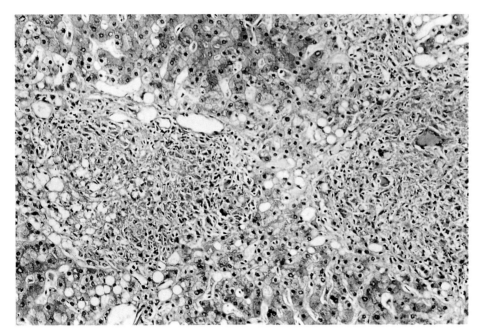

Figure 15.10. *Tuberculosis.* Two granulomas are seen within fatty liver tissue. The lesion to the right contains multinucleated giant cells. Needle biopsy, H & E.

infection without typical granulomas, or may form tuberculous abscesses.[102] In all patients in whom tuberculosis is suspected, part of the liver biopsy specimen should be cultured. Lesions similar to those of tuberculosis have been reported in patients given BCG immunotherapy.[103–105]

Leprosy

In lepromatous leprosy specific granuloma-like lesions composed of foam cells are found in the liver and often contain acid-fast bacilli.[106] Organisms are also seen in Kupffer cells. Epithelioid-cell granulomas of tuberculoid type, rare in lepromatous leprosy, are found in the livers of some patients with the tuberculoid form of the disease. Either type of granuloma is seen in borderline leprosy.[107]

Spirochaetal Infection

Syphilis

In congenital syphilis there is widespread fibrosis separating small groups of hepatocytes and spirochaetes are numerous. In early infections in adults, liver biopsies are normal or show non-specific changes.[108] Spirochaetes may be demonstrable histologically. In patients with secondary syphilis and jaundice or abnormal liver function tests, there is a variable degree of focal parenchymal inflammation, granuloma formation,[109] hepatocellular necrosis and portal inflammation. The portal reaction may mimic that of biliary obstruction,[110] and there may be inflammation of bile-duct epithelium as well as of the walls of small arteries and veins.[111,112] Because patients with syphilis often have other infections as well, lesions cannot always be confidently attributed to the syphilis itself.[113]

The typical lesion of tertiary syphilis is the gumma, an area of necrosis surrounded by granulomatous tissue in which there is endarteritis. Healing is by fibrosis.

Leptospirosis

Most studies of the pathology of leptospirosis have dealt with autopsy material, in which disorganization of liver-cell plates is a prominent feature. This is usually absent from liver biopsies.[114] Hepatocytes are swollen, especially in perivenular areas, and there is an increase in mitotic figures. A few acidophil bodies and fat vacuoles may be seen. Kupffer cells are prominent and there is a mild mononuclear-cell infiltrate in portal tracts. Cholestasis is common and may persist after resolution of the other changes.[115] The diagnosis can be confirmed by demonstrating leptospiral antigen in paraffin sections by immunocytochemistry.[116]

Lyme Disease

Hepatomegaly, elevated serum aminotransferase activity and biopsy features resembling viral hepatitis may be seen in patients infected with the tick-borne spirochaete *Borrelia burgdorferi*.[117] Liver-cell ballooning and numerous mitoses are accompanied by sinusoidal inflammation (hyperplastic Kupffer cells, lymphocytes, plasma cells and neutrophilic leucocytes). The organism can be identified in liver tissue by Dieterle silver stain.

Candidiasis

The most common hepatic manifestations of candidiasis in immunocompromised hosts are **microabscesses** and **granulomas**.[118,119] The more acute lesions show microabscess formation with central necrosis, visible on gross examination as 1–2 mm yellow–white nodules. Yeasts and pseudohyphae can be seen in some, but not all, cases with diastase-PAS and Gomori methenamine silver stains. The predominantly neutrophilic infiltrates are replaced by epithelioid histiocytes and granulomas as the lesions evolve, sometimes surrounded by reactive fibrosis. Candidiasis is most often diagnosed post-mortem but should be suspected in the presence of fever, abdominal symptoms and elevated serum alkaline phosphatase activity. Systemic candidiasis has been noted as an important cause of mortality in patients with zone 3 or multilobular hepatic necrosis due to **exertional heatstroke**.[120]

Histoplasmosis

Hepatomegaly is common in disseminated histoplasmosis due to *Histoplasma capsulatum*. The disease is very occasionally seen in countries where it is not endemic.[121] The liver may rarely be the only organ clinically involved.[122] Liver biopsy shows non-specific inflammation as well as granulomas which may be mistaken for the lesions of tuberculosis.[123,124] The organisms may be scanty or abundant, and are found in Kupffer cells and granulomas. They are round or oval, 1–5 μm across, and have a capsule and central chromatin mass. Diastase-PAS and other stains for fungi can be used for their demonstration and differentiation from Leishman–Donovan bodies; the latter are PAS-negative in tissues.[125] Disseminated infection with *H. duboisii*, seen in Africa, also involves the liver. Nodular lesions contain the much larger and easily demonstrable organisms.[126]

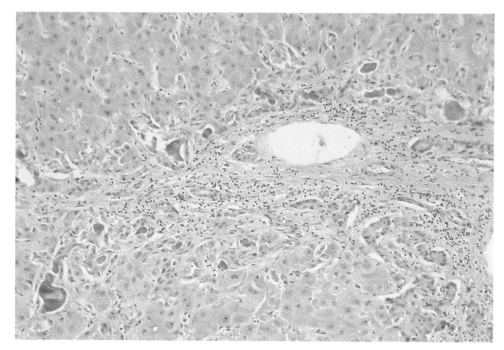

Figure 15.11. *Bile ductular cholestasis in sepsis.* Proliferated bile ductules at the edge of the portal tract contain inspissated bile. The patient died of septicaemia. Post-mortem liver, H & E.

Fibrous, calcified and even bony nodules are sometimes found in and deep to the liver capsule in long-standing histoplasmosis. The nodules, 1–3 mm in diameter, may have a necrotic core surrounded by granulomatous tissue and the organism is demonstrable in some instances.[127]

The Liver in Sepsis

Hepatic changes in sepsis are the result of infection of the liver itself, of circulating toxins, of ischaemia or of a combination of these factors. In many patients the exact cause cannot be established.

Infective lesions include **liver abscess** and **bacterial cholangitis**, the pathology of which is described on p. 45. Less commonly, infection produces a diffuse **bacterial hepatitis** in which bacterial colonization of the liver is associated with portal inflammation.[128] Infection in areas drained by the portal venous system can give rise to **pylephlebitis**. Post-mortem liver sections from septic patients may show neutrophils aggregated within sinusoids and in sparse numbers dispersed throughout the connective tissue of portal tracts.

Patients with extrahepatic sepsis are often jaundiced, especially when the infection is due to Gram-negative organisms.[129] Three histological patterns have been described in such patients. The commonest is **canalicular cholestasis**, most severe in perivenular areas. This is associated with various degrees of Kupffer-cell activation, fatty change and portal inflammation, but usually little or no hepatocellular necrosis.[130]

The second pattern is one of **ductular cholestasis and inflammation**.[129,131] Bile ductules and canals of Hering at the margins of portal tracts are dilated and filled with bile, often in the form of dense, highly pigmented deposits, and neutrophils are seen within and around the affected ductules (Fig. 15.11). Perivenular cholestasis is usually present. Periportal canalicular bile is also sometimes present. These changes are not seen in uncomplicated bile-duct obstruction. They are common in the terminal stages of fatal acute or chronic liver disease complicated by sepsis. Damage to bile-duct epithelium has been reported,[132] but in most instances the interlobular bile ducts are not affected. Patients with the ductular cholestasis pattern have a disproportionately elevated serum bilirubin compared to alkaline phosphatase and aminotransferases.[133] Because of its dire implications, this biopsy finding should be communicated rapidly to the clinician and sepsis should be investigated.

The third pattern is **non-bacterial cholangitis**, seen in the **toxic shock syndrome**.[134] The histological features are similar to those of bacterial cholangitis, but the biliary tree is anatomically normal and the lesion is attributed to a circulating staphylococcal toxin rather than to bacteraemia. In many, but not all patients, the underlying lesion is a staphylococcal vaginitis associated with the use of tampons.

PARASITIC DISEASES

Toxoplasmosis

Toxoplasma gondii is occasionally responsible for neonatal liver injury. In adults, hepatic changes include extensive lymphocytic infiltration of sinusoids, evidence of mild liver-cell damage and granuloma formation.[4,135] Trophozoites may be seen within necrotic hepatocytes and can be identified by specific immunocytochemical methods.[136,137]

Malaria

In non-immune patients with malaria there is hypertrophy of Kupffer cells and these contain malarial pigment (haemozoin) in the form of fine, dark-brown or black pigment granules (Fig. 15.12). In acute malaria due to *Plasmodium falciparum* they also contain erythrocytes, parasites and iron. Malarial pigment closely resembles schistosomal pigment. It often gives pin-point birefringence and, like formalin pigment, is soluble in alcoholic picric acid. This distinguishes it from carbon, with which it may be confused.[138] Following an attack of malaria the pigment clears from the acini but can be found in portal macrophages.

The **tropical splenomegaly syndrome** probably represents an abnormal response of the patient to the malarial parasite.[139] Large numbers of small lymphocytes are seen in dilated hepatic sinusoids (Fig. 15.13). Kupffer cells are enlarged but hepatocytes remain normal. Malarial pigment is scanty or absent. The differential histological diagnosis is from leukaemia, hepatitis C virus infection, infectious mononucleosis, cytomegalovirus infection and toxoplasmosis.

Visceral Leishmaniasis (Kala-Azar)

Infection by *Leishmania donovani* produces striking hypertrophy of Kupffer cells and portal macrophages. These cells contain variable, sometimes very large numbers of Leishman–Donovan bodies, easily visible in haematoxylin and eosin-stained sections (Fig. 15.14). The PAS stain after diastase digestion is negative, in contrast to the positive staining obtained with *Histoplasma*. In some patients the liver contains epithelioid-cell granulomas, which heal by fibrosis.[4,140]

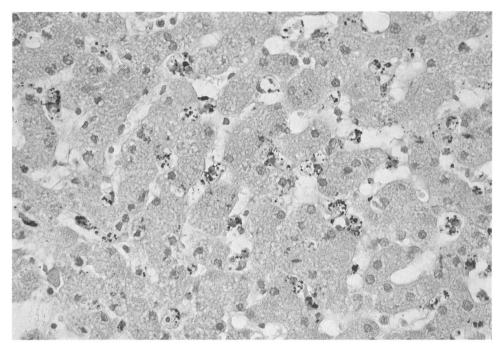

Figure 15.12. *Malaria.* Kupffer cells contain abundant dark granules of malarial pigment. Needle biopsy, H & E.

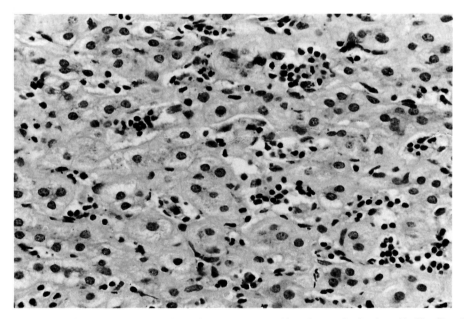

Figure 15.13. *Tropical splenomegaly syndrome.* There are groups of lymphocytes in the sinusoids. Kupffer cells are enlarged. Hepatocytes appear normal. Needle biopsy, H & E.

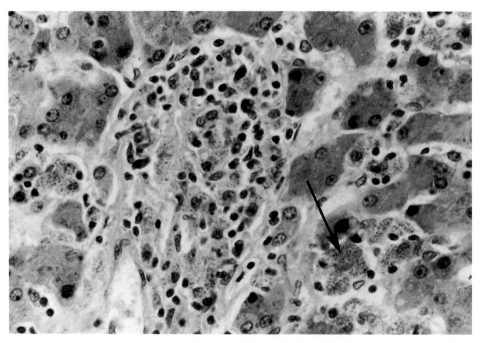

Figure 15.14. *Kala-azar.* There are many Leishman–Donovan bodies in Kupffer cells (arrow) as well as in macrophages in the portal tract. The parasites are just large enough to be seen at this magnification, and give the cells a stippled appearance. Post-mortem liver, H & E.

Amoebiasis

In patients with liver abscesses due to *Entamoeba histolytica*[141] the amoebae may be found at the margins of the lesion or, less often, within the necrotic debris. They may also be seen in the adjacent liver tissue (Fig. 15.15). They are most easily demonstrated by the PAS or Giemsa methods.

Schistosomiasis

Liver lesions are usually caused by *Schistosoma mansoni* or *S. japonicum*, and less commonly by other species.[142] In acute schistosomiasis due to *S. mansoni* the portal tracts are infiltrated by eosinophils, lymphocytes and macrophages. Kupffer cells are enlarged and there is focal hepatocellular necrosis. Granulomas around ova are rare.[143]

More commonly schistosomiasis is chronic. Ova, initially containing live miracidia, are trapped in portal tracts where they excite a granulomatous reaction. This is composed of epithelioid cells, multinucleated giant cells, eosinophils and lymphocytes (Fig. 15.16). Healing is by fibrosis. When ova are scanty and granulomas are no longer seen, step sections may need to be searched. Ziehl–Neelsen staining is then helpful, because the ova of species other than *S. haematobium* are acid-fast.[34] Schistosomal pigment, found in portal tracts in some patients with chronic or past schistosomiasis, is a fine dark granular material closely resembling malarial pigment.

There are lesions in portal-vein branches of all sizes.[143] The smallest contain ova and granulomas. Angiomatoids, wide irregular thin-walled vascular channels, are characteristically found in fibrotic and enlarged portal tracts. Medium-sized veins show intimal thickening which may be eccentric and polypoid, and in large veins there are thrombi and adult worms. In the course of portal scarring, isolated smooth muscle cells may become

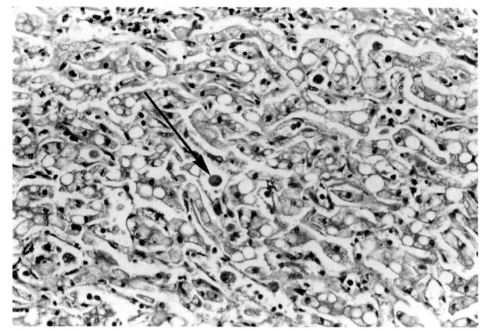

Figure 15.15. *Amoebic abscess.* Rounded amoebae (arrow) are seen among fatty hepatocytes near the edge of an abscess. Post-mortem liver, H & E.

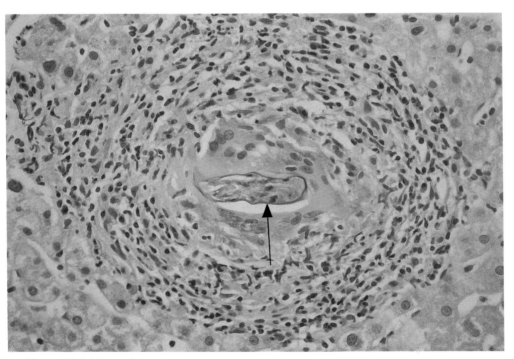

Figure 15.16. *Schistosomiasis.* An ovum (arrow) surrounded by giant cells is seen at the centre of a granuloma. The infiltrate is rich in eosinophil leucocytes. Needle biopsy, H & E.

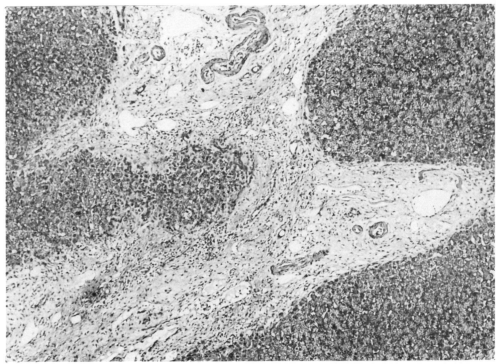

Figure 15.17. *Schistosomiasis.* Serpiginous septa contain many small blood vessels in this example of "pipestem" fibrosis. Wedge biopsy, H & E.

separated from the portal vein wall and entrapped in fibrous tissue, a helpful diagnostic feature.[144] Diffuse hyaline thickening and tortuosity of veins with surrounding fibrosis constitute "clay pipestem fibrosis" in which hepatic artery branches and bile ducts are preserved[144] (Fig. 15.17).

Acinar changes are usually slight, but sinusoidal lining cells are prominent and there is an increase in fibre within the space of Disse.[145,146] Portal tract lymphocytic infiltrates and piecemeal necrosis are likely to reflect the presence of chronic hepatitis, as hepatitis B virus infection is increased in patients with hepatosplenic schistosomiasis,[147,148] as is hepatitis C.

Liver Flukes

Invasion of the biliary tree by the trematodes *Clonorchis sinensis* (the Chinese liver fluke), *Opisthorchis viverrini* and *O. felineus* is followed by proliferation of duct-like structures around the large bile ducts (Fig. 15.18). The duct epithelium may undergo goblet-cell metaplasia.[149] Smaller ducts are surrounded by an eosinophil-rich infiltrate. Complications include bile-duct obstruction, infection, portal fibrosis and hypertension, and bile-duct carcinoma.[150] Infestation may present several years after the patient has left an endemic area.[151]

The liver fluke *Fasciola hepatica* enters the liver from the peritoneal cavity and reaches the biliary tree some weeks later. White nodules are seen on the liver surface at the points of entry and may be mistaken for tumour. Migration tracks extend into the liver. Histologically capsular and subcapsular lesions are composed of serpiginous areas of necrosis containing eosinophils and Charcot–Leyden crystals and bordered by palisaded histiocytes[152] (Fig. 15.19). Elsewhere in the liver, portal tracts are infiltrated with eosinophils. The biliary phase of the infestation is marked by cholangitis with rather less

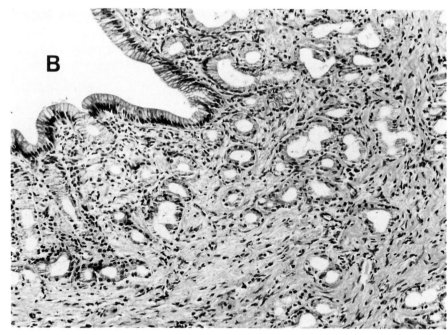

Figure 15.18. *Clonorchiasis.* There has been proliferation of duct-like structures around a large bile-duct (B). Wedge biopsy, H & E.

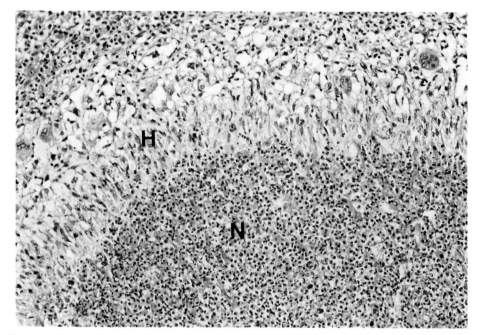

Figure 15.19. *Fascioliasis.* Part of a nodule near the surface of the liver. A central area of necrosis (N) filled with leucocytes is bordered by palisaded histiocytes (H). Wedge biopsy, H & E.

bile-duct hyperplasia than in *Clonorchis* or *Opisthorchis* infections, and both arterial and venous thrombosis. Features of bile-duct obstruction, periductal fibrosis and an ovum within a granuloma have also been reported.[153]

Ascariasis

Focal areas of necrosis with infiltration by eosinophils and neutrophils are seen in the migratory phase, when larvae travel to the lungs via the liver. Adult worms may enter the biliary tree from the duodenum, giving rise to bile-duct obstruction, cholangitis and abscess formation.[34]

Larval Diseases

In several parasitic diseases with larval stages, including infestation by *Toxocara*, the larvae may reach the liver and give rise to eosinophil-rich abscesses or granulomas. Larvae are sometimes seen within these lesions.[4] White capsular and subcapsular liver nodules composed of mature fibrous tissue with calcification and few infiltrating cells surround larval remnants in long-standing disease due to *Toxocara* or to arthropod larvae.[154]

GASTROINTESTINAL DISORDERS AND THE LIVER

Patients with **coeliac disease** sometimes have evidence of liver injury.[155] Lesions reported range from portal inflammation and fatty liver to chronic hepatitis, cirrhosis and hepatocellular carcinoma.[156] Isolated cases of coeliac disease associated with primary biliary cirrhosis[157–159] and primary sclerosing cholangitis[160] are also described. In **Whipple's disease** the characteristic foamy PAS-positive macrophages may be found in the liver[161] and epithelioid-cell granulomas have been reported.[162] Granulomas, associated with a heavy infiltration by eosinophils, have also been described in **eosinophilic gastroenteritis**.[163]

Chronic Inflammatory Bowel Disease

The spectrum of liver lesions is generally similar in ulcerative colitis and Crohn's disease. In Crohn's disease, serious hepatic complications such as sclerosing cholangitis are much less common and there may be granulomas in the liver[164] or amyloid deposition.[165] Gallstones are more common in Crohn's disease than in the general population. In both Crohn's disease and ulcerative colitis, malnutrition, anaemia and toxaemia can lead to steatosis.[166]

A minority of patients with ulcerative colitis have persistent abnormalities of liver function tests.[167] Careful examination including cholangiography shows that most of these patients have primary sclerosing cholangitis, the pathology of which has already been described in detail on p. 47. Bile-duct carcinoma, sometimes accompanied by diffuse dysplasia of biliary epithelium,[168] is increased in patients with ulcerative colitis, probably reflecting underlying sclerosing cholangitis.[169,170] Portal inflammatory lesions with or without periductal fibrosis in ulcerative colitis have occasioned use of the term "pericholangitis". However, patients with such portal inflammation have largely been shown to have typical primary sclerosing cholangitis[171] or its small-duct variant.[172] Furthermore, some examples of so-called pericholangitis probably represent a non-specific inflammatory response to the colitis. The term pericholangitis should therefore be discarded.[172] While liver biopsies from patients with ulcerative colitis may show features of chronic hepatitis, this may be due to intercurrent viral hepatitis (for example, following blood transfusion). However, it should be noted that piecemeal necrosis is also common in primary sclerosing cholangitis (see p. 49). From a practical point of view it therefore seems wise to consider the possibility of sclerosing cholangitis in all patients with ulcerative colitis and chronic liver disease.

HAEMATOLOGICAL DISORDERS AND THE LIVER

One of the most common findings in liver biopsies from patients with haematological disorders is diffuse **Kupffer cell siderosis**, usually reflecting prior transfusion (see Chapter 14). In **reactive haemophagocytic syndrome**,[173] diffuse Kupffer cell hyperplasia with siderosis and phagocytosis of erythrocytes may be seen in patients with systemic infections, disseminated carcinoma, leukaemia and lymphoma. Phagocytosed red blood cells are well demonstrated on chromotrope aniline blue stain and the histiocytes stain much less intensely on diastase-PAS than those engaged in necrotizing processes such as viral hepatitis. Hepatic involvement by leukaemias and lymphomas is discussed in Chapter 11, the effects of thrombosis and sickle-cell disease in Chapter 12, and graft-versus-host disease following bone marrow transplantation in Chapter 16.

Haemophilia

Hepatitis viruses are readily transmitted in blood products, and hepatitis is therefore common in patients with haemophilia.[174-177] Hepatitis C virus and possibly other putative non-A, non-B hepatitis viruses are the most important agents involved, but markers of infection with hepatitis B virus are also present in some patients. Liver histopathology is most often that of a mild chronic hepatitis, on the border of chronic persistent hepatitis and mild chronic active hepatitis;[177] cirrhosis is infrequent.

Extramedullary Haemopoiesis

Haemopoiesis in the liver sinusoids is normal in fetal and neonatal life. In adults it is seen mainly in the myeloproliferative disorders and when bone marrow is invaded by tumours. Foci of haemopoiesis may also be seen in the congested liver of patients with cardiac failure,[178] in transplant livers with zone 3 necrosis[179] or in the rare situation of graft-versus-host disease in liver transplant recipients.[180] The sinusoids and spaces of Disse of the enlarged liver contain discrete clumps of haemopoietic cells (Fig. 15.20), and there are similar cells in portal tracts. Features which distinguish haemopoiesis from the infiltrates of leukaemias, infectious mononucleosis, other infections and the tropical splenomegaly syndrome are the variety of cells in the aggregates and the presence of recognizable marrow cells such as normoblasts and eosinophil myelocytes. Megakaryocytes are commonly seen and are sometimes the only marrow elements found (Fig. 15.21). Owing to the restraints of space, these cells are more elongated than in a section or smear of bone marrow. In the liver of neonates or stillborn infants, if megakaryocytes are the predominant form of extramedullary haemopoiesis, **Down syndrome** should be considered.[181,182]

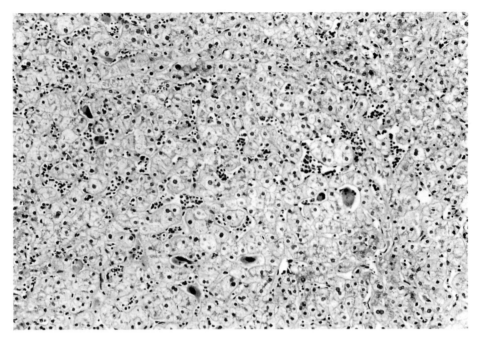

Figure 15.20. *Extramedullary haemopoiesis.* Clumps of haemopoietic cells in the sinusoids. Several megakaryocytes are seen. Needle biopsy, H & E.

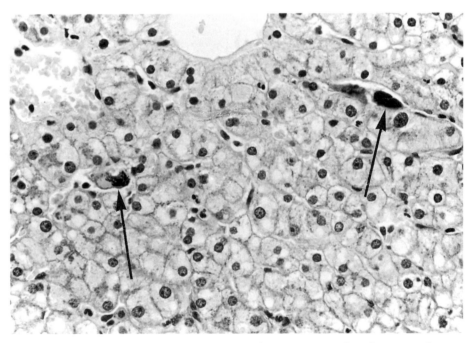

Figure 15.21. *Extramedullary haemopoiesis.* Megakaryocytes (arrows) are present but other marrow elements are not seen. Needle biopsy, H & E.

THE LIVER IN RHEUMATOID, IMMUNE-COMPLEX AND COLLAGEN DISEASES

Polyarteritis nodosa in small hepatic arteries can lead to infarction. Immune complexes containing hepatitis B surface antigen are sometimes demonstrable in vessel walls in this disease.[183] Both hepatitis B and C virus antigen–antibody complexes have been implicated in the pathogenesis of **essential (type II) mixed cryoglobulinae-mia**.[184-186] In the **polymyalgia rheumatica–giant cell arteritis syndrome** the liver may contain granulomas.[187,188] Other findings reported include fatty change, venous congestion, non-specific hepatitis and prominent lipocytes.[189,190]

Patients with **rheumatoid arthritis** often have abnormal liver function tests, but liver biopsy more often shows non-specific changes or normal liver than definitive liver disease.[191-193] Amyloidosis or necrotizing arteritis may be found and rheumatoid nodules in the liver like those typically found in subcutaneous tissue have been reported.[194] Nodular regenerative hyperplasia (p. 155) is common in **Felty's syndrome**[195] (rheumatoid arthritis, leukopenia and splenomegaly). The nodular lesions may be attributable to arteritis involving small intrahepatic vessels.[196]

Scleroderma and the **CRST syndrome** (calcinosis, Raynaud's phenomenon, sclero-dactyly and telangiectasia) may be associated with primary biliary cirrhosis.[197,198] Giant, dense mitochondria on electron microscopy, with normal liver or non-specific changes on light microscopy, have been described in patients with **systemic sclerosis**.[199]

The majority of patients with **systemic lupus erythematosus (SLE)** do not have significant liver pathology. However, cirrhosis, chronic hepatitis or hepatic granulomas have been reported in several series.[200,201] Abnormal liver function tests may be present without serious lesions.[202,203] Steatosis, cholestasis, nodular regenerative hyperplasia, and necrotizing arteritis involving arteries of 100–400 μm diameter have also been reported.[201] An unusual case of **malacoplakia** involving the liver in a steroid-treated patient with SLE and Gram-negative bacterial infection showed aggregates of histiocytes with typical Michaelis–Gutmann bodies.[204] There appears to be no close relationship between systemic lupus and autoimmune (lupoid) hepatitis. A patient with chronic active hepatitis and **mixed connective tissue disease** has been reported.[205]

AMYLOIDOSIS AND LIGHT CHAIN DEPOSITION

The liver is commonly involved in systemic amyloidosis. "Primary" (AL) and reactive (AA) amyloidosis cannot reliably be distinguished by the pattern of liver involve-ment.[206,207] This distinction is made by the resistance of AL amyloid to potassium permanganate before Congo red staining[208] and by immunohistochemistry.[207,209] In most patients the amyloid is deposited in portal arteries (Fig. 15.22) or diffusely in the perisinusoidal space of Disse (Fig. 15.23). The two patterns are often combined. The perisinusoidal deposits compress both the sinusoids and the liver-cell plates, occasionally leading to portal hypertension or to cholestasis.[210-212] Rarely, the amyloid is in the form of globular deposits[213-215] (Fig. 15.24), when it may be difficult to detect in haematoxylin and eosin-stained sections.

Amorphous perisinusoidal and portal deposits somewhat like amyloid are seen when the liver is involved in light chain deposit disease.[216] Immunoglobulin light chains, usually kappa, can be identified immunochemically. The characteristic green birefringence of amyloid after Congo red staining is absent. Occasionally amyloid and light chain deposits are found in the same patient.[217,218]

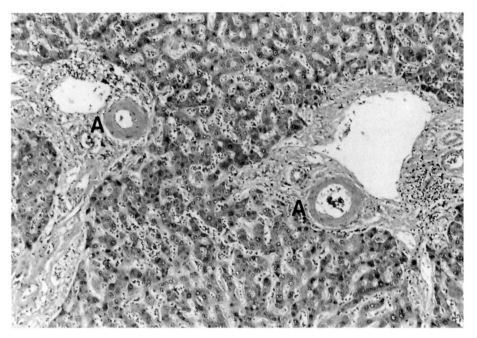

Figure 15.22. *Amyloidosis*. Two small arteries (A) are thickened by amyloid deposits. Needle biopsy, H & E.

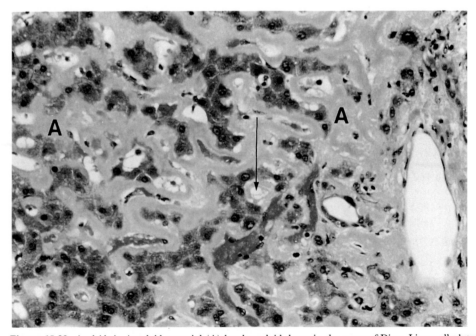

Figure 15.23. *Amyloidosis*. Amyloid material (A) has been laid down in the space of Disse. Liver-cell plates have undergone atrophy, and sinusoids (arrow) are narrowed. Needle biopsy, H & E.

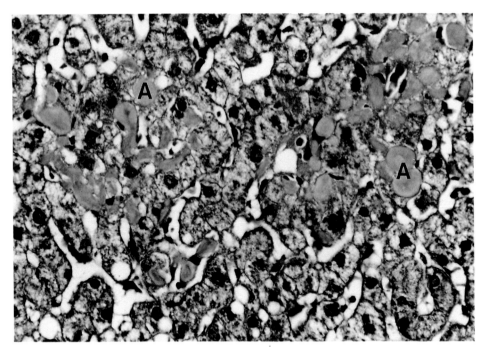

Figure 15.24. *Globular amyloid.* There are rounded deposits of amyloid (A) in the space of Disse. Needle biopsy, H & E.

THE LIVER IN THE PORPHYRIAS

Liver lesions are found in **porphyria cutanea tarda** and **protoporphyria**.[219] Red porphyrin fluorescence can be demonstrated in both diseases using unfixed liver tissue.

In **porphyria cutanea tarda** (**PCT**) hepatocytes contain needle-shaped birefringent porphyrin crystals, sufficiently water-soluble to make their demonstration difficult or impossible in routinely prepared paraffin sections. They can be seen in unstained paraffin sections, and in haematoxylin and eosin-stained sections prepared with minimal exposure to water.[220] Fatty change and hepatocellular siderosis are common. There are characteristic intra-acinar clumps of iron- and ceroid-containing macrophages, fat droplets and inflammatory cells.[221] Alcohol contributes to the pathogenesis of PCT and biopsies should be critically examined for alcohol-related injury. More importantly, **chronic hepatitis** and **cirrhosis** are common in patients with PCT and the majority have hepatitis C virus infection.[222–224] The prevalence of chronic hepatitis C in this population may also explain the development of **hepatocellular carcinoma**.[219]

In **protoporphyria** (erythropoietic or erythrohepatic protoporphyria) dense, dark brown deposits of poorly soluble protoporphyrin accumulate in the liver. These give a diagnostic red birefringence under polarized light.[225] There may be serious liver damage, with cholestasis, perisinusoidal and perivenular fibrosis and cirrhosis developing in some patients.[226,227]

NON-SPECIFIC REACTIVE CHANGES

A variety of changes including portal and acinar inflammation, fat accumulation and Kupffer-cell hypertrophy are seen in extrahepatic conditions, especially febrile,

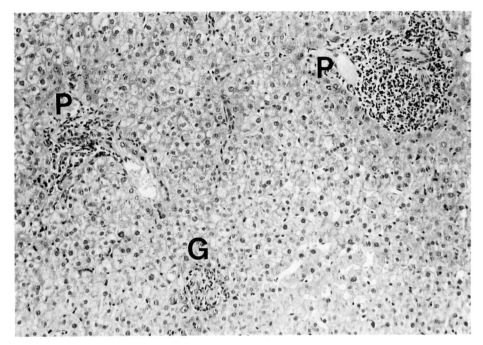

Figure 15.25. *Non-specific reactive changes.* Portal tracts (P) are infiltrated with mononuclear cells. A small granuloma (G) is seen below. Needle biopsy, H & E.

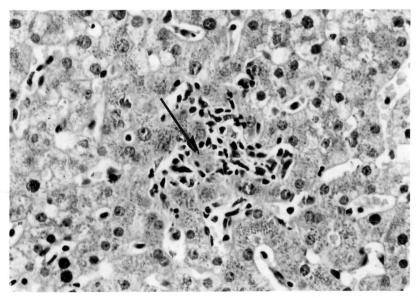

Figure 15.26. *Focal liver-cell necrosis.* A necrotic liver cell (arrow) among inflammatory cells, from the biopsy with non-specific reactive changes shown in Figure 15.25. Needle biopsy, H & E.

inflammatory or widespread neoplastic diseases. Focal hepatocellular necroses may be found in the parenchyma (Figs 15.25 and 15.26). The distinction of these reactive changes from a mild form of chronic viral hepatitis or from residual acute hepatitis

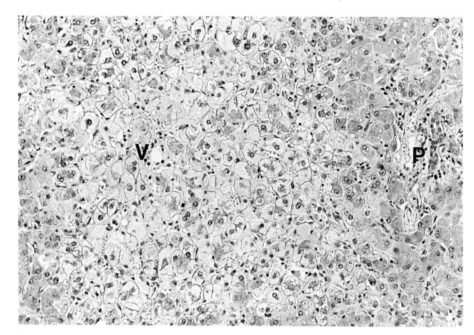

Figure 15.27. *Acute fatty liver of pregnancy.* Swollen pale-staining hepatocytes around a terminal hepatic venule (V) contrast with the rim of normal cells near a portal tract (P). No large fat vacuoles are seen. The lesion resembles that of Reye's syndrome, shown in Figure 13.17 (p. 210). Post-mortem liver, H & E.

requires clinical information. The latter may sometimes be suspected from a predominantly perivenular location of inflammation and liver-cell loss. Reactive changes near space-occupying lesions such as metastatic tumours are discussed on p. 3 and illustrated in Fig. 1.5 (p. 4).

THE LIVER IN PREGNANCY

In normal pregnancy there are no specific light microscopic abnormalities in the liver. Electron microscopic changes reported in late pregnancy include giant mitochondria with paracrystalline inclusions, increase in the number of peroxisomes and proliferation of smooth endoplasmic reticulum.[228]

Liver disease in pregnancy is rare and falls into three categories:[229]

1. **Liver disease unique to pregnancy**. The four conditions included in this category are **acute fatty liver of pregnancy (AFLP)**, **pre-eclampsia/eclampsia**, the **HELLP syndrome (haemolysis, elevated liver enzymes, and low platelets)** and **intrahepatic cholestasis of pregnancy (ICP)**.
2. **Intercurrent liver disease during pregnancy**. Viral hepatitis and cholelithiasis are examples. Hepatocellular carcinoma, including the fibrolamellar variety,[230] occurs rarely. **Viral hepatitis** is the most common form of liver disease encountered in pregnancy.
3. **Pre-existing liver disease in the pregnant patient**. Chronic hepatitis B viral infection and autoimmune hepatitis with or without cirrhosis are examples of this category.

Jaundice and elevated serum aminotransferases are important aspects of the clinical

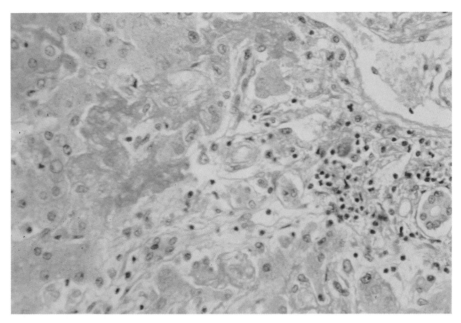

Figure 15.28. *Pre-eclampsia/eclampsia.* The periportal sinusoids at left contain strands of fibrin. Post-mortem liver, H & E.

presentation of liver disease in pregnancy. The following discussion is limited to those diseases unique to pregnancy.

Acute Fatty Liver of Pregnancy

This uncommon and serious complication of pregnancy develops in the last weeks of gestation.[229,231,232] Fatty change involves the greater part of each acinus, usually leaving a thin and incomplete rim of normal hepatocytes around the portal tracts.[233,234] The fat is mainly in the form of fine droplets, as in Reye's syndrome (p. 210) and other examples of microvesicular steatosis.[235] Large fat vacuoles of the kind seen in alcoholic liver disease are scanty, and the cause of the hepatocellular swelling and pallor may not be readily apparent on examination of paraffin sections (Fig. 15.27). Fat staining of frozen sections makes the diagnosis clear, and a piece of the biopsy specimen should therefore be kept for frozen sectioning in patients with unexplained jaundice in late pregnancy. Inflammatory cells, mostly lymphocytes, are prominent in some examples and may lead to confusion with acute viral hepatitis,[236] in which microsteatosis is not seen. In more severe examples of AFLP there is loss of hepatocytes leading to approximation of portal tracts. Fibrin deposits are occasionally demonstrable in hepatic sinusoids. One series noted cholestasis, extramedullary haemopoiesis and giant mitochondria[234] in some patients. With rare exception,[237] acute fatty liver does not recur in subsequent pregnancies.

Pre-eclampsia/Eclampsia

Hypertension, proteinuria, peripheral oedema and occasional coagulation abnormalities in pregnancy constitute pre-eclampsia, or eclampsia if convulsions and hyperreflexia are also present. Liver involvement is unusual, but may be manifested by elevated serum aminotransferases and/or alkaline phosphatase. The incidence of pre-eclampsia is increased in patients with acute fatty liver.[236] The liver in pre-eclampsia shows fibrin thrombi in portal vessels and periportal sinusoids (Fig. 15.28) associated with necrosis and haemorrhage in more severe cases.[238,239] The identity of the fibrin can be established by phosphotungstic acid-haematoxylin (PTAH) staining or immunofluorescence.[240] These changes are not seen in all patients. Infarction, haematoma and rupture of the liver[241] are complications.

HELLP Syndrome

This syndrome is exceedingly uncommon in pregnancy and is seen in pre-eclamptic women.[229,242] Periportal haemorrhage and necrosis (sometimes confluent) with periportal sinusoidal fibrin deposition appear to be the characteristic lesions.[243] Non-specific portal inflammation and glycogenated hepatocyte nuclei have also been reported.[229,244-246]

Intrahepatic Cholestasis of Pregnancy

Pruritus, with or without cholestatic jaundice, may develop in late pregnancy and recur in subsequent pregnancies. It regresses after delivery. Liver biopsy shows little apart from canalicular cholestasis, most severe in perivenular areas.[238] Minor hepatocellular changes and inflammation are attributable to the cholestasis itself. Portal inflammation is absent or mild. No histological abnormalities are detectable between pregnancies but the jaundice has been shown to return on administration of oral contraceptives.[247] Concomitant ICP and acute fatty liver has been reported.[248]

REFERENCES

1. Holtz T, Moseley RH, Scheiman JM. Liver biopsy in fever of unknown origin. *J Clin Gastroenterol* 1993; **17**: 29–32.
2. Fauci AS, Wolff SM. Granulomatous hepatitis. In Popper H, Schaffner F (eds): Progress in Liver Diseases, Vol. V. New York: Grune and Stratton, 1976, pp 609–621.
3. Guckian JC, Perry JE. Granulomatous hepatitis: an analysis of 63 cases and review of the literature. *Ann Intern Med* 1966; **65**: 1081–1100.
4. Ishak KG. Granulomas of the liver. In Ioachim HL (ed): Pathology of Granulomas. New York: Raven Press, 1983, pp 307–369.
5. Israel HL, Margolis ML, Rose LJ. Hepatic granulomatosis and sarcoidosis. Further observations. *Dig Dis Sci* 1984; **29**: 353–356.
6. Hercules HD, Bethlem NM. Value of liver biopsy in sarcoidosis. *Arch Pathol Lab Med* 1984; **108**: 831–834.
7. Epstein MS, Devaney KO, Goodman ZD, Zimmerman HJ, Ishak KG. Liver disease in sarcoidosis. *Hepatology* 1990; **12**: 839A.
7a. Devaney K, Goodman ZD, Epstein MS, Zimmerman HJ, Ishak KG. Hepatic sarcoidosis. Clinicopathologic features in 100 patients. *Am J Surg Pathol* 1993; **17**: 1272–1280.
8. Maddrey WC, Johns CJ, Boitnott JK, Iber FL. Sarcoidosis and chronic hepatic disease: a clinical and pathologic study of 20 patients. *Medicine* 1970; **49**: 375–395.
9. Tekeste H, Latour F, Levitt RE. Portal hypertension complicating sarcoid liver disease: case report and review of the literature. *Am J Gastroenterol* 1984; **79**: 389–396.
10. Rudzki C, Ishak KG, Zimmerman HJ. Chronic intrahepatic cholestasis of sarcoidosis. *Am J Med* 1975; **59**: 373–387.
11. Bridges RA, Berendes H, Good RA. A fatal granulomatous disease of childhood. *Am J Dis Child* 1959; **97**: 387–408.
12. Ishak KG, Sharp HL. Metabolic errors and liver disease. In MacSween RNM, Anthony PP, Scheuer PJ, Portmann BC, Burt AD (eds): Pathology of the Liver, 3rd edn. Edinburgh: Churchill Livingstone, 1994.
13. Nakhleh RE, Glock M, Snover DC. Hepatic pathology of chronic granulomatous disease of childhood. *Arch Pathol Lab Med* 1992; **116**: 71–75.
14. Dilworth JA, Mandell GL. Adults with chronic granulomatous disease of "childhood". *Am J Med* 1977; **63**: 233–243.
15. McMaster KR, Hennigar GR. Drug-induced granulomatous hepatitis. *Lab Invest* 1981; **44**: 61–73.
16. Kurumaya H, Kono N, Nakanuma Y, Tomoda F, Takazakura E. Hepatic granulomata in long-term hemodialysis patients with hyperaluminumemia. *Arch Pathol Lab Med* 1989; **113**: 1132–1134.

17. Leong AS-Y, Disney APS, Gove DW. Spallation and migration of silicone from blood-pump tubing in patients on hemodialysis. *N Engl J Med* 1982; **306**: 135–140.

18. Yao-Chang L, Tomashefski J, McMahon JT, Petrelli M. Mineral-associated hepatic injury: a report of seven cases with X-ray microanalysis. *Hum Pathol* 1991; **22**: 1120–1127.

19. Bernstein M, Edmondson HA, Barbour BH. The liver lesion in Q-fever. Clinical and pathologic features. *Arch Intern Med* 1965; **116**: 491–498.

20. Pellegrin M, Delsol G, Auvergnat JC, Familiades J, Faure H, Guiu M. Granulomatous hepatitis in Q fever. *Hum Pathol* 1980; **11**: 51–57.

21. Hofmann CE, Heaton JW Jr. Q fever hepatitis: clinical manifestations and pathological findings. *Gastroenterology* 1982; **83**: 474–479.

22. Qizilbash AH. The pathology of Q fever as seen on liver biopsy. *Arch Pathol Lab Med* 1983; **107**: 364–367.

23. Srigley JR, Vellend H, Palmer N et al. Q-fever. The liver and bone marrow pathology. *Am J Surg Pathol* 1985; **9**: 752–758.

24. Marazuela M, Moreno A, Yebra M, Cerezo E, Gomez-Gesto C, Vargas JA. Hepatic fibrin-ring granulomas. A clinicopathologic study of 23 patients. *Hum Pathol* 1991; **22**: 607–613.

25. Vanderstigel M, Zafrani ES, Lejonc JL, Schaeffer A, Portos JL. Allopurinol hypersensitivity syndrome as a cause of hepatic fibrin-ring granulomas. *Gastroenterology* 1986; **90**: 188–190.

26. Lobdell DH. "Ring" granulomas in cytomegalovirus hepatitis. *Arch Pathol Lab Med* 1987; **111**: 881–882.

27. Nenert M, Mavier P, Dubuc N, Deforges L, Zafrani ES. Epstein–Barr virus infection and hepatic fibrin-ring granulomas. *Hum Pathol* 1988; **19**: 608–610.

28. Moreno A, Marazuela M, Yebra M et al. Hepatic fibrin-ring granulomas in visceral leishmaniasis. *Gastroenterology* 1988; **95**: 1123–1126.

29. Ponz E, García-Pagán JC, Bruguera M, Bruix J, Rodés J. Hepatic fibrin-ring granulomas in a patient with hepatitis A. *Gastroenterology* 1991; **100**: 268–270.

30. Ruel M, Sevestre H, Henry-Biabaud E, Courouce AM, Capron JP, Erlinger S. Fibrin ring granulomas in hepatitis A. *Dig Dis Sci* 1992; **37**: 1915–1917.

30a. De Bayso L, Roblot P, Ramassamy A et al. Hepatic fibrin-ring granulomas in giant cell arteritis. *Gastroenterology* 1993; **105**: 272–273.

31. Murphy E, Griffiths MR, Hunter JA, Burt AD. Fibrin-ring granulomas: a non-specific reaction to liver injury? *Histopathology* 1991; **19**: 91–93.

32. Simon HB, Wolff SM. Granulomatous hepatitis and prolonged fever of unknown origin: a study of 13 patients. *Medicine* 1973; **52**: 1–21.

33. Zoutman DE, Ralph ED, Frei JV. Granulomatous hepatitis and fever of unknown origin. An 11-year experience of 23 cases with three years' follow-up. *J Clin Gastroenterol* 1991; **13**: 69–75.

34. Lucas SB. Other viral and infectious diseases. In MacSween RNM, Anthony PP, Scheuer PJ, Portmann BC, Burt AD (eds): Pathology of the Liver, 3rd edn. Edinburgh: Churchill Livingstone, 1994.

35. Kuo C-H, Tai D-I, Chang-Chien C-S, Lan C-K, Chiou S-S, Liaw Y-F. Liver biochemical tests and Dengue fever. *Am J Trop Med Hyg* 1992; **47**: 265–270.

36. Elisaf M, Stefanaki S, Repanti M, Korakis H, Tsianos E, Siamopoulos KC. Liver involvement in hemorrhagic fever with renal syndrome. *J Clin Gastroenterol* 1993; **17**: 33–37.

37. Vieira WT, Gayotto LC, de Lima CP, De Brito T. Histopathology of the human liver in yellow fever with special emphasis on the diagnostic role of the Councilman body. *Histopathology* 1983; **7**: 195–208.

38. Goodman ZD, Ishak KG, Sesterhenn IA. Herpes simplex hepatitis in apparently immunocompetent adults. *Am J Clin Pathol* 1986; **85**: 694–699.

39. Jacques SM, Qureshi F. Herpes simplex virus hepatitis in pregnancy: a clinicopathologic study of three cases. *Hum Pathol* 1992; **23**: 183–187.

40. Carmichael GP Jr, Zahradnik JM, Moyer GH, Porter DD. Adenovirus hepatitis in an immunosuppressed adult patient. *Am J Clin Pathol* 1979; **71**: 352–355.

41. Varki NM, Bhuta S, Drake T, Porter DD. Adenovirus hepatitis in two successive liver transplants in a child. *Arch Pathol Lab Med* 1990; **114**: 106–109.

42. Phillips MJ, Glendis LM, Paucell S et al. Syncytial giant-cell hepatitis. Sporadic hepatitis with distinctive pathologic features, a severe clinical course, and paramyxoviral features. *N Engl J Med* 1991; **324**: 455–460.

43. Devaney K, Goodman ZD, Ishak KG. Postinfantile giant-cell transformation in hepatitis. *Hepatology* 1992; **16**: 327–333.

44. Lau J, Koukoulis G, Mieli-Vergani G, Portmann BC, Williams R. Syncytial giant-cell hepatitis – a specific disease entity? *J Hepatol* 1992; **15**: 216–219.

45. Finegold MJ, Carpenter RJ. Obliterative cholangitis due to cytomegalovirus: a possible precursor of paucity of intrahepatic bile ducts. *Hum Pathol* 1982; **13**: 662–665.

46. Chang M-H, Huang H-H, Huang E-S, Kao C-L, Hsu H-Y, Lee C-Y. Polymerase chain reaction to detect human cytomegalovirus in livers of infants with neonatal hepatitis. *Gastroenterology* 1992; **103**: 1022–1025.

47. Theise ND, Conn M, Thung SN. Localization of cytomegalovirus antigens in liver allografts over time. *Hum Pathol* 1993; **24**: 103–108.

48. Vanstapel MJ, Desmet VJ. Cytomegalovirus hepatitis: a histological and immunohistochemical study. *Appl Pathol* 1983; **1**: 41–49.

49. Clarke J, Craig RM, Saffro R, Murphy P, Yokoo H. Cytomegalovirus granulomatous hepatitis. *Am J Med* 1979; **66**: 264–269.

50. Snover DC, Horwitz CA. Liver disease in cytomegalovirus mononucleosis: a light microscopical and immunoperoxidase study of six cases. *Hepatology* 1984; **4**: 408–412.

51. Kilpatrick ZM. Structural and functional abnormalities of liver in infectious mononucleosis. *Arch Intern Med* 1966; **117**: 47–53.
52. Chang MY, Campbell WG Jr. Fatal infectious mononucleosis. Association with liver necrosis and herpes-like virus particles. *Arch Pathol* 1975; **99**: 185–191.
53. Lebovics E, Thung SN, Schaffner F, Radensky PW. The liver in the acquired immunodeficiency syndrome: a clinical and histologic study. *Hepatology* 1985; **5**: 293–298.
54. Glasgow BJ, Anders K, Layfield LJ, Steinsapir KD, Gitnick GL, Lewin KJ. Clinical and pathologic findings of the liver in the acquired immune deficiency syndrome (AIDS). *Am J Clin Pathol* 1985; **83**: 582–588.
55. Dworkin BM, Stahl RE, Giardina MA et al. The liver in acquired immune deficiency syndrome: emphasis on patients with intravenous drug abuse. *Am J Gastroenterol* 1987; **82**: 231–236.
56. Schneiderman DJ, Arenson DM, Cello JP, Margaretten W, Weber TE. Hepatic disease in patients with the acquired immune deficiency syndrome (AIDS). *Hepatology* 1987; **7**: 925–930.
57. Lebovics E, Dworkin BM, Heier SK, Rosenthal WS. The hepatobiliary manifestations of human immunodeficiency virus infection. *Am J Gastroenterol* 1988; **83**: 1–7.
58. Wilkins MJ, Lindley R, Dourakis SP, Goldin RD. Surgical pathology of the liver in HIV infection. *Histopathology* 1991; **18**: 459–464.
59. Comer GM. Hepatobiliary disease in AIDS. In Kotler DP (ed): Gastrointestinal and Nutritional Manifestations of AIDS. New York: Raven Press Ltd, 1991, pp 119–140.
60. Bach N, Theise ND, Schaffner F. Hepatic histopathology in the acquired immunodeficiency syndrome. *Semin Liver Dis* 1992; **12**: 205–212.
61. Housset C, Boucher O, Girard PM et al. Immunohistochemical evidence for human immunodeficiency virus-1 infection of liver Kupffer cells. *Hum Pathol* 1990; **21**: 404–408.
62. Steffan A-M, Lafon M-E, Gendrault J-L et al. Primary cultures of endothelial cells from the human liver sinusoid are permissive for human immunodeficiency virus type 1. *Proc Natl Acad Sci USA* 1992; **89**: 1582–1586.
63. Lafon M-E, Kirn A. Human immunodeficiency virus infection of the liver. *Semin Liver Dis* 1992; **12**: 197–204.
63a. Houssett C, Lamas E, Courgnaud V et al. Presence of HIV-1 in human parenchymal and non-parenchymal liver cells in vivo. *J Hepatol.* 1993; **19**: 252–258.
64. Kahn DG, Garfinkle JM, Klonoff DC, Pembrook LJ, Morrow DJ. Cryptosporidial and cytomegaloviral hepatitis and cholecystitis. *Arch Pathol Lab Med* 1987; **111**: 879–881.
65. Beaugerie L, Teilhac M-F, Deluol A-M et al. Cholangiopathy associated with Microsporidia infection of the common bile duct mucosa in a patient with HIV infection. *Ann Intern Med* 1992; **117**: 401–402.
66. Pol S, Romana C, Richard S et al. Enterocytozoon bieneusi infection in acquired-immunodeficiency syndrome-related sclerosing cholangitis. *Gastroenterology* 1992; **102**: 1778–1781.
67. Pol S, Romana CA, Richard S et al. Microsporidia infection in patients with the human immunodeficiency virus and unexplained cholangitis. *N Engl J Med* 1993; **328**: 95–99.
68. Poblete RB, Rodgriguez K, Foust RT, Reddy R, Saldana MJ. Pneumocystis carinii hepatitis in the acquired immunodeficiency syndrome (AIDS). *Ann Intern Med* 1989; **110**: 737–738.
69. Caccamo D, Pervez NK, Marchevsky A. Primary lymphoma of the liver in the acquired immuno-deficiency syndrome. *Arch Pathol Lab Med* 1986; **110**: 553–555.
70. Beral V, Peterman T, Berkelman R, Jaffe H. AIDS-associated non-Hodgkin lymphoma. *Lancet* 1991; **337**: 805–809.
71. Greene JB, Sidhu GS, Lewin S et al. Mycobacterium avium-intracellulare: a cause of disseminated life-threatening infection in homosexuals and drug abusers. *Ann Intern Med* 1982; **97**: 539–546.
72. Orenstein MS, Tavitian A, Yonk B, Dincsoy HP, Zerega J, Iyer SK. Granulomatous involvement of the liver in patients with AIDS. *Gut* 1985; **26**: 1220–1225.
73. Gordon SC, Reddy KR, Gould EE et al. The spectrum of liver disease in the acquired immunodeficiency syndrome. *J Hepatol* 1986; **2**: 475–484.
74. Nakanuma Y, Liew CT, Peters RL, Govindarajan S. Pathologic features of the liver in acquired immune deficiency syndrome (AIDS). *Liver* 1986; **6**: 158–166.
75. Stevens A. Micro-organisms. In Bancroft JD, Stevens A (eds): Theory and Practice of Histological Techniques, 2nd edn. Edinburgh: Churchill Livingstone, 1982, pp 278-297.
76. Kuper SWA, May JR. Detection of acid-fast-organisms in tissue sections by fluorescence microscopy. *J Pathol Bacteriol* 1960; **79**: 59–68.
77. Margulis SJ, Honig CL, Soave R, Govoni AF, Mouradian JA, Jacobson IM. Biliary tract obstruction in the acquired immunodeficiency syndrome. *Ann Intern Med* 1986; **105**: 207–210.
78. Cello J. Human immunodeficiency virus-associated biliary tract disease. *Semin Liver Dis* 1992; **12**: 213–218.
79. Bouche H, Housset C, Dumont J-L et al. AIDS-related cholangitis: diagnostic features and course in 15 patients. *J Hepatol* 1993; **17**: 34–39.
80. Czapar CA, Weldon-Linne CM, Moore DM, Rhone DP. Peliosis hepatis in the acquired immuno-deficiency syndrome. *Arch Pathol Lab Med* 1986; **110**: 611–613.
81. Boylston AW, Cook HT, Francis ND, Goldin RD. Biopsy pathology of acquired immune deficiency syndrome (AIDS). *J Clin Pathol* 1987; **40**: 1–8.
82. Perkocha LA, Geaghan SM, Yen TSB et al. Clinical and pathological features of bacillary peliosis hepatis in association with human immunodeficiency virus infection. *N Engl J Med* 1990; **323**: 1581–1586.
83. Garcia-Tsao G, Panzini L, Yoselevitz M, West AB. Bacillary peliosis hepatis as a cause of acute anemia in a patient with the acquired immunodeficiency syndrome. *Gastroenterology* 1992; **102**: 1065–1070.

84. Tappero JW, Koehler JE, Berger TG et al. Bacillary angiomatosis and bacillary splenitis in immunocompetent adults. *Ann Intern Med* 1993; **118**: 363–365.

85. Lichtenstein DR, Makadon HJ, Chopra S. Fulminant hepatitis B and delta virus coinfection in AIDS. *Am J Gastroenterol* 1992; **87**: 1643–1647.

86. Housset C, Pol S, Carnot F et al. Interactions between human immunodeficiency virus-1, hepatitis delta virus and hepatitis B virus infections in 260 chronic carriers of hepatitis B virus. *Hepatology* 1992; **15**: 578–583.

87. Fernandez-Miranda C, Colina F, Delgado JM, Lopez-Carreira M. Diffuse nodular regenerative hyperplasia of the liver associated with human immunodeficiency virus and visceral leishmaniasis. *Am J Gastroenterol* 1993; **88**: 433–435.

88. Kossaifi T, Dupon M, Le Bail B, Lacut Y, Balabaud C, Bioulac-Sage P. Perisinusoidal cell hypertrophy in a patient with acquired immunodeficiency syndrome. *Arch Pathol Lab Med* 1990; **114**: 876–879.

89. Witzleben CL, Marshall GS, Wenner W, Piccoli DA, Barbour SD. HIV as a cause of giant cell hepatitis. *Hum Pathol* 1988; **19**: 603–605.

90. Kahn E, Greco A, Daum F et al. Hepatic pathology in pediatric acquired immunodeficiency syndrome. *Hum Pathol* 1991; **22**: 1111–1119.

91. Duffy LF, Daum F, Kahn E et al. Hepatitis in children with acquired immune deficiency syndrome. Histopathologic and immunocytologic features. *Gastroenterology* 1986; **90**: 173–181.

92. Ross JS, Del Rosario A, Bui HX, Sonbati H, Solis O. Primary hepatic leiomyosarcoma in a child with the acquired immunodeficiency syndrome. *Hum Pathol* 1992; **23**: 69–72.

93. Turck WP, Howitt G, Turnberg LA et al. Chronic Q fever. *Quart J Med* 1976; **45**: 193–217.

94. Cervantes F, Bruguera M, Carbonell J, Force L, Webb S. Liver disease in brucellosis. A clinical and pathological study of 40 cases. *Postgrad Med J* 1982; **58**: 346–350.

95. Khosla SN. Typhoid hepatitis. *Postgrad Med J* 1990; **66**: 923–925.

96. De Brito T, Trench Vieira W, D'Agostino Dias M. Jaundice in typhoid hepatitis: a light and electron microscopy study based on liver biopsies. *Acta Hepato-Gastroenterol* 1977; **24**: 426–433.

97. Nasrallah SM, Nassar VH. Enteric fever: a clinicopathologic study of 104 cases. *Am J Gastroenterol* 1978; **69**: 63–69.

98. Pais P. A hepatitis like picture in typhoid fever. *Br Med J* 1984; **289**: 225–226.

99. Asada Y, Hayashi T, Sumiyoshi A, Aburaya M, Shishime E. Miliary tuberculosis presenting as fever and jaundice with hepatic failure. *Hum Pathol* 1991; **22**: 92–94.

100. Alvarez SZ, Carpio R. Hepatobiliary tuberculosis. *Dig Dis Sci* 1983; **28**: 193–200.

101. Essop AR, Posen JA, Hodkinson JH, Segal I. Tuberculosis hepatitis: a clinical review of 96 cases. *Quart J Med* 1984; **53**: 465–477.

102. Pottipati AR, Dave PB, Gumaste V, Vieux U. Tuberculous abscess of the liver in acquired immunodeficiency syndrome. *J Clin Gastroenterol* 1991; **13**: 549–553.

103. Hunt JS, Silverstein MJ, Sparks FC, Haskell CM, Pilch YH, Morton DL. Granulomatous hepatitis: a complication of BCG immunotherapy. *Lancet* 1973; **2**: 820–821.

104. Bodurtha A, Kim YH, Laucius JF, Donato RA, Mastrangelo MJ. Hepatic granulomas and other hepatic lesions associated with BCG immunotherapy for cancer. *Am J Clin Pathol* 1974; **61**: 747–752.

105. Proctor DD, Chopra S, Rubenstein SC, Jokela JA, Uhl L. Mycobacteremia and granulomatous hepatitis following initial intravesical bacillus Calmette–Guerin instillation for bladder carcinoma. *Am J Gastroenterol* 1993; **88**: 1112–1115.

106. Karat AB, Job CK, Rao PS. Liver in leprosy: histological and biochemical findings. *Br Med J* 1971; **1**: 307–310.

107. Chen TS, Drutz DJ, Whelan GE. Hepatic granulomas in leprosy. Their relation to bacteremia. *Arch Pathol Lab Med* 1976; **100**: 182–185.

108. Terry SI, Hanchard B, Brooks SE, McDonald H, Siva S. Prevalence of liver abnormality in early syphilis. *Br J Venereal Dis* 1984; **60**: 83–86.

109. Murray FE, O'Loughlin S, Dervan P, Lennon JR, Crowe J. Granulomatous hepatitis in secondary syphilis. *Irish J Med Sci* 1990; **159**: 53–54.

110. Sobel HJ, Wolf EH. Liver involvement in early syphilis. *Arch Pathol* 1972; **93**: 565–568.

111. Fehér J, Somogyi T, Timmer M, Jozsa L. Early syphilitic hepatitis. *Lancet* 1975; **2**: 896–899.

112. Romeu J, Rybak B, Dave P, Coven R. Spirochetal vasculitis and bile ductular damage in early hepatic syphilis. *Am J Gastroenterol* 1980; **74**: 352–354.

113. Veeravahu M. Diagnosis of liver involvement in early syphilis. A critical review. *Arch Intern Med* 1985; **145**: 132–134.

114. De Brito T, Machado MM, Montans SD, Hoshino S, Freymuller E. Liver biopsy in human leptospirosis: a light and electron microscopy study. *Virchows Archiv Pathol Anat Physiol Klin Med* 1967; **342**: 61–69.

115. De Brito T, Penna DO, Hoshino S, Pereira VG, Caldas ACPG, Rothstein W. Cholestasis in human leptospirosis: a clinical, histochemical, biochemical and electron microscopy study based on liver biopsies. *Beiträge zur Pathologie* 1970; **140**: 345–361.

116. Ferreira Alves VA, Vianna MR, Yasuda PH, De Brito T. Detection of leptospiral antigen in the human liver and kidney using an immunoperoxidase staining procedure. *J Pathol* 1987; **151**: 125–131.

117. Goellner MH, Agger WA, Burgess JH, Duray PH. Hepatitis due to recurrent Lyme disease. *Ann Intern Med* 1988; **108**: 707–708.

118. Thaler M, Pastakia B, Shawker TH, O'Leary T, Pizzo PA. Hepatic candidiasis in cancer patients: the evolving picture of the syndrome. *Ann Intern Med* 1988; **108**: 88–100.

119. Lewis JH, Patel HR, Zimmerman HJ. The spectrum of hepatic candidiasis. *Hepatology* 1982; **2**: 479–487.
120. Hassanein T, Perper JA, Tepperman L, Starzl TE, Van Thiel DH. Liver failure occurring as a component of exertional heatstroke. *Gastroenterology* 1991; **100**: 1442–1447.
121. Jariwalla A, Tulloch BR, Fox H, Kelly J, Davies R. Disseminated histoplasmosis in an English patient with diabetes mellitus. *Br Med J* 1977; **1**: 1002–1004.
122. Lanza FL, Nelson RS, Somayaji BN. Acute granulomatous hepatitis due to histoplasmosis. *Gastroenterology* 1970; **58**: 392–396.
123. Smith JW, Utz JP. Progressive disseminated histoplasmosis. A prospective study of 26 patients. *Ann Intern Med* 1972; **76**: 557–565.
124. Edmondson RP, Eykyn S, Davies DR, Fawcett IW, Phillips I. Disseminated histoplasmosis successfully treated with amphotericin B. *J Clin Pathol* 1974; **27**: 308–310.
125. Ridley DS. The laboratory diagnosis of tropical diseases with special reference to Britain: a review. *J Clin Pathol* 1974; **27**: 435–444.
126. Williams AO, Lawson EA, Lucas AO. African histoplasmosis due to Histoplasma duboisii. *Arch Pathol* 1971; **92**: 306–318.
127. Okudaira M, Straub M, Schwarz J. The etiology of discrete splenic and hepatic calcifications in an endemic area of histoplasmosis. *Am J Pathol* 1961; **39**: 599–611.
128. Weinstein L. Bacterial hepatitis: a case report on an unrecognized cause of fever of unknown origin. *N Engl J Med* 1978; **299**: 1052–1054.
129. Banks JG, Foulis AK, Ledingham IM, MacSween RN. Liver function in septic shock. *J Clin Pathol* 1982; **35**: 1249–1252.
130. Zimmerman HJ, Fang M, Utili R, Seeff LB, Hoofnagle J. Jaundice due to bacterial infection. *Gastroenterology* 1979; **77**: 362–374.
131. Lefkowitch JH. Bile ductular cholestasis: an ominous histopathologic sign related to sepsis and "cholangitis lenta". *Hum Pathol* 1982; **13**: 19–24.
132. Vyberg M, Poulsen H. Abnormal bile duct epithelium accompanying septicaemia. *Virchows Archiv A Pathol Anat Histopathol* 1984; **402**: 451–458.
133. Riely CA, Dean PJ, Park AL, Levinson MJ. A distinct syndrome of liver disease with multisystem organ failure associated with bile ductular cholestasis. *Hepatology* 1989; **10**: 739A.
134. Ishak KG, Rogers WA. Cryptogenic acute cholangitis – association with toxic shock syndrome. *Am J Clin Pathol* 1981; **76**: 619–626.
135. Weitberg AB, Alper JC, Diamond I, Fligiel Z. Acute granulomatous hepatitis in the course of acquired toxoplasmosis. *N Engl J Med* 1979; **300**: 1093–1096.
136. Andres TL, Dorman SA, Winn W Jr, Trainer TD, Perl DP. Immunohistochemical demonstration of Toxoplasma gondii. *Am J Clin Pathol* 1981; **75**: 431–434.
137. Conley FK, Jenkins KA, Remington JS. Toxoplasma gondii infection of the central nervous system. Use of the peroxidase-antiperoxidase method to demonstrate toxoplasma in formalin fixed, paraffin embedded tissue sections. *Hum Pathol* 1981; **12**: 690–698.
138. Pounder DJ. Malarial pigment and hepatic anthracosis. *Am J Surg Pathol* 1983; **7**: 501–502.
139. Lancet. Annotation: tropical splenomegaly syndrome. *Lancet* 1976; **i**: 1058–1059.
140. Daneshbod K. Visceral leishmaniasis (kala-azar) in Iran: a pathologic and electron microscopic study. *Am J Clin Pathol* 1972; **57**: 156–166.
141. Maltz G, Knauer CM. Amebic liver abscess: a 15-year experience. *Am J Gastroenterol* 1991; **86**: 704–710.
142. Dunn MA, Kamel R. Hepatic schistosomiasis. *Hepatology* 1981; **1**: 653–661.
143. Andrade ZA. Hepatic schistosomiasis. Morphological aspects. In Popper H, Schaffner F (eds): Progress in Liver Diseases, Vol. II. New York: Grune and Stratton, 1965, pp 228–242.
144. Andrade ZA, Peixoto E, Guerret S, Grimaud J-A. Hepatic connective tissue changes in hepatosplenic schistosomiasis. *Hum Pathol* 1992; **23**: 566–573.
145. Canto AL, Sesso A, De Brito T. Human chronic Mansonian schistosomiasis-cell proliferation and fibre formation in the hepatic sinusoidal wall: a morphometric, light and electron-microscopy study. *J Pathol* 1977; **123**: 35–44.
146. Grimaud JA, Borojevic R. Chronic human schistosomiasis mansoni. Pathology of the Disse's space. *Lab Invest* 1977; **36**: 268–273.
147. Lyra LG, Reboucas G, Andrade ZA. Hepatitis B surface antigen carrier state in hepatosplenic schistosomiasis. *Gastroenterology* 1976; **71**: 641–645.
148. Nash TE, Cheever AW, Ottesen EA, Cook JA. Schistosome infections in humans: perspectives and recent findings. *Ann Intern Med* 1982; **97**: 740–754.
149. Sun T. Pathology and immunology of clonorchis sinensis infection in the liver. *Ann Clin Lab Sci* 1984; **14**: 208–215.
150. Ona FV, Dytoc JNT. Clonorchis-associated cholangiocarcinoma: a report of two cases with unusual manifestations. *Gastroenterology* 1991; **101**: 831–839.
151. Hartley JP, Douglas AP. A case of clonorchiasis in England. *Br Med J* 1975; **3**: 575.
152. Acosta–Ferreira W, Vercelli-Retta J, Falconi LM. Fasciola hepatica human infection. Histopathological study of sixteen cases. *Virchows Archiv A Pathol Anat Histol* 1979; **383**: 319–327.
153. Jones EA, Kay JM, Milligan HP, Owens D. Massive infection with Fasciola hepatica in man. *Am J Med* 1977; **63**: 836–842.
154. Drury RAB. Larval granulomata in the liver. *Gut* 1962; **3**: 289–294.
155. Hagander B, Berg NO, Brandt L, Norden A, Sjolund K, Stenstam M. Hepatic injury in adult coeliac disease. *Lancet* 1977; **2**: 270–272.

156. Pollock DJ. The liver in coeliac disease. *Histopathology* 1977; **1**: 421–430.
157. Gabrielsen TO, Hoel PS. Primary biliary cirrhosis associated with coeliac disease and dermatitis herpetiformis. *Dermatologica* 1985; **170**: 31–34.
158. Fouin-Fortunet H, Duprey F, Touchais O et al. Coeliac disease associated with primary biliary cirrhosis. *Gastroenterol Clin Biol* 1985; **9**: 641–642.
159. Behr W, Barnert J. Adult coeliac disease and primary biliary cirrhosis. *Am J Gastroenterol* 1986; **81**: 796–799.
160. Hay JE, Wiesner RH, Shorter RG, LaRusso NF, Baldus WP. Primary sclerosing cholangitis and celiac disease. *Ann Intern Med* 1988; **109**: 713–717.
161. Burt AD, MacSween RNM. Liver pathology associated with diseases of other organs. In MacSween RNM, Anthony PP, Scheuer PJ, Portmann BC, Burt AD (eds): Pathology of the Liver, 3rd edn. Edinburgh: Churchill Livingstone, 1994.
162. Saint-Marc Girardin MF, Zafrani ES, Chaumette MT, Delchier JC, Metreau JM, Dhumeaux D. Hepatic granulomas in Whipple's disease. *Gastroenterology* 1984; **86**: 753–756.
163. Everett GD, Mitros FA. Eosinophilic gastroenteritis with hepatic eosinophilic granulomas. Report of a case with 30-year follow-up. *Am J Gastroenterol* 1980; **74**: 519–521.
164. Eade MN, Cooke WT, Brooke BN, Thompson H. Liver disease in Crohn's colitis. A study of 21 consecutive patients having colectomy. *Ann Intern Med* 1971; **74**: 518–528.
165. Shorvon PJ. Amyloidosis and inflammatory bowel disease. *Am J Dig Dis* 1977; **22**: 209–213.
166. Quigley EMM, Zetterman RK. Hepatobiliary complications of malabsorption and malnutrition. *Semin Liver Dis* 1988; **8**: 218–228.
167. Shepherd HA, Selby WS, Chapman RW, Nolan D, Barbatis C, McGee JO. Ulcerative colitis and persistent liver dysfunction. *Quart J Med* 1983; **52**: 503–513.
168. Haworth AC, Manley PN, Groll A, Pace R. Bile duct carcinoma and biliary tract dysplasia in chronic ulcerative colitis. *Arch Pathol Lab Med* 1989; **113**: 434–436.
169. Wee A, Ludwig J, Coffey RJ Jr, LaRusso NF, Wiesner RH. Hepatobiliary carcinoma associated with primary sclerosing cholangitis and chronic ulcerative colitis. *Hum Pathol* 1985; **16**: 719–726.
170. Mir-Madjlessi SH, Farmer RG, Sivak MV Jr. Bile duct carcinoma in patients with ulcerative colitis. Relationship to sclerosing cholangitis: report of six cases and review of the literature. *Dig Dis Sci* 1987; **32**: 145–154.
171. Blackstone MO, Nemchausky BA. Cholangiographic abnormalities in ulcerative colitis associated pericholangitis which resemble sclerosing cholangitis. *Am J Dig Dis* 1978; **23**: 579–585.
172. Wee A, Ludwig J. Pericholangitis in chronic ulcerative colitis: primary sclerosing cholangitis of the small bile ducts? *Ann Intern Med* 1985; **102**: 581–587.
173. Tsui WMS, Wong KF, Tse CCH. Liver changes in reactive haemophagocytic syndrome. *Liver* 1992; **12**: 363–367.
174. Aledort LM, Levine PH, Hilgartner M et al. A study of liver biopsies and liver disease among hemophiliacs. *Blood* 1985; **66**: 367–372.
175. Colombo M, Mannucci PM, Carnelli V et al. Transmission of non-A, non-B hepatitis by heat-treated factor VIII concentrate. *Lancet* 1985; **ii**: 1–4.
176. Hay CR, Preston FE, Triger DR, Underwood JC. Progressive liver disease in haemophilia: an understated problem? *Lancet* 1985; **1**: 1495–1498.
177. Bianchi L, Desmet VJ, Popper H, Scheuer PJ, Aledort LM, Berk PD. Histologic patterns of liver disease in hemophiliacs, with special reference to morphologic characteristics of non-A, non-B hepatitis. *Semin Liver Dis* 1987; **7**: 203–209.
178. Lefkowitch JH, Mendez L. Morphologic features of hepatic injury in cardiac disease and shock. *J Hepatol* 1986; **2**: 313–327.
179. Ludwig J, Gross JB, Perkins JD, Moore SB. Persistent centrilobular necroses in hepatic allografts. *Hum Pathol* 1990; **21**: 656–661.
180. Collins RH, Anastasi J, Terstappen LWMM et al. Brief report: donor-derived long-term multilineage hematopoiesis in a liver-transplant recipient. *N Engl J Med* 1993; **328**: 762–765.
181. Gilson TP, Bendon RW. Megakaryocytosis of the liver in a trisomy 21 stillbirth. *Arch Pathol Lab Med* 1993; **117**: 738–739.
182. Ruchelli ED, Uri A, Dimmick JE et al. Severe perinatal liver disease and Down syndrome: an apparent relationship. *Hum Pathol* 1991; **22**: 1274–1280.
183. Gocke DJ, Hsu K, Morgan C, Bombardieri S, Lockshin M, Christian CL. Association between polyarteritis and Australia antigen. *Lancet* 1970; **2**: 1149–1153.
184. Levo Y, Gorevic PD, Kassab HJ, Tobias H, Franklin EC. Liver involvement in the syndrome of mixed cryoglobulinemia. *Ann Intern Med* 1977; **87**: 287–292.
185. Misiani R, Bellavita P, Fenili D et al. Hepatitis C virus' infection in patients with essential mixed cryoglobulinemia. *Ann Intern Med* 1992; **117**: 573–577.
186. Agnello V, Chung RT, Kaplan LM. A role for hepatitis C virus infection in type II cryoglobulinemia. *N Engl J Med* 1992; **327**: 1490–1495.
187. Long R, James O. Polymyalgia rheumatica and liver disease. *Lancet* 1974; **1**: 77–79.
188. Litwack KD, Bohan A, Silverman L. Granulomatous liver disease and giant cell arteritis. Case report and literature review. *J Rheumatol* 1977; **4**: 307–312.
189. Gossmann HH, Dölle W, Korb G, Gerdes H, Martini GA. Leberveränderungen bei Riesenzellarteriitis. Arteriitis temporalis und Polymyalgia rheumatica. *Deutsche Med Wochenschr* 1979; **104**: 1199–1202.
190. Leong AS, Alp MH. Hepatocellular disease in the giant-cell arteritis/polymyalgia rheumatica syndrome. *Ann Rheum Dis* 1981; **40**: 92–95.

191. Rao R, Pfenniger K, Boni A. Liver function tests and liver biopsies in patients with rheumatoid arthritis. *Ann Rheum Dis* 1975; **34**: 198–199.

192. Mills PR, MacSween RN, Dick WC, More IA, Watkinson G. Liver disease in rheumatoid arthritis. *Scottish Med J* 1980; **25**: 18–22.

193. Mills PR, Sturrock RD. Clinical associations between arthritis and liver disease. *Ann Rheum Dis* 1982; **41**: 295–307.

194. Smits JG, Kooijman CD. Rheumatoid nodules in liver. *Histopathology* 1986; **10**: 1211–1213.

195. Thorne C, Urowitz MB, Wanless I, Roberts E, Blendis LM. Liver disease in Felty's syndrome. *Am J Med* 1982; **73**: 35–40.

196. Reynolds WJ, Wanless IR. Nodular regenerative hyperplasia of the liver in a patient with rheumatoid vasculitis: a morphometric study suggesting a role for hepatic arteritis in the pathogenesis. *J Rheumatol* 1984; **11**: 838–842.

197. Murray-Lyon IM, Thompson RP, Ansell ID, Williams R. Scleroderma and primary biliary cirrhosis. *Br Med J* 1970; **1**: 258–259.

198. Reynolds TB, Denison EK, Frankl HD, Lieberman FL, Peters RL. Primary biliary cirrhosis with scleroderma, Raynaud's phenomenon and telangiectasia. New syndrome. *Am J Med* 1971; **50**: 302–312.

199. Feldmann G, Maurice M, Husson JM, Fiessinger JN, Camilleri JP, Housset E. Hepatocyte giant mitochondria: an almost constant lesion in systemic scleroderma. *Virchows Archiv A Pathol Anat Histol* 1977; **374**: 215–227.

200. Runyon BA, LaBrecque DR, Anuras S. The spectrum of liver disease in systemic lupus erythematosus. Report of 33 histologically-proved cases and review of the literature. *Am J Med* 1980; **69**: 187–194.

201. Matsumoto T, Yoshimine T, Shimouchi K et al. The liver in systemic lupus erythematosus: pathologic analysis of 52 cases and review of Japanese autopsy registry data. *Hum Pathol* 1992; **23**: 1151–1158.

202. Gibson T, Myers AR. Subclinical liver disease in systemic lupus erythematosus. *J Rheumatol* 1981; **8**: 752–759.

203. Miller MH, Urowitz MB, Gladman DD, Blendis LM. The liver in systemic lupus erythematosus. *Quart J Med* 1984; **53**: 401–409.

204. Robertson SJ, Higgins RB, Powell C. Malacoplakia of liver: a case report. *Hum Pathol* 1991; **22**: 1294–1295.

205. Marshall JB, Ravendhran N, Sharp GC. Liver disease in mixed connective tissue disease. *Arch Intern Med* 1983; **143**: 1817–1818.

206. Chopra S, Rubinow A, Koff RS, Cohen AS. Hepatic amyloidosis. A histopathologic analysis of primary (AL) and secondary (AA) forms. *Am J Pathol* 1984; **115**: 186–193.

207. Buck FS, Koss MN. Hepatic amyloidosis: morphologic differences between systemic AL and AA types. *Hum Pathol* 1991; **22**: 904–907.

208. Wright JR, Calkins E, Humphrey RL. Potassium permanganate reaction in amyloidosis. A histologic method to assist in differentiating forms of this disease. *Lab Invest* 1977; **36**: 274–281.

209. Shirahama T, Skinner M, Cohen AS. Immunocytochemical identification of amyloid in formalin-fixed paraffin sections. *Histochemistry* 1981; **72**: 161–171.

210. Rubinow A, Koff RS, Cohen AS. Severe intrahepatic cholestasis in primary amyloidosis: a report of four cases and a review of the literature. *Am J Med* 1978; **64**: 937–946.

211. Finkelstein SD, Fornasier VL, Pruzanski W. Intrahepatic cholestasis with predominant pericentral deposition in systemic amyloidosis. *Hum Pathol* 1981; **12**: 470–472.

212. Case records of the Massachusetts General Hospital. Case 50-1987. *N Engl J Med* 1987; **317**: 1520–1531.

213. Livni N, Behar AJ, Lafair JS. Unusual amyloid bodies in human liver. Ultrastructural and freeze-etching studies. *Israel J Med Sci* 1977; **13**: 1163–1170.

214. French SW, Schloss GT, Stillman AE. Unusual amyloid bodies in human liver. *Am J Clin Pathol* 1981; **75**: 400–402.

215. Kanel GC, Uchida T, Peters RL. Globular hepatic amyloid – an unusual morphologic presentation. *Hepatology* 1981; **1**: 647–652.

216. Droz D, Noel LH, Carnot F, Degos F, Ganeval D, Grunfeld JP. Liver involvement in nonamyloid light chain deposits disease. *Lab Invest* 1984; **50**: 683–689.

217. Kirkpatrick CJ, Curry A, Galle J, Melzner I. Systemic kappa light chain deposition and amyloidosis in multiple myeloma: novel morphological observations. *Histopathology* 1986; **10**: 1065–1076.

218. Smith NM, Malcolm AJ. Simultaneous AL-type amyloid and light chain deposit disease in a liver biopsy: a case report. *Histopathology* 1986; **10**: 1057–1064.

219. Bruguera M. Liver involvement in porphyria. *Sem Dermatology* 1986; **5**: 178–185.

220. Cortés JM, Oliva H, Paradinas FJ, Hernandez-Guio C. The pathology of the liver in porphyria cutanea tarda. *Histopathology* 1980; **4**: 471–485.

221. Lefkowitch JH, Grossman ME. Hepatic pathology in porphyria cutanea tarda. *Liver* 1983; **3**: 19–29.

222. Fargion S, Piperno A, Cappellini MD et al. Hepatitis C virus and porphyria cutanea tarda: evidence of a strong association. *Hepatology* 1992; **16**: 1322–1326.

223. Herrero C, Vicente A, Bruguera M et al. Is hepatitis C virus infection a trigger of porphyria cutanea tarda? *Lancet* 1993; **341**: 788–789.

224. DeCastro M, Sánchez J, Herrera JF et al. Hepatitis C virus antibodies and liver disease in patients with porphyria cutanea tarda. *Hepatology* 1993; **17**: 551–557.

225. Klatskin G, Bloomer JR. Birefringence of hepatic pigment deposits in erythropoietic protoporphyria. Specificity of polarization microscopy in the identification of hepatic protoporphyrin deposits. *Gastroenterology* 1974; **67**: 294–302.

226. Bloomer JR, Phillips MJ, Davidson DL, Klatskin G. Hepatic disease in erythropoietic protoporphyria. *Am J Med* 1975; **58**: 869–882.
227. Bonkovsky HL, Schned AR. Fatal liver failure in protoporphyria. Synergism between ethanol excess and the genetic defect. *Gastroenterology* 1986; **90**: 191–201.
228. Pérez V, Gorodisch S, Casavilla F, Maruffo C. Ultrastructure of human liver at the end of normal pregnancy. *Am J Obs Gyn* 1971; **110**: 428–431.
229. Schorr-Lesnick B, Lebovics E, Dworkin B, Rosenthal WS. Liver diseases unique to pregnancy. *Am J Gastroenterol* 1991; **86**: 659–670.
230. Kroll D, Mazor M, Zirkin H, Schulman H, Glezerman M. Fibrolamellar carcinoma of the liver in pregnancy. A case report. *J Reprod Med* 1991; **36**: 823–827.
231. Samuels P, Cohen AW. Pregnancies complicated by liver disease and liver dysfunction. *Obstet Gynecol Clin N Amer* 1992; **19**: 745–763.
232. Kaplan MM. Acute fatty liver of pregnancy. *N Engl J Med* 1985; **313**: 367–370.
233. Burroughs AK, Seong NH, Dojcinov DM, Scheuer PJ, Sherlock SV. Idiopathic acute fatty liver of pregnancy in 12 patients. *Quart J Med* 1982; **51**: 481–497.
234. Rolfes DB, Ishak KG. Acute fatty liver of pregnancy: a clinicopathologic study of 35 cases. *Hepatology* 1985; **5**: 1149–1158.
235. Sherlock S. Acute fatty liver of pregnancy and the microvesicular fat diseases. *Gut* 1983; **24**: 265–269.
236. Riely CA. Acute fatty liver of pregnancy. *Semin Liver Dis* 1987; **7**: 47–54.
237. Schoeman MN, Batey RG, Wilcken B. Recurrent acute fatty liver of pregnancy associated with a fatty-acid oxidation defect in the offspring. *Gastroenterology* 1991; **100**: 544–548.
238. Rolfes DB, Ishak KG. Liver disease in toxemia of pregnancy. *Am J Gastroenterol* 1986; **81**: 1138–1144.
239. Rolfes DB, Ishak KG. Liver disease in pregnancy. *Histopathology* 1986; **10**: 555–570.
240. Arias F, Mancilla-Jimenez R. Hepatic fibrinogen deposits in pre-eclampsia. Immunofluorescent evidence. *N Engl J Med* 1976; **295**: 578–582.
241. Cheung H, Hamzah H. Liver rupture in pregnancy: a typical case? *Singapore Med J* 1992; **33**: 89–91.
242. Schorr-Lesnick B, Dworkin B, Rosenthal WS. Hemolysis, elevated liver enzymes, and low platelets in pregnancy (HELLP syndrome). A case report and literature review. *Dig Dis Sci* 1991; **36**: 1649–1652.
243. Barton JR, Riely CA, Adamec TA et al. Hepatic histopathologic condition does not correlate with laboratory abnormalities in HELLP syndrome (hemolysis, elevated liver enzymes, and low platelet count). *Am J Obstet Gynecol* 1992; **167**: 1538–1543.
244. Weinstein L. Syndrome of hemolysis, elevated liver enzymes, and low platelet count: a severe consequence of hypertension in pregnancy. *Am J Obs Gyn* 1982; **142**: 159–167.
245. Weinstein L. Preeclampsia/eclampsia with hemolysis, elevated liver enzymes, and thrombocytopenia. *Obstet Gynecol* 1985; **66**: 657–660.
246. Baca L, Gibbons RB. The HELLP syndrome: a serious complication of pregnancy with hemolysis, elevated levels of liver enzymes, and low platelet count. *Am J Med* 1988; **85**: 590–591.
247. Adlercreutz H, Tenhunen R. Some aspects of the interaction between natural and synthetic female sex hormones and the liver. *Am J Med* 1970; **49**: 630–648.
248. Vanjak D, Moreau R, Roche-Sicot J, Soulier A, Sicot C. Intrahepatic cholestasis of pregnancy and acute fatty liver of pregnancy. An unusual but favorable association? *Gastroenterology* 1991; **100**: 1123–1125.

GENERAL READING

Burt AD, MacSween RNM. Liver pathology associated with diseases of other organs. In MacSween RNM, Anthony PP, Scheuer PJ, Portmann BC, Burt AD (eds): Pathology of the Liver, 3rd edn. Edinburgh: Churchill Livingstone, 1994.

Ferrell LD. Hepatic granulomas: a morphologic approach to diagnosis. *Surgical Pathol* 1990; **3**: 87–106.

Lefkowitch JH. Pathologic aspects of the liver in human immunodeficiency virus (HIV) infection. In McIntyre N, Benhamou J-P, Bircher J, Rizzetto M, Rodes J (eds): Oxford Textbook of Clinical Hepatology. Oxford: Oxford University Press, 1991, pp 630–634.

Lucas SB. Other viral and infectious diseases. In MacSween RNM, Anthony PP, Scheuer PJ, Portmann BC, Burt AD (eds): Pathology of the Liver, 3rd edn. Edinburgh: Churchill Livingstone, 1994.

Sartin JS, Walker RC. Granulomatous hepatitis: a retrospective review of 88 cases at the Mayo Clinic. *Mayo Clin Proc* 1991; **66**: 914–918.

16

THE LIVER IN ORGAN TRANSPLANTATION

Orthotopic liver transplantation is now an established procedure in the treatment of severe acute and chronic liver disease, second only to renal transplantation in frequency of transplant procedures.[1] The growth of regional centres for liver transplantation has resulted in an increased demand on pathologists for their expertise in diagnosing rejection and other potential perioperative or postoperative complications. Liver biopsy remains the diagnostic "gold standard" when jaundice and allograft dysfunction develop, as biochemical tests do not adequately discriminate between rejection and other conditions that may develop in the allograft.[2] This chapter reviews the histopathological features of liver transplant rejection and other forms of disease affecting the donor liver. The concluding portions of the chapter discuss liver disease in recipients of renal and bone marrow transplants.

LIVER TRANSPLANTATION

General Considerations

Percutaneous liver biopsies are obtained as part of a liver transplantation protocol or because of clinical deterioration.[3] In appropriate settings, fine needle aspiration biopsy of the liver may also provide diagnostic information.[4] Biopsy specimens taken at the time of transplantation provide a useful baseline and give an indication of the state of the donor liver. Frozen section may be requested to exclude pre-existing disease such as fatty liver, which is associated with an increased incidence of **primary graft dysfunction**.[5] When special studies such as immunofluorescent microscopy, immunohistochemistry, *in situ* hybridization, or polymerase chain reaction are anticipated, a portion of the biopsy sample should be snap-frozen. These techniques are helpful in documenting infection of the donor liver by cytomegalovirus[6–8] or hepatitis viruses.[9–12] Discussion with the clinical team and careful review of pertinent radiographic, biochemical and microbiological findings are critical to biopsy interpretation and institution of appropriate therapy. Serial biopsies may be necessary to resolve difficult diagnostic problems.

There are many causes of allograft injury in addition to rejection (Table 16.1). For several weeks following transplantation, **functional cholestasis** may be present and must, if possible, be distinguished from the cholestasis of cellular (acute) rejection, bile-duct obstruction, hepatitis, drug toxicity and sepsis. Bile is present within hepatocytes and canaliculi. This impairment of bile flow can be explained by exposure of the donor liver to

Table 16.1. Pathological Considerations in the Transplant Liver

Graft rejection
  Hyperacute
  Cellular
  Ductopenic
Functional cholestasis
Preservation injury
Bile-duct obstruction
Thrombosis of hepatic artery or portal vein
Infections and sepsis
Drug toxicity
Recurrence of original disease
Neoplastic disease
  Post-transplant lymphoproliferative disease
  Hepatocellular carcinoma

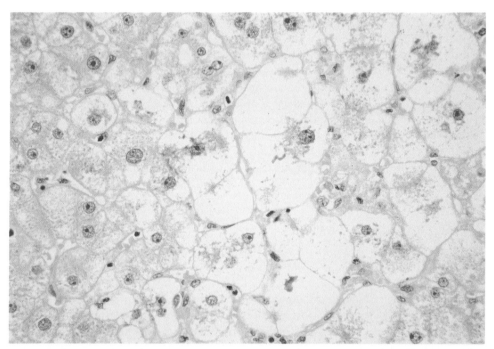

Figure 16.1. *Liver-cell ballooning after transplantation.* A liver biopsy obtained in week 2 following transplant shows ballooning of hepatocytes in a perivenular area. Intracellular cholestasis is visible. Needle biopsy, H & E.

cold ischaemia ("preservation injury") with resultant damage to liver-cell organelles.[13] Cholestasis may be accompanied by **hepatocellular ballooning** in zone 3 (Fig. 16.1) or in a diffuse distribution.[14,15] In the absence of frank zone 3 necrosis, ballooning does not confer an unfavourable prognosis.[14] Hypoperfusion liver damage in the perioperative period may result in necrosis in zones 1 or 3 and sometimes an irregular subcapsular band of infarction.[16]

In evaluating post-transplant biopsies, special attention should be paid to the portal tracts, the major sites of rejection lesions. The type of cellular infiltrate, the bile ducts, portal vein branches and hepatic arterioles are examined to distinguish rejection from other conditions with portal tract pathology, particularly **bile-duct obstruction**, **recurrent viral hepatitis**, **drug toxicity** and immunosuppression-related **lympho-**

proliferative disease (see "Differential diagnosis in transplant biopsies", p. 274). The lobular parenchyma shows few alterations in rejection apart from cholestasis, occasional acidophilic bodies and scattered liver-cell mitoses. As a result, in cases where confusion arises in the interpretation of portal changes, it is important to evaluate the lobular parenchyma carefully for evidence of intercurrent diseases such as viral or drug hepatitis.

Graft Rejection

The histopathological lesions of liver allograft rejection have been well characterized[17-26] and can be classified as **hyperacute**, **cellular** and **ductopenic rejection**. These diagnostic categories have also been applied in special circumstances such as baboon-to-human liver xenografts.[27] Cellular and ductopenic rejection are the most common forms of rejection to be encountered by the pathologist. The terms "acute rejection" and "chronic rejection" have not proven to be as applicable to liver transplantation as to other organ transplants because of variations observed in the timing of rejection episodes. These terms are used in the description below only to provide an approximate time frame for the several forms of rejection.

Hyperacute (antibody-mediated) rejection is rare after liver transplantation, developing in patients who receive ABO blood group-incompatible donor livers. Microvascular damage evolves over the first few hours after transplantation, consisting of sinusoidal infiltrates of neutrophilic leucocytes, fibrin and red blood cells associated with focal haemorrhages. This progresses to haemorrhagic infarction over the ensuing several days.[28] Immunofluorescent studies show focal IgM and complement fraction C1q deposits in arterial walls.[28] The graft may remain stable in some patients for the first few days, however, possibly because of Kupffer cell protection against the effects of circulating antibodies.[29] Graft failure within 2–4 weeks is associated with a progressive marked rise in serum aminotransferase activity. The liver appears mottled and cyanotic at gross examination.

Cellular (acute) rejection, the most common form of rejection, is a cell-mediated immune injury directed at bile-duct epithelium and the endothelium of portal vein branches, and terminal hepatic venules. This usually occurs within the first 15 days after transplantation but may be seen later if immunosuppression is lowered or discontinued. The characteristic histological **triad** of cellular rejection includes **portal inflammation**, **bile duct damage** and **endotheliitis (endothelialitis)**. Endotheliitis is not present in all cases. The portal inflammatory lesion consists of large lymphoid cells, some in mitosis, plasmacytoid cells, macrophages and neutrophilic leucocytes (Fig. 16.2). Eosinophils may be abundant (Fig. 16.3). Bile ducts are surrounded and infiltrated by immune cells and damage to their epithelium takes the form of variation in nuclear size, vacuolation of cytoplasm, regions of cell stratification or cell loss, and irregularity of duct outlines (Figs 16.2–16.4). Endotheliitis comprises attachment of lymphoid cells to the endothelium of portal-vein branches or terminal hepatic venules, variable degrees of endothelial damage and lifting off of endothelial cells from the underlying vein wall (Fig. 16.5). Vein walls may be infiltrated by lymphocytes (phlebitis). Mild focal endotheliitis is sometimes found in association with hypoperfusion damage in baseline biopsies but extensive endotheliitis in the post-operative period is very characteristic of rejection.[17]

Ductopenic (chronic) rejection is manifested as graft dysfunction unresponsive to immunosuppression which most commonly occurs 2–6 months or later after transplantation, although it can occur earlier.[26] The incidence of ductopenic rejection in liver transplant patients is of the order of 10–20%.[25,26] The diagnosis of ductopenic rejection can be problematic even for experienced hepatic pathologists.[30,31] It is morphologically characterized by **progressive loss of bile ducts** ("ductopenia", "vanishing bile duct

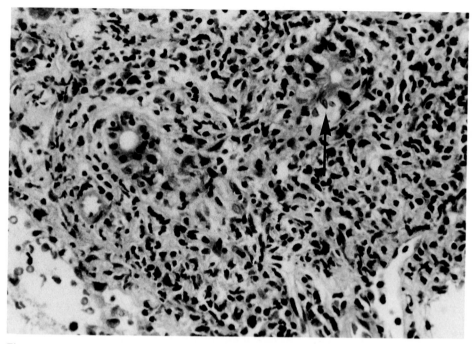

Figure 16.2. *Cellular rejection.* A damaged bile duct (arrow) infiltrated with lymphocytes is seen in a densely infiltrated portal tract. Needle biopsy, H & E.

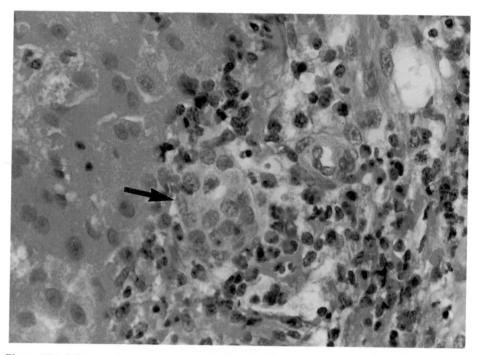

Figure 16.3. *Cellular rejection.* The portal tract infiltrate is rich in eosinophils. The bile duct (arrow) shows epithelial stratification. Needle biopsy, H & E.

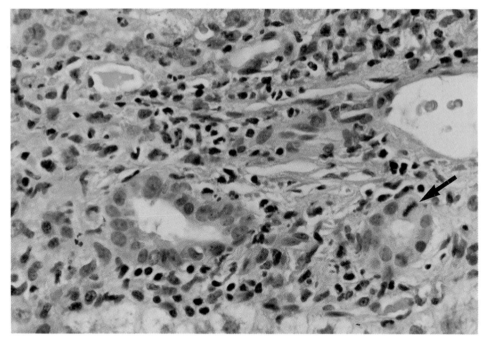

Figure 16.4. *Cellular rejection.* A damaged bile duct, cut twice in this portal tract, shows irregular epithelium with mild nuclear pleomorphism. Neutrophils are admixed with lymphocytes around and above the duct at left. The duct profile at right shows a mitotic figure (arrow). Needle biopsy, H & E. Case kindly provided by Dr Jurgen Ludwig, Rochester, Minnesota.

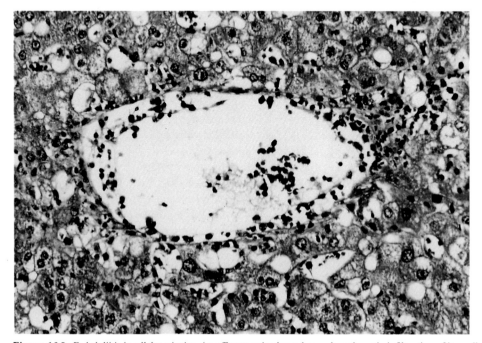

Figure 16.5. *Endotheliitis in cellular rejection.* An efferent vein shows heavy lymphocytic infiltration of its wall, with partial endothelial destruction. Needle biopsy, H & E.

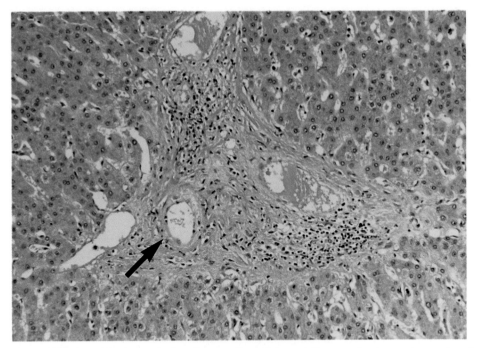

Figure 16.6. *Ductopenic rejection.* An hepatic artery branch (arrow) is present in the portal tract but the corresponding interlobular bile duct has disappeared as a result of rejection. A sparse lymphocytic infiltrate remains. Explanted donor liver, H & E. Case kindly provided by Dr Jurgen Ludwig, Rochester, Minnesota.

syndrome" [32–37]) or **loss of bile ducts in combination with obliterative arterio-pathy**[38] ("foam cell arteriopathy", "rejection arteriopathy"). Ductopenic rejection usually leads to irreversible graft failure but some patients with ductopenia may recover.[25,37]

Progressive bile duct loss results from a destructive cholangitis which in some cases stems from early bouts of acute rejection that are not controlled by immunosuppression. Over time, portal inflammation becomes sparse and bile ducts disappear from the majority of portal tracts (Fig. 16.6). Cytokeratin immunostaining may help identify remnants of bile duct epithelium and proliferating ductular structures.[25]

Rejection arteriopathy has been studied in failed grafts at autopsy or at the time of re-transplantation. Large-calibre arteries of the liver hilum typically are involved and show subintimal accumulations of foamy histiocytes and myointimal cells[38] (Fig. 16.7). Portal veins and sinusoids (Fig. 16.8) may also show foam cell lesions. The small and medium-sized arterioles present in needle biopsy specimens infrequently show foam cell change. As a consequence, the presence of arteriopathy in most cases must be inferred when zone 3 ischaemic necrosis and fibrosis are seen in liver biopsies obtained in the appropriate time frame of chronic rejection. Demonstration of perivenular necrosis in repeated biopsies indicates a poor prognosis.[39] Mismatch of recipient and donor histocompatibility antigens and persistent cytomegalovirus infection in the allograft have been invoked in the pathogenesis of bile duct loss and arteriopathy.[25,33,35,36]

Other Causes of Graft Dysfunction

Infection

Cytomegalovirus (CMV) is a common pathogen in liver allografts. Typical intra-nuclear and cytoplasmic CMV inclusions (see Chapter 15, p. 233) can be found in

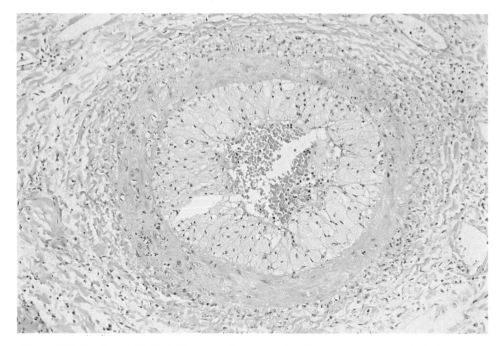

Figure 16.7. *Rejection arteriopathy.* A hilar artery from a transplant liver removed because of rejection shows an accumulation of subintimal foam cells. Explanted donor liver, H & E. Case kindly provided by Dr Jurgen Ludwig, Rochester, Minnesota.

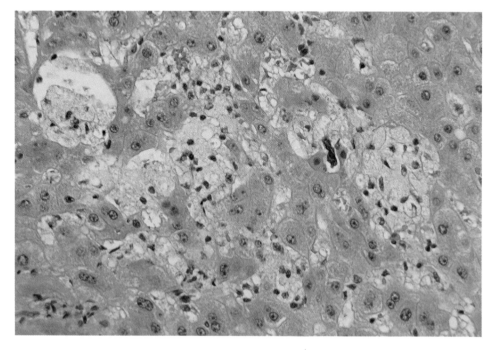

Figure 16.8. *Sinusoidal foam cells in transplant rejection.* Months after transplantation, foam cells may be deposited in large-calibre arteries and also within hepatic sinuoids. Needle biopsy, H & E.

hepatocytes, bile duct epithelium (Fig. 15.5), and endothelial cells. CMV infection should be suspected when small microabscess-like foci of necrosis with an infiltrate of neutrophilic leucocytes are present. Epithelioid granulomas may also be seen. Immunohistochemical staining for CMV antigens is a sensitive method of demonstrating occult infection.[8] **Epstein–Barr Virus (EBV)** infection should be considered if portal tracts and sinusoids contain a preponderance of atypical lymphocytes and immunoblasts.[39a]

Infection by **Gram-negative bacilli** may produce hepatocellular and canalicular cholestasis or, with sepsis, the more unusual picture of inspissated bile in periportal bile ductules ("bile ductular cholestasis" (see Chapter 15, p. 241 and Fig. 15.11). Cholestasis due to infection and/or sepsis must be distinguished from that seen in bile duct obstruction and rejection. Assessment of portal tract changes as well as results of microbiological studies are important in making these distinctions. The diagnosis of fungal and other opportunistic infections is best established by culture and special stains of the liver biopsy specimen.

Vascular Thrombosis

Thrombosis of the hepatic artery[22] or portal vein[40] (the latter particularly in children) may develop in the first 10 days after transplantation, leading to haemorrhagic infarction of the liver (see Chapter 12, p. 182). Needle biopsy specimens may not be representative owing to the irregular distribution of infarcted liver parenchyma. Thrombosis, stricture or foam cell arteriopathy of perihilar arteries may cause necrosis, stricture, or cholangiectases of perihilar bile ducts due to impaired duct perfusion.[41] Liver biopsy in such cases may show features of biliary obstruction.[41]

Drug Toxicity

The therapeutic regimen for immunosuppression in liver transplant patients includes several potentially hepatotoxic agents. **Azathioprine** hepatotoxicity has been reported primarily in renal transplant patients (see "Renal transplantation"). Elevated activities of serum aminotransferases with **sinusoidal congestion** and **zone 3 necrosis** have been described in liver transplant patients treated with the drug.[42] There may also be **fibrosis of terminal hepatic venules**, particularly in patients with cellular rejection and endotheliitis.[43] **Cyclosporin A** may cause **cholestasis**[44] by inhibition of ATP-dependent bile salt transport.[45,46] Although a similar mechanism of cholestasis obtains for **FK 506**, hepatotoxicity is rare, probably due to the lower dose of FK 506 required for immunosuppression.[47,48]

Recurrent Viral Hepatitis

Although the incidence of recurrent viral hepatitis in patients transplanted for severe liver disease due to hepatitis B, C and D varies at different transplantation centres, it is an expected outcome in many cases. There are varied histopathological expressions of **recurrent hepatitis B**, including acute hepatitis, chronic hepatitis, cirrhosis, a carrier state with minimal histological disease and fibrosing cholestatic hepatitis[49,50] (see below). Recurrent hepatitis B may evolve from chronic hepatitis to cirrhosis within a year after transplantation.[51] Hepatitis B and D (delta) antigens can be demonstrated by immunohistochemistry in allografts as early as 1–3 weeks after transplantation.[51] For patients with **co-infection by hepatitis B and hepatitis D** in the native liver, recurrence may follow a variable course. In some patients, delta virus recurs without demonstrable hepatitis B

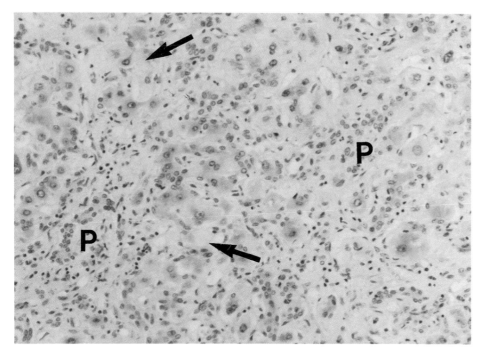

Figure 16.9. *Fibrosing cholestatic hepatitis.* Recurrence of hepatitis B virus infection in a transplant liver is associated with a network of fibrosis extending into the surrounding parenchyma from two portal tracts (*P*) and ground-glass inclusions in hepatocytes (arrows). Explanted donor liver, H & E. Illustration kindly provided by Dr Bernard Portmann, London.

virus replication (absence of HBV core antigen on immunohistochemistry) or histological evidence of hepatitis.[52] Once HBV replication recurs and core antigen is present in the allograft, chronic hepatitis may then be seen on biopsy.[53] A minority of patients with recurrent hepatitis B infection may show a **fibrosing cholestatic hepatitis** with large numbers of ground-glass inclusions, "cytopathic" liver-cell ballooning, cholestasis and a network of periportal fibrosis[50,54–58] (Figs 16.9 and 16.10). This pattern of disease recurrence is associated with a high rate of graft failure. **Hepatitis C**, either recurrent or acquired through blood transfusion or the donor liver, may result in lymphoid aggregates in portal tracts and other characteristic features[11,12] (see Chapter 9, p. 127). Recurrent hepatitis C in the allograft is often mild.[11]

Recurrent Primary Biliary Cirrhosis

Following transplantation for primary biliary cirrhosis (PBC), serum anti-mitochondrial antibodies may persist or recur, liver function tests (particularly serum alkaline phosphatase activity) may worsen and liver biopsy may demonstrate recurrent damage to bile ducts.[59,60,60a] Florid bile duct lesions and adjacent epithelioid granulomas are the most useful histological signs of recurrent disease. Bile ductular proliferation and progressive copper deposition are other helpful features. There may also be portal lymphoid aggregates and mononuclear inflammation as well as ductopenia, but these can also be seen in hepatitis C virus infection and rejection. If there is uncertainty, hepatitis C virus infection should be excluded by antibody testing and/or polymerase chain reaction. Recurrent PBC can progress to cirrhosis within several years.[60]

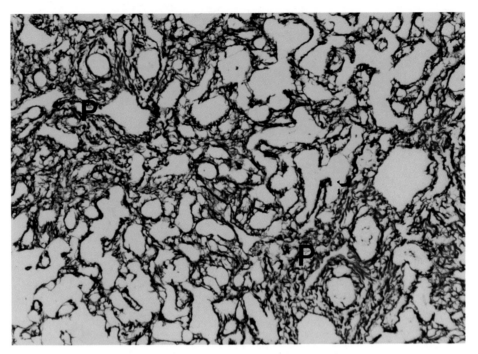

Figure 16.10. *Fibrosing cholestatic hepatitis.* Reticulin stain from the case depicted in Figure 16.9 shows an intricate network of fibrosis around portal tracts (P). Explanted donor liver, reticulin. Illustration kindly provided by Dr Bernard Portmann, London.

Neoplastic Disease

Post-transplant lymphoproliferative disease (PTLD), chiefly B-cell lymphomas in lymph nodes and extranodal sites, is a complication of immunosuppression in patients with organ transplants. B-cell lymphoma in the liver has been reported as early as 2 months after liver transplantation.[61] Lymphoma usually originates in recipient lymphoid tissue but rarely it may be derived from donor lymphoid tissue present in the allograft.[62] Hepatic involvement consists of diffuse lymphoma nodules or portal tract infiltration by lymphoma cells. *De novo*[63] or recurrent[64] **hepatocellular carcinoma** has also developed in patients transplanted for chronic hepatitis B.

Differential Diagnosis in Transplant Biopsies

Most problems in biopsy interpretation after liver transplantation arise in distinguishing rejection from other conditions (Table 16.2). It should be kept in mind that rejection and other allograft disorders can co-exist. Difficult pathological problems are usually resolved by discussion with clinicians, assessment of viral serologies and microbial culture results, and review of drug therapy. When necessary, patency of vascular or biliary anastomoses may need to be radiologically demonstrated.

While **endotheliitis** may be seen in several forms of liver disease,[65] when it is found in combination with bile duct damage and a mixed portal inflammatory infiltrate, the diagnosis of acute rejection is usually clear. **Bile duct damage** represents a more difficult histological problem, because it is a feature seen in rejection, chronic hepatitis C and PBC. Portal tract lymphoid aggregates, frequent acidophilic bodies and prominent sinusoidal inflammation support the diagnosis of chronic hepatitis C. As noted earlier, the presence of a granulomatous, destructive cholangitis in a hepatitis C-seronegative patient transplanted for PBC is important evidence of disease recurrence.

Neutrophilic leucocytes may be seen in the vicinity of damaged bile ducts in

Table 16.2. Differential Diagnostic Features in Transplant Biopsies

Histological Feature	Rejection	Recurrent HBV	Recurrent HCV	Biliary Obstruction	Ischaemia
			Condition		
Cholestasis	+/−	Unusual (except in fibrosing cholestatic hepatitis)	Unusual	Yes	No
Portal inflammation					
Mixed (L,P,N,E)*	Yes	+/−	+/−	No	No
Lymphocytes, plasma cells	+/−	Yes	Yes	No	No
Neutrophils	+/−	No	No	Yes	No
Bile duct damage	Yes	Unusual	Yes	No	No
Endotheliitis	Yes	Unusual	Unusual	No	Occasional
Zone 3 necrosis	Yes, if chronic	No	No	No	Yes
Sinusoidal inflammation	No	+/−	++	No	No
Acidophilic bodies	+/−	+	+++	No	No

+/− indicates a feature which is not characteristic, but which may sometimes be present.
* Mixed portal inflammation includes lymphocytes (L), plasma cells (P), neutrophils (N) and eosinophils (E).

rejection (Fig. 16.4) and should not be mistaken as evidence of biliary obstruction. Obstruction can usually be excluded if portal tract oedema and proliferation of bile ductules are absent. **Cholestasis** may pose significant diagnostic problems because of several potential causes, including biliary obstruction, rejection and sepsis. In biopsies obtained early (1–2 weeks) after transplantation, cholestasis is usually functional in nature. Cholestasis accompanied by portal oedema and bile ductular proliferation should prompt an assessment of the biliary anastomosis. The distinctive pattern of "bile ductular cholestasis" is usually associated with sepsis.

RENAL TRANSPLANTATION

Patients who have undergone renal transplantation are exposed to many viruses capable of causing acute or chronic hepatitis, particularly hepatitis B[66] and hepatitis C.[67] Steatosis, chronic persistent hepatitis, chronic active hepatitis and cirrhosis are often found on biopsy.[68] There may be lesions related to administration of potentially hepatotoxic drugs such as azathioprine, which may cause cholestasis, veno-occlusive disease, nodular regenerative hyperplasia and other lesions.[42,69–71] Cirrhosis develops in a small proportion of patients. Incrimination of a single aetiological agent is often difficult. Transfusions may cause substantial siderosis involving both hepatocytes and macrophages.[72,73] This can lead to cirrhosis, and therefore requires treatment. Vascular lesions following renal transplantation include narrowing or occlusion of efferent veins,[74] peliosis hepatis[75] and non-cirrhotic portal hypertension.[76] Portal hypertension associated with dilatation of sinusoids in acinar zones 2 and 3, with eventual development of fibrosis or cirrhosis has also been reported.[77]

Patients who have been treated by **haemodialysis** may have birefringent material, probably derived from silicone tubing, in portal tracts. In some instances this material gives rise to a giant-cell or granulomatous reaction.[78–80]

BONE MARROW TRANSPLANTATION

Graft recipients are liable to liver damage from graft-versus-host disease, infection and idiosyncratic drug jaundice. **Graft-versus-host disease** (**GVHD**) involving the liver has varying histological features depending on the stage of evolution.[81–83] The most characteristic features of acute (less than 90 days after transplant) GVHD are **bile duct damage** and **cholestasis**.[81,82] The duct epithelium becomes irregular, with vacuolated or acidophilic cytoplasm, nuclear pleomorphism and multilayering, and increased nuclear–cytoplasmic ratio[81,84] (Fig. 16.11). Lymphocytes infiltrate the portal tracts and duct epithelium, but are sparse. In early GVHD (less than 35 days), duct changes are less apparent and numerous parenchymal acidophilic bodies may be present.[81] Histological features of GVHD resemble those seen in hepatitis C virus (HCV) infection and serological testing to exclude HCV may be required. More severe degrees of bile duct atypia and duct destruction favour the diagnosis of GVHD over HCV infection. Other findings include endotheliitis (see "Graft rejection") and siderosis. Venous occlusion by loose or mature connective tissue is common.[85–88] In chronic GVHD (after 90 days) there is progressive bile duct dropout (ductopenia) with portal fibrosis.[81,83] The clinical and radiological picture may mimic intrahepatic primary sclerosing cholangitis.[89] Cirrhosis of biliary type may finally develop.[90] Eosinophilic cytoplasmic inclusions in hepatocytes of patients dying after bone marrow transplantation have been described.[91]

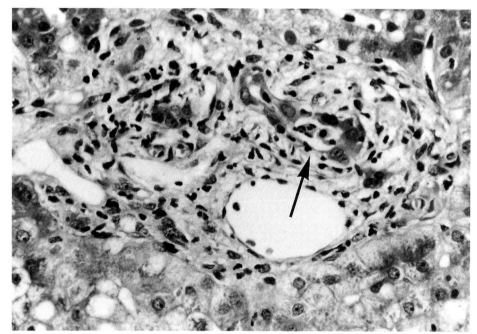

Figure 16.11. *Graft-versus-host disease.* A small bile duct (arrow) has irregular, attenuated epithelium. Inflammation is relatively mild. Needle biopsy, H & E.

REFERENCES

1. Murray JE. Human organ transplantation: background and consequences. *Science* 1992; **256**: 1411–1416.
2. Henley KS, Lucey MR, Appelman HD et al. Biochemical and histopathological correlation in liver transplant: the first 180 days. *Hepatology* 1992; **16**: 688–693.
3. Eggink HF, Hofstee N, Gips CH, Krom RA, Houthoff HJ. Histopathology of serial graft biopsies from liver transplant recipients. *Am J Pathol* 1984; **114**: 18–31.
4. Kubota K, Ericzon B-G, Reinholt FP. Comparison of fine-needle aspiration biopsy and histology in human liver transplants. *Transplantation* 1991; **51**: 1010–1013.
5. Ploeg RJ, D'Allessandro AM, Knechtle SJ et al. Risk factors for primary dysfunction after liver transplantation – a multivariate analysis. *Transplantation* 1993; **55**: 807–813.
6. Masih AS, Linder J, Shaw BW et al. Rapid identification of cytomegalovirus in liver allograft biopsies by in situ hybridization. *Am J Surg Pathol* 1988; **12**: 362–367.
7. Naoumov NV, Alexander GJM, O'Grady JG, Aldis P, Portmann BC, Williams R. Rapid diagnosis of cytomegalovirus infection by in-situ hybridisation in liver grafts. *Lancet* 1988; **1**: 1361–1364.
8. Theise ND, Conn M, Thung SN. Localization of cytomegalovirus antigens in liver allografts over time. *Hum Pathol* 1993; **24**: 103–108.
9. König V, Bauditz J, Lobeck H et al. Hepatitis C virus reinfection in allografts after orthotopic liver transplantation. *Hepatology* 1992; **16**: 1137–1143.
10. Wright TL, Donegan E, Hsu HH et al. Recurrent and acquired hepatitis C viral infection in liver transplant recipients. *Gastroenterology* 1992; **103**: 317–322.
11. Ferrell LD, Wright TL, Roberts J, Ascher N, Lake J. Hepatitis C viral infection in liver transplant recipients. *Hepatology* 1992; **16**: 865–876.
12. Thung SN, Shim K-S, Shieh C et al. Hepatitis C in liver allografts. *Arch Pathol Lab Med* 1993; **117**: 145–149.
13. Williams JW, Vera S, Peters TG et al. Cholestatic jaundice after hepatic transplantation. A nonimmunologically mediated event. *Am J Surg* 1986; **151**: 65–70.
14. Ng IOL, Burroughs AK, Rolles K, Belli LS, Scheuer PJ. Hepatocellular ballooning after liver transplantation: a light and electronmicroscopic study with clinicopathological correlation. *Histopathology* 1991; **18**: 323–330.
15. Goldstein NS, Hart J, Lewin KJ. Diffuse hepatocyte ballooning in liver biopsies from orthotopic liver transplant patients. *Histopathology* 1991; **18**: 331–338.
16. Russo PA, Yunis EJ. Subcapsular hepatic necrosis in orthotopic liver allografts. *Hepatology* 1986; **6**: 708–713.
17. Snover DC, Sibley RK, Freese DK, Sharp HL, Bloomer JR, Najarian JS. Orthotopic liver transplantation: a pathological study of 63 serial liver biopsies from 17 patients with special reference to the diagnostic features and natural history of rejection. *Hepatology* 1984; **4**: 1212–1222.
18. Demetris AJ, Lasky S, Van Thiel DH, Starzl TE, Dekker A. Pathology of hepatic transplantation: A review

of 62 adult allograft recipients immunosuppressed with a cyclosporine/steroid regimen. *Am J Pathol* 1985; **118**: 151–161.

19. Ray RA, Lewin KJ, Colonna J, Goldstein LI, Busuttil RW. The role of liver biopsy in evaluating acute allograft dysfunction following liver transplantation: a clinical histologic correlation of 34 liver transplants. *Hum Pathol* 1988; **19**: 835–848.

20. Gouw ASH, Snover DC, Grond J et al. Acute rejection in human liver grafts: a comparative histologic study of cases maintained on azathioprine and prednisone versus cyclosporine A and low-dose steroids. *Hum Pathol* 1988; **19**: 1036–1042.

21. Kemnitz J, Ringe B, Cohnert TR, Gubernatis G, Choritz H, Georgii A. Bile duct injury as a part of diagnostic criteria for liver allograft rejection. *Hum Pathol* 1989; **20**: 132–143.

22. Hertzler GL, Millikan WJ. The surgical pathologist's role in liver transplantation. *Arch Pathol Lab Med* 1991; **115**: 273–282.

23. Colina F, Mollejo M, Moreno E et al. Effectiveness of histopathological diagnoses in dysfunction of hepatic transplantation. Review of 146 histopathological studies from 53 transplants. *Arch Pathol Lab Med* 1991; **115**: 998–1005.

24. Hubscher SG. Histological findings in liver allograft rejection – new insights into the pathogenesis of hepatocellular damage in liver allografts. *Histopathology* 1991; **18**: 377–383.

25. Freese DK, Snover DC, Sharp HL, Gross CR, Savick SK, Payne WD. Chronic rejection after liver transplantation: a study of clinical, histopathological and immunological features. *Hepatology* 1991; **13**: 882–891.

26. Wiesner RH, Ludwig J, Krom RAF, Hay JE, van Hoek B. Hepatic allograft rejection: new developments in terminology, diagnosis, prevention, and treatment. *Mayo Clin Proc* 1993; **68**: 69–79.

27. Starzl TE, Fung J, Tzakis A et al. Baboon-to-human liver transplantation. *Lancet* 1993; **341**: 65–71.

28. Demetris AJ, Jaffe R, Tzakis A et al. Antibody-mediated rejection of human orthotopic liver allografts. A study of liver transplantation across ABO blood group barriers. *Am J Pathol* 1988; **132**: 489–502.

29. Wardle EN. Kupffer cells and their function. *Liver* 1987; **7**: 63–75.

30. Demetris AJ, Belle SH, Hart J et al. Intraobserver and interobserver variation in the histopathological assessment of liver allograft rejection. *Hepatology* 1991; **14**: 751–755.

31. Thung SN, Gerber MA. Histological features of liver allograft rejection: do you see what I see? *Hepatology* 1991; **14**: 949–951.

32. Ludwig J, Wiesner RH, Batts KP, Perkins JD, Krom RAF. The acute vanishing bile duct syndrome (acute irreversible rejection) after orthotopic liver transplantation. *Hepatology* 1987; **7**: 476–483.

33. Arnold JC, Portmann BC, O'Grady JG, Naoumov NV, Alexander GJM, Williams R. Cytomegalovirus infection persists in the liver graft in the vanishing bile duct syndrome. *Hepatology* 1992; **16**: 285–292.

34. Wright TL. Cytomegalovirus infection and vanishing bile duct syndrome: culprit or innocent bystander? *Hepatology* 1992; **16**: 494–496.

35. Donaldson PT, Alexander GJM, O'Grady J et al. Evidence for an immune response to HLA Class I antigens in the vanishing-bileduct syndrome after liver transplantation. *Lancet* 1987; **1**: 945–948.

36. O'Grady JG, Alexander GJM, Sutherland S et al. Cytomegalovirus infection and donor/recipient HLA antigens: interdependent co-factors in pathogenesis of vanishing bileduct syndrome after liver transplantation. *Lancet* 1988; **2**: 302–305.

37. Hubscher SG, Buckels JAC, Elias E, McMaster P, Neuberger J. Vanishing bile-duct syndrome following liver transplantation – is it reversible? *Transplantation* 1991; **51**: 1004–1010.

38. Liu G, Butany J, Wanless IR, Cameron R, Greig P, Levy G. The vascular pathology of human hepatic allografts. *Hum Pathol* 1993; **24**: 182–188.

39. Ludwig J, Gross JB, Perkins JD, Moore SB. Persistent centrilobular necroses in hepatic allografts. *Hum Pathol* 1990; **21**: 656–661.

39a. Alshak NS, Jimenez AM, Gedebou M et al. Epstein–Barr virus infection in liver transplantation patients: correction of histopathology and semiquantitative Epstein–Barr virus-DNA recovery using polymerase chain reaction. *Hum Pathol* 1993; **24**: 1306–1312.

40. Harper PL, Edgar PR, Luddington RJ et al. Protein C deficiency and portal thrombosis in liver transplantation in children. *Lancet* 1988; **2**: 924–927.

41. Ludwig J, Batts KP, MacCarty RL. Ischemic cholangitis in hepatic allografts. *Mayo Clin Proc* 1992; **67**: 519–526.

42. Sterneck M, Wiesner R, Ascher N et al. Azathioprine hepatotoxicity after liver transplantation. *Hepatology* 1991; **14**: 806–810.

43. Dhillon AP, Burroughs AK, Hudson M, Shah N, Rolles K, Scheuer PJ. Hepatic venular stenosis after orthotopic liver transplantation. *Hepatology* 1994; **19**: 106–11.

44. Gulbis B, Adler M, Ooms HA, Desmet JM, Leclerc JL, Primo G. Liver-function studies in heart-transplant recipients treated with cyclosporin A. *Clin Chem* 1988; **34**: 1772–1774.

45. Kadmon M, Klünemann C, Böhme M et al. Inhibition by Cyclosporin A of adenosine triphosphate-dependent transport from the hepatocyte into bile. *Gastroenterology* 1993; **104**: 1507–1514.

46. Arias IM. Cyclosporin, the biology of the bile canaliculus, and cholestasis. *Gastroenterology* 1993; **104**: 1558–1560.

47. Thomson AW. FK-506 enters the clinic. *Immunol Today* 1990; **11**: 35–36.

48. Fung JJ, Todo S, Tzakis A et al. Current status of FK 506 in liver transplantation. *Transplant Proc* 1991; **23**: 1902–1905.

49. Walker N, Apel R, Kerlin P et al. Hepatitis B virus infection in liver allografts. *Am J Surg Pathol* 1993; **17**: 666–677.

50. Lucey MR, Graham DM, Martin P et al. Recurrence of hepatitis B and delta hepatitis after orthotopic liver transplantation. *Gut* 1992; **33**: 1390–1396.

51. ten Kate FJW, Schalm SW, Willemse PJA, Blok APR, Heijtink RA, Terpstra OT. Course of hepatitis B and D virus infection in auxiliary liver grafts in hepatitis B-positive patients. A light-microscopic and immunohistochemical study. *J Hepatol* 1992; **14**: 168–175.

52. Ottobrelli A, Marzano A, Smedile A et al. Patterns of hepatitis delta virus reinfection and disease in liver transplantation. *Gastroenterology* 1991; **101**: 1649–1655.

53. David E, Rahier J, Pucci A et al. Recurrence of hepatitis D (delta) in liver transplants: histopathological aspects. *Gastroenterology* 1993; **104**: 1122–1128.

54. Davies SE, Portmann BC, O'Grady JG et al. Hepatic histological findings after transplantation for chronic hepatitis B virus infection, including a unique pattern of fibrosing cholestatic hepatitis. *Hepatology* 1991; **13**: 150–157.

55. O'Grady JG, Smith HM, Davies SE et al. Hepatitis B virus reinfection after orthotopic liver transplantation. Serological and clinical implications. *J Hepatol* 1992; **14**: 104–111.

56. Benner KG, Lee RG, Keeffe EB, Lopez RR, Sasaki AW, Pinson CW. Fibrosing cytolytic liver failure secondary to recurrent hepatitis B after liver transplantation. *Gastroenterology* 1992; **103**: 1307–1312.

57. Lau JYN, Bain VG, Davies SE et al. High-level expression of hepatitis B viral antigens in fibrosing cholestatic hepatitis. *Gastroenterology* 1992; **102**: 956–962.

58. Phillips MJ, Cameron R, Flowers MA et al. Post-transplant recurrent hepatitis B viral liver disease. Viral-burden, steatoviral, and fibroviral hepatitis B. *Am J Pathol* 1992; **140**: 1295–1308.

59. Wong PYN, Portmann B, O'Grady JG et al. Recurrence of primary biliary cirrhosis after liver transplantation following FK506-based immunosuppression. *J Hepatol* 1993; **17**: 284–287.

60. Hubscher SG, Elias E, Buckels JAC, Mayer AD, McMaster P, Neuberger JM. Primary biliary cirrhosis. Histological evidence of disease recurrence after liver transplantation. *J Hepatol* 1993; **18**: 173–184.

60a. Balan V, Batts KP, Porayko MK et al. Histological evidence for recurrence of primary biliary cirrhosis after liver transplantation. *Hepatology* 1993; **18**: 1392–1398.

61. Palazzo JP, Lundquist K, Mitchell D et al. Rapid development of lymphoma following liver transplantation in a recipient with hepatitis B and primary hemochromatosis. *Am J Gastroenterol* 1991; **88**: 102–104.

62. Spiro IJ, Yandell DW, Li C et al. Brief report: lymphoma of donor origin occurring in the porta hepatis of a transplanted liver. *N Engl J Med* 1993; **329**: 27–29.

63. Luketic VA, Shiffman ML, McCall JB, Posner MP, Mills AS, Carithers RL. Primary hepatocellular carcinoma after orthotopic liver transplantation for chronic hepatitis B infection. *Ann Intern Med* 1991; **114**: 212–213.

64. McPeake JR, O'Grady JG, Zaman S et al. Liver transplantation for primary hepatocellular carcinoma: tumor size and number determine outcome. *J Hepatol* 1993; **18**: 226–234.

65. Nonomura A, Mizukami Y, Matsubara F, Kobayashi K. Clinicopathological study of lymphocyte attachment to endothelial cells (endothelialitis) in various liver diseases. *Liver* 1991; **11**: 78–88.

66. Degos F, Degott C. Hepatitis in renal transplant recipients. *J Hepatol* 1989; **9**: 114–123.

67. Chan T-M, Lok ASF, Cheng IKP, Chan RT. A prospective study of hepatitis C virus infection among renal transplant recipients. *Gastroenterology* 1993; **104**: 862–868.

68. Rao KV, Anderson WR, Kasiske BL, Dahl DC. Value of liver biopsy in the evaluation and management of chronic liver disease in renal transplant recipients. *Am J Med* 1993; **94**: 241–250.

69. Sopko J, Anuras S. Liver disease in renal transplant recipients. *Am J Med* 1978; **64**: 139–146.

70. Ware AJ, Luby JP, Hollinger B et al. Etiology of liver disease in renal-transplant patients. *Ann Intern Med* 1979; **91**: 364–371.

71. Weir MR, Kirkman RL, Strom TB, Tilney NL. Liver disease in recipients of long-functioning renal allografts. *Kidney Int* 1985; **28**: 839–844.

72. Rao KV, Anderson WR. Hemosiderosis: an unrecognized complication in renal allograft recipients. *Transplantation* 1982; **33**: 115–117.

73. Rao KV, Anderson WR. Hemosiderosis and hemochromatosis in renal transplant recipients. Clinical and pathological features, diagnostic correlations, predisposing factors, and treatment. *Am J Nephrol* 1985; **5**: 419–430.

74. Marubbio AT, Danielson B. Hepatic veno-occlusive disease in a renal transplant patient receiving azathioprine. *Gastroenterology* 1975; **69**: 739–743.

75. Degott C, Rueff B, Kreis H, Duboust A, Potet F, Benhamou JP. Peliosis hepatis in recipients of renal transplants. *Gut* 1978; **19**: 748–753.

76. Nataf C, Feldmann G, Lebrec D, Degott C, Descamps JM, Rueff B. Idiopathic portal hypertension (perisinusoidal fibrosis) after renal transplantation. *Gut* 1979; **20**: 531–537.

77. Gerlag PG, Lobatto S, Driessen WM et al. Hepatic sinusoidal dilatation with portal hypertension during azathioprine treatment after kidney transplantation. *J Hepatol* 1985; **1**: 339–348.

78. Krempien B, Bommer J, Ritz E. Foreign body giant cell reaction in lungs, liver and spleen. A complication of long term haemodialysis. *Virchows Archiv A Pathol Anat Histol* 1981; **392**: 73–80.

79. Leong AS, Disney AP, Gove DW. Refractile particles in liver of haemodialysis patients. *Lancet* 1981; **1**: 889–890.

80. Parfrey PS, O'Driscoll JB, Paradinas FJ. Refractile material in the liver of haemodialysis patients. *Lancet* 1981; **1**: 1101–1102.

81. Shulman HM, Sharma P, Amos D, Fenster LF, McDonald GB. A coded histologic study of hepatic graft-versus-host disease after human bone marrow transplantation. *Hepatology* 1988; **8**: 463–470.

82. McDonald GB, Shulman HM, Sullivan KM, Spencer GD. Intestinal and hepatic complications of human bone marrow transplantation. Part I. *Gastroenterology* 1986; **90**: 460–477.

83. McDonald GB, Shulman HM, Sullivan KM, Spencer GD. Intestinal and hepatic complications of human bone marrow transplantation. Part II. *Gastroenterology* 1986; **90**: 770–784.

84. Snover DC, Weisdorf SA, Ramsay NK, McGlave P, Kersey JH. Hepatic graft versus host disease: a study of the predictive value of liver biopsy in diagnosis. *Hepatology* 1984; **4**: 123–130.

85. Berk PD, Popper H, Krueger GR, Decter J, Herzig G, Graw RG Jr. Veno-occlusive disease of the liver after allogeneic bone marrow transplantation: possible association with graft-versus-host disease. *Ann Intern Med* 1979; **90**: 158–164.

86. Sloane JP, Farthing MJ, Powles RL. Histopathological changes in the liver after allogeneic bone marrow transplantation. *J Clin Pathol* 1980; **33**: 344–350.

87. Farthing MJ, Clark ML, Sloane JP, Powles RL, McElwain TJ. Liver disease after bone marrow transplantation. *Gut* 1982; **23**: 465–474.

88. McDonald GB, Sharma P, Matthews DE, Shulman HM, Thomas ED. Venocclusive disease of the liver after bone marrow transplantation: diagnosis, incidence, and predisposing factors. *Hepatology* 1984; **4**: 116–122.

89. Geubel AP, Cnudde A, Ferrant A, Latinne D, Rahier J. Diffuse biliary tract involvement mimicking primary sclerosing cholangitis after bone marrow transplantation. *J Hepatol* 1990; **10**: 23–28.

90. Knapp AB, Crawford JM, Rappeport JM, Gollan JL. Cirrhosis as a consequence of graft-versus-host disease. *Gastroenterology* 1987; **92**: 513–519.

91. Zubair I, Herrera GA, Pretlow TG, Roper M, Zornes SL. Cytoplasmic inclusions in hepatocytes of bone marrow transplant patients: light and electron microscopic characterization. *Am J Clin Pathol* 1985; **83**: 65–68.

GENERAL READING

Hertzler GL, Millikan WJ. The surgical pathologist's role in liver transplantation. *Arch Pathol Lab Med* 1991; **115**: 273–282.

Ludwig J, Batts KP. Transplantation pathology, including liver injury in graft versus host disease and in recipients of renal and other allografts. In MacSween RNM, Anthony PP, Scheuer PJ, Portmann BC, Burt AD (eds): Pathology of the Liver, 3rd edn. Edinburgh: Churchill Livingstone, 1994.

Wiesner RH, Ludwig J, Krom RAF, Hay JE, van Hoek B. Hepatic allograft rejection: new developments in terminology, diagnosis, prevention, and treatment. *Mayo Clin Proc* 1993; **68**: 69–79.

17

ELECTRON MICROSCOPY AND OTHER TECHNIQUES

During the past decade, traditional diagnostic histopathology has emerged as a hybrid species, with routine light microscopy now linked to an increasingly varied repertoire of immunohistochemical stains, electron microscopy, computer-driven analytical techniques and molecular diagnostic methods. The polymerase chain reaction, flow cytometry and confocal laser scanning microscopy are only a few of the more recent techniques which have augmented the diagnostic and research potential of liver tissue obtained by biopsy, at autopsy or from explanted livers at the time of orthotopic transplantation. While many of the newer procedures are primarily used in research, some have already had an impact on daily practice, as, for example, in using the polymerase chain reaction to evaluate the effects of interferon therapy in chronic viral hepatitis on liver tissue expression of hepatitis C viral RNA.

This chapter will focus primarily on the role of transmission electron microscopy in the assessment of liver ultrastructure and disease. It also describes, in brief, the principles and uses of newer methodologies. While some of these are not universally available in pathology departments, other departments at one's institution or at other centres of investigation may be consulted in cases of particular diagnostic or research interest. In considering some of these procedures there should be careful advance planning for optimal processing of the specimen. Brief guidelines for preparing liver tissue are shown in Table 17.1. Procedures for fixation and processing for transmission electron microscopy are outlined in the chapter's Appendix. Additional details are provided in the references listed at the end of the chapter.

ELECTRON MICROSCOPY OF LIVER BIOPSIES

Transmission electron microscopy (TEM) continues to provide important information about the normal cellular and extracellular constituents of the liver and their alterations in disease. Recent interest in the relationships between the various sinusoidal cells of the liver has benefited from TEM studies.[1,2] Similarly, since the advent of the acquired immune deficiency syndrome, electron microscopy of hepatic and intestinal biopsy material has been critical in identifying "new" pathogens such as cryptosporidia and microsporidia. Data from standard TEM studies can be enhanced by the application of immunohistochemical stains (see "Immunoelectron microscopy"), digitized three-dimensional computer reconstructions[3,4] and morphometry. Transmission electron microscopy is sometimes limited by the lack of specificity of certain ultrastructural changes and the

Table 17.1. Liver Tissue Processing for Various Techniques

Technique	Tissue Preparation
Transmission electron microscopy	Glutaraldehyde fixation
Scanning electron microscopy	Perfusion-fixation; critical point drying; coating with gold or platinum
Immunoelectron microscopy	Glutaraldehyde/paraformaldehyde fixation
Immunoperoxidase of paraffin sections	Fixation in 10% neutral formalin or alternative fixative
Immunoperoxidase and immunofluorescence of frozen sections	Snap-freeze after embedding in OCT compound
In situ hybridization	Snap-freeze after embedding in OCT compound
Flow cytometry	Fresh tissue
Confocal laser scan microscopy	Snap-freeze after embedding in OCT compound

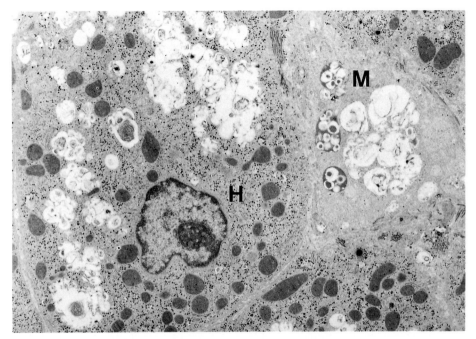

Figure 17.1. *Liver tissue from a patient with Niemann–Pick disease.* Macrophages (*M*) and hepatocytes (*H*) contain abundant vacuoles in which there are lamellar lipid inclusions. Needle biopsy, lead citrate, × 4600.

problem of sampling error in lesions that may not be uniformly distributed. The first of these limitations is well illustrated in cholestasis; various features of cholestasis such as loss of canalicular microvilli are easily recognized under the electron microscope but many causes produce these changes. Sampling error can sometimes be reduced by the combination of light and electron microscopy in a single instrument.[5]

In diagnostic work TEM should be considered seriously under five circumstances:

1. *To establish the nature of an inborn error of metabolism.* In a number of storage diseases the ultrastructural changes are diagnostic or give an indication of the type of disease to be considered.[6,7] Specific features are seen, for example, in type II glycogenosis, in Gaucher's disease and in Niemann–Pick disease (Fig. 17.1). Storage diseases can and should often be diagnosed by other, usually biochemical methods but even then electron microscopy can reduce the period of investigation by drawing attention to a likely diagnosis. Electron microscopy may show whether a liver-cell pigment is lipofuscin or the pigment of the Dubin–Johnson syndrome (Fig. 17.2), and can

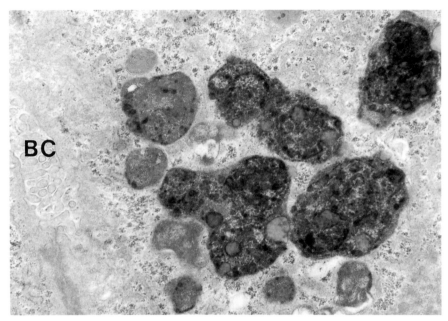

Figure 17.2. *Dubin–Johnson syndrome.* Large, characteristically complex dense bodies are seen near a bile canaliculus *(BC)*. Needle biopsy, lead citrate, × 18,900.

therefore be helpful when this syndrome is suspected but not fully proved by light microscopy.[8] In some patients with Wilson's disease characteristic changes may be seen in liver-cell mitochondria (see below).

2. *To establish the presence of viral infection.* Electron microscopy of liver biopsies may prove to be important when serological test results or cultures for suspected viral infection are unavailable or incomplete. Both intranuclear and intracytoplasmic virions may be identified by the appearances of their spherical or hexagonal capsids, dense core material, surface envelopes and paracrystalline and lattice-like arrays. These features can be compared to published micrographs for identification of the candidate virion.[9,10] For example, some adult patients with the unusual finding of giant-cell hepatitis on routine light microscopy have been shown to have paramyxovirus-like particles in the liver as a result of electron microscopic studies of biopsy material.[11] Glutaraldehyde fixation of biopsy specimens is preferred, but viral particles can also be identified in formalin-fixed tissues which are washed and then processed for electron microscopy.

3. *To establish the nature of a tumour of doubtful histogenesis.* The ultrastructural features of many tumours, including neuroendocrine tumours and malignant melanomas, help in making a firm diagnosis. The more obvious features such as neurosecretory granules in neuroendocrine tumours survive paraffin embedding; re-embedding of paraffin material for electron microscopy should therefore be considered.

4. *To establish the presence of specific drug-related changes.* In liver damage due to a small number of drugs, including perhexiline maleate[12] and amiodarone[13–16] hepatocytes contain lysosomes filled with lamellar phospholipid material (Fig. 17.3).

5. *To provide material for research.* Electron microscopy offers wide potential for research into human liver disease and it may be that future research will increase the diagnostic value of electron microscopy in this field. If liver biopsy is performed in a patient having a disease with potentially helpful or interesting ultrastructural features, small pieces of the specimen can be embedded for electron microscopy and stored indefinitely in block form. The extent to which this is done clearly depends on the resources of the particular laboratory.

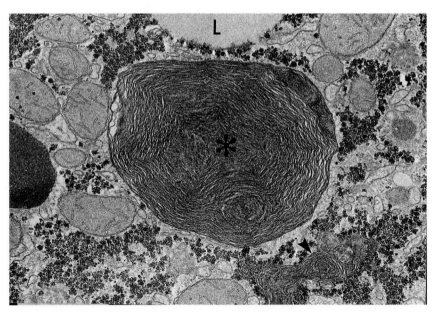

Figure 17.3. *Amiodarone-induced phospholipidosis.* An enlarged lysosome (asterisk), resembling a myelin figure, contains densely packed, concentrically arranged osmiophilic lipids, thought to represent drug-lipid complexes. A smaller membranous whorl (arrowhead) is seen in the cytoplasm. L = lipid. Illustration kindly provided by Dr S. Poucell and Professor M.J. Phillips, Toronto. Ferrocyanide, × 38,000.

Whenever electron microscopy of a liver biopsy specimen is considered, the laboratory should be contacted beforehand and arrangements made for collection and fixation of the specimen at the bedside. Proper processing of the tissue, including optimal fixation, provides the basis for accurate analysis of ultrastructural changes. The methods for appropriate fixation and processing of tissue specimens for transmission electron microscopy are described at the end of this chapter.

THE NORMAL LIVER AND EXAMPLES OF ULTRASTRUCTURAL CHANGES IN DISEASE

The following description of the liver under the transmission electron microscope is a general one. It should be noted that the quality of fixation will influence the appearance of cells and organelles. The letters in the description of normal liver refer to Figs 17.4 and 17.5.

Several cell types are found in the hepatic acini. The hepatocytes or parenchymal cells (PC) are separated from the sinusoidal endothelial cells (EC) by the space of Disse (SD), in which there are collagen fibres and lipocytes (LC), also known as perisinusoidal cells, Ito cells or fat-storing cells. Within the sinusoidal lumen are Kupffer cells (KC), the hepatic macrophages and large granular lymphocytes (also called pit cells) with natural killer activity.

Hepatocyte (Liver Cell, Parenchymal Cell)

Hepatocytes have similar features in different acinar zones but vary in detailed structure. For example, there are more lysosomes and mitochondria in periportal than in perivenular (acinar zone 3) hepatocytes, while the converse is true for the smooth-surfaced endoplasmic reticulum. The hepatocyte is a highly polarized cell with surfaces facing the space of Disse, other hepatocytes and the bile canaliculus. The plasma

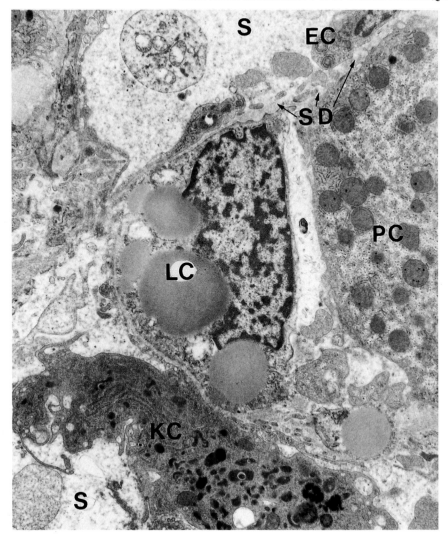

Figure 17.4. *Normal human liver.* At the edge of a liver-cell plate the parenchymal cell (PC) is separated from the sinusoidal lumen (S) by an endothelial cell (EC) and Kupffer cell (KC). LC = lipocyte; SD = space of Disse. Needle biopsy, lead citrate, × 10,000.

membrane is specialized in these three areas. Many microvilli project into the space of Disse and into the bile canaliculus. This is a potential space formed by two or three hepatocytes in normal liver, and sometimes more in disease. The intercellular membrane of the hepatocyte is relatively smooth and forms several types of intercellular junctions.

The nucleus (N)

The nucleus is normally limited by a double membrane, the nuclear envelope, which is continuous with the rough-surfaced endoplasmic reticulum. The nuclear envelope has small pores which are thought to serve as a route of communication between the nucleoplasm and the cytoplasm. Within the nucleus there is irregularly distributed chromatin, and a nucleolus is often visible.

Structural changes. Large amounts of monoparticulate glycogen are seen in some hepatocyte nuclei in diabetes mellitus, in children and also in normal subjects. In type B hepatitis, core virus particles are seen (Fig. 17.6). Intranuclear virions are also seen in infections due to cytomegalovirus, herpesvirus, echovirus and adenovirus.

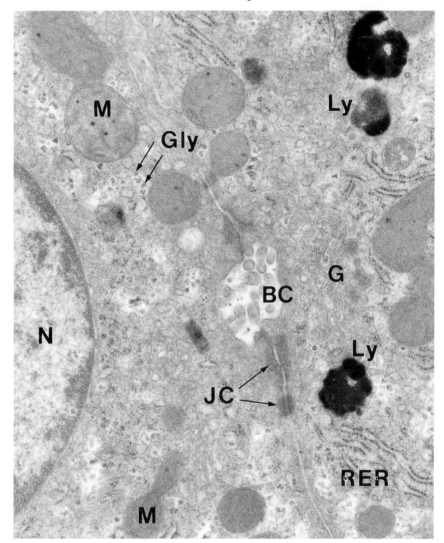

Figure 17.5. *Normal human liver.* Two parenchymal cells have formed a bile canaliculus (BC) delimited by junctional complexes (JC). Lysosomes (Ly) have varying density, the darker ones corresponding to lipofuscin as seen under the light microscope. N = nucleus; M = mitochondria; Gly = glycogen; RER = rough-surfaced endoplasmic reticulum; G = Golgi apparatus. Needle biopsy, lead citrate, × 24,000.

Mitochondria (M)

These are the sites of oxidative enzyme activity, and are involved in the metabolism of amino acids, lipids and carbohydrates. There are approximately 2000 mitochondria within the hepatocyte.[17] A smooth outer limiting membrane and an inner membrane with deep infoldings, the cristae, give the mitochondria a characteristic appearance. The inner membrane surrounds the mitochondrial matrix which contains many dense granules.

Structural changes. Cristae of atypical shape, crystalline inclusions and enlarged or unusually scanty granules are found in a wide variety of conditions, and sometimes also in normal liver. Giant mitochondria are seen most often in alcoholic liver disease[18] but are not diagnostic of alcohol excess.[19] They are frequently found in patients with systemic sclerosis.[20] In early stages of Wilson's disease mitochondria show variation in shape, increased electron density, widening of the spaces between membranes, vacuolation, enlargement of matrix granules and deposition of crystalline material[21,22] (Fig. 17.7).

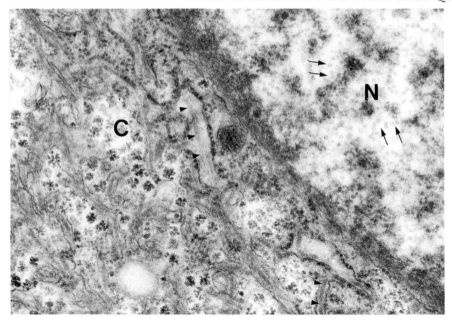

Figure 17.6. *Hepatocyte in HBsAg-positive chronic active hepatitis.* In the nucleus (N) there are numerous core particles (arrows). The cytoplasm (C) contains irregularly shaped cisternae of the endoplasmic reticulum in which there are tubules (arrowheads), the morphological *in situ* counterpart of surface antigen. Needle biopsy, lead citrate, × 45,000.

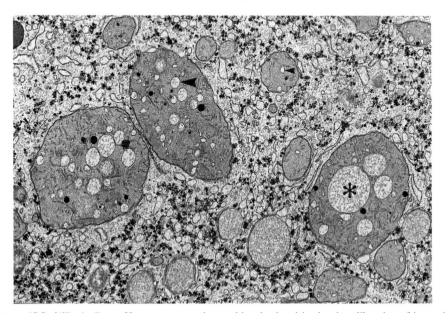

Figure 17.7. *Wilson's disease.* Hepatocyte cytoplasm with mitochondria showing dilatation of intracristal spaces (arrowheads). Some are microcystic and their contents finely granular (asterisk). Dense granules are prominent. Illustration kindly supplied by Professor M.J. Phillips and Ms J.S. Patterson, Toronto. Ferrocyanide, × 11,400.

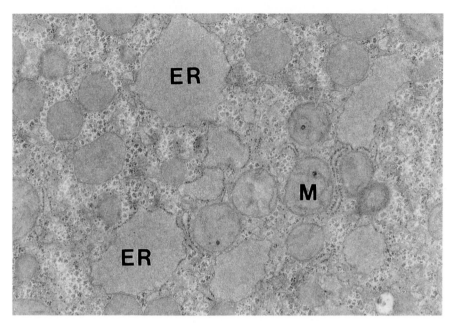

Figure 17.8. α₁-*Antitrypsin deficiency*. In this parenchymal cell the cisternae of the endoplasmic reticulum (*ER*) are dilated and filled with finely granular material. *M* = mitochondrion. Needle biopsy, lead citrate, × 16,000.

Three types of Wilsonian mitochondria are described which show intrafamilial concordance.[23] Abnormal, swollen and irregular mitochondria are found in hepatocytes in Reye's syndrome.[24]

Endoplasmic reticulum

This is an important site of protein synthesis and transport. It also contains enzymes involved in drug and steroid metabolism. Morphologically the endoplasmic reticulum is a cisternal membrane-bound system continuous with the nuclear envelope. It is the morphological counterpart of the microsomes. Two main types of endoplasmic reticulum can be recognized. The **rough-surfaced endoplasmic reticulum (RER)** is studded with ribosomes and is often arranged in a lamellar pattern. The **smooth-surfaced endoplasmic reticulum (SER)** lacks ribosomes and has a tubular or vesicular appearance.

Structural changes. Dilatation, degranulation, vesiculation and proliferation of the endoplasmic reticulum can be seen in many conditions. Some of these "changes" are also influenced by the fixation procedure, making them difficult to evaluate. Their accurate quantification requires carefully controlled processing conditions and morphometric analysis. However, in α₁-antitrypsin deficiency the dilatation of endoplasmic reticulum is striking, and finely granular material accumulates in the cisternae (Fig. 17.8). In chronic type B hepatitis the cisternae are also dilated and contain tubular structures representing the surface material of the hepatitis B virus (Fig. 17.6), and sometimes complete Dane particles.

Lysosomes (Ly)

These organelles carry many different lytic enzymes and are involved in the breakdown of proteins, carbohydrates and lipids. **Primary lysosomes** are small vesicles containing enzymes, but not yet involved in catabolic processes. **Secondary lysosomes** are membrane-bound, often irregularly shaped electron-dense bodies in which the breakdown processes take place. When undigested residues accumulate and enzyme activity is diminished, the secondary lysosomes are called residual bodies. These are the lipofuscin granules. All types of secondary lysosomes tend to be concentrated around the bile canaliculi.

Structural changes. Lysosomes accumulate iron pigment in various forms of iron overload, including genetic haemochromatosis. They can be strikingly enlarged in inborn errors of metabolism, such as Niemann–Pick disease (Fig. 17.1) and type II glycogenosis, or show characteristic changes as in the Dubin–Johnson syndrome (Fig. 17.2). Lamellar and reticular inclusions are seen within them in acquired, drug-related phospholipidosis.[12-16]

Peroxisomes

These are round or oval bodies with an even, granular matrix bounded by a single membrane. Human peroxisomes infrequently have a nucleoid, whereas this is seen in other species. They are most numerous in acinar zone 3 hepatocytes. They contain numerous oxidative enzymes and are involved in β-oxidation of long-chain fatty acids, and synthesis of bile acids and prostaglandins. Their catalase enzyme mediates conversion of peroxidase to water.

Structural changes. Peroxisomes are absent in Zellweger's syndrome (cerebro-hepato-renal syndrome).[25] In alcoholic and drug hepatitis, catalase content of peroxisomes is decreased[26] and they show irregular shapes.[26,27] Increased numbers of peroxisomes are seen in alcoholic and drug hepatitis as well as in cirrhosis.[28]

Golgi system (G)

This is a membranous system involved in excretory functions of the cell. It contains enzymes such as glycosyl transferases and is involved in glycoprotein metabolism. Morphologically it is composed of small groups of flattened sacs with associated vesicles.

Structural changes. The appearance of the Golgi system is influenced by fixation, and changes are therefore difficult to quantify, but dilatation is evident in regenerating liver and in hepatocellular carcinoma. Electron-dense liposomes accumulate in the system during the development of fatty liver.

Cell sap (cytosol)

The soluble portion of the cytoplasm (cell sap) contains variable amounts of glycogen, free ribosomes, microtubules, intermediate filaments and microfilaments. A few lipid droplets and scanty iron-containing granules are also seen.

Structural changes. Ferritin particles accumulate in iron storage disorders. Fat droplets are numerous in fatty liver, but the amount of fat varies greatly with the patient's state of nutrition. Core particles of hepatitis B virus can be identified in the cytoplasm in many cases of chronic type B hepatitis. Cytoplasmic crystalline inclusions are seen both in normal and in diseased livers. In alcoholic hepatitis, the Mallory bodies found in ballooned hepatocytes are composed of accumulations of cytokeratin and other proteins in the form of filaments (Fig. 17.9).

Bile canaliculus (BC)

The bile canaliculus measures approximately 0.75 μm and is formed by membranes of several contiguous hepatocytes which are joined by tight junctions.[29] Surface microvilli

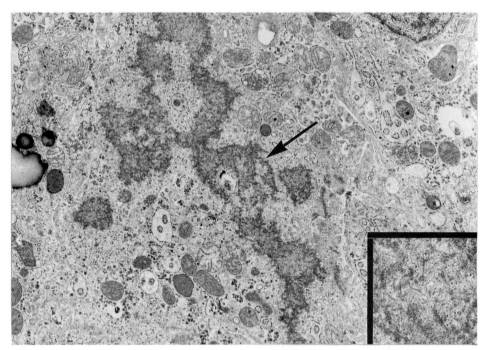

Figure 17.9. *Mallory bodies.* Irregular electron-dense material (arrow) is seen in the cytoplasm of a hepatocyte. The fibrillar nature of the material is evident at the higher magnification shown in the inset. Needle biopsy, uranyl acetate and lead citrate, × 8600 (inset × 27,000).

covered with a thin glycoprotein coat project into the canalicular lumen. Actin filaments are present within the microvilli and extend downward into a pericanalicular web also composed of actin, functioning in canalicular contraction.

Structural changes. Alterations in the bile canaliculus are similar in many forms of cholestasis. There is loss of microvilli, formation of surface membrane blebs and disorganization of the pericanalicular actin filament web. Intracanalicular bile appears as electron-dense filamentous material.

Kupffer Cell (KC)

The Kupffer cell has an irregular outline, with many finger-like protrusions of the cell surface by which it anchors to endothelial cells. It is rich in phagocytic vacuoles (phagosomes), lysosomes and mitochondria, while the endoplasmic reticulum is only moderately well developed. The nucleus is irregular in shape, with a tendency for the chromatin to be concentrated at the nuclear periphery.

Structural changes. Hypertrophied Kupffer cells can be seen in all conditions of parenchymal cell destruction (e.g. hepatitis) and in pigment overload (e.g. cholestasis, haemosiderosis). Many storage disorders affect the Kupffer cells; in Niemann–Pick disease, for example, both Kupffer cells and hepatocytes are enlarged and filled with vacuoles containing accumulated sphingomyelin (Fig. 17.1).

Endothelial Cell (EC)

This is a flattened cell with a smooth surface, showing small fenestrations which provide direct communication between the sinusoidal lumen and the space of Disse.[30] The cytoplasmic volume is relatively small. Many micropinocytotic vesicles can be seen beneath the plasma membrane.

Structural changes. In hepatitis and other conditions, endothelial cells undergo several changes, including the accumulation of iron-rich siderosomes and the formation of basement membrane material on the aspect of the cells facing the space of Disse.[31] In patients with chronic viral hepatitis and acquired immune deficiency syndrome, **tubulo-reticular structures** and **cylindrical confronting cisternae** develop within the rough endoplasmic reticulum of endothelial cells and sometimes within Kupffer cells, lipocytes (see below) and lymphocytes.[32,33] Tubuloreticular structures are reticular aggregates of branching tubules within the cisternae of the endoplasmic reticulum and sometimes the perinuclear envelope. Cylindrical confronting cisternae are cylinders of fused membranous lamellae derived from two or more cisternae of endoplasmic reticulum, one inside the other. They appear to be a result of increased endogenous levels of α- and β-interferon.

Lipocyte (LC)

This cell, also known as the Ito cell, fat-storing cell, perisinusoidal cell or stellate cell, is a major storage site for vitamin A. In liver injury, it becomes a transitional cell or myofibroblast-like cell capable of synthesizing collagen type I, III and IV as well as laminin.[34] Lipocytes are located within the space of Disse and have conspicuous rough endoplasmic reticulum, a large Golgi apparatus and large lipid droplets containing vitamin A. In alcoholic liver disease, hypervitaminosis A and methotrexate toxicity lipocytes undergo hyperplasia and are associated with increased collagen fibres within the space of Disse.

Pit Cell (Large Granular Lymphocyte)

This cell is located within the sinusoidal lumen. Its surface uropodia and pseudopodia are often in close contact with endothelial cells or Kupffer cells. The nucleus is dense, eccentrically located in the cell and indented. The cell's name derives from its characteristic electron-dense, membrane-bound granules of cytotoxic enzymes which resemble "pits" or pips in fruit. The cytoplasm contains profiles of rough endoplasmic reticulum, a well-developed Golgi apparatus, centrioles and occasional rod-cored vesicles. Pit cells function as natural killer cells and have been identified in autoimmune hepatitis and in increased numbers in livers with malignant tumours.[35]

Immunoelectron Microscopy

The principles employed in immunohistochemical staining of liver biopsy sections for light microscopy (see "Immunohistochemistry") can be adapted for use in electron microscopy.[36] Following fixation of the specimen in a mixture of glutaraldehyde and paraformaldehyde, the tissue is treated with borohydride, cryoprotected and frozen for storage. Thick sections of 20–40 μm are later cut from the thawed samples and stained by either a direct or indirect immunoperoxidase method.[37] The stained sections are then post-fixed in osmium tetroxide, dehydrated and embedded in epon. Under the electron microscope, electron-dense immunoreactive material is seen at the site of the targeted antigen.

Availability of a wide variety of monoclonal and polyclonal antibodies to tissue antigens and receptors has greatly expanded investigations of interactions of hepatocytes with immune cells and with the extracellular matrix. Intercellular adhesion molecules, histocompatibility antigens and interferon receptors are among the potential list of

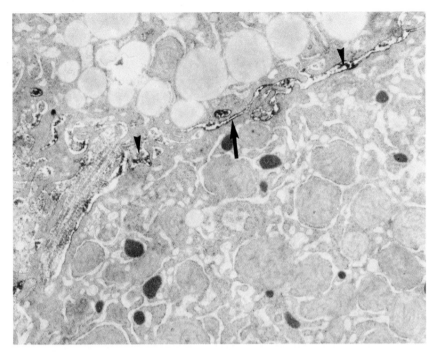

Figure 17.10. *Type A receptor for tumour necrosis factor (TNF).* A case of hepatitis B virus-positive chronic hepatitis stained with monoclonal antibody utr-1 (directed against type A receptor of TNF) shows positive staining on the membranes of two adjacent hepatocytes in a discontinuous pattern (arrow) and in the intercellular space (arrowheads). Illustration kindly provided by Drs V.J. Desmet, R. Volpes, J. Van den Oord and R. De Vos, Leuven. Immunoelectron microscopy, × 18,400.

antigens that can be studied by immunoelectron microscopy.[38–40] Examples of this technique are shown in Figs 17.10 and 17.11 which demonstrate the up-regulation of the type A receptor for tumour necrosis factor on hepatocyte membranes and in mononuclear cells in a patient with hepatitis B virus-related chronic active hepatitis.[41]

Scanning Electron Microscopy

The three-dimensional structure of the liver can be assessed by scanning electron microscopy (SEM) of specially prepared tissues,[42] or even of sections from paraffin blocks.[43] X-ray microanalysis may be combined with the scanning technique and is useful in elemental analysis. Laboratories with scanning electron microscopes are best equipped to provide details on appropriate tissue fixation, critical point drying and coating of specimens with gold or platinum. SEM is particularly useful in examining resin casts of hepatic vasculature.[44–47]

IMMUNOHISTOCHEMISTRY

Immunohistochemical techniques are now widely available in pathology laboratories and the methods for both immunoperoxidase stains and immunofluorescence microscopy are covered in standard textbooks.[37] Both direct and indirect labelling methods are used to detect antigens in liver biopsy tissue; the indirect method is the more popular and more sensitive. Important variables that may affect results include the type and duration of

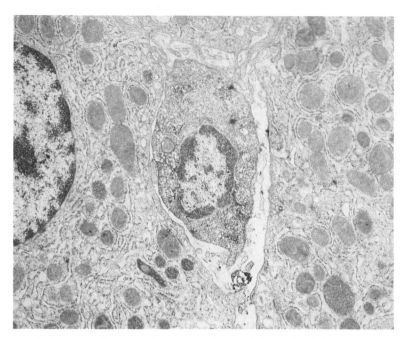

Figure 17.11. *Type A receptor for TNF.* The same case depicted in Figure 17.10 shows immunoreactivity for type A receptor for TNF in the hyaloplasm of a mononuclear cell surrounded by hepatocytes. Illustration kindly provided by Drs V.J. Desmet, R. Volpes, J. Van den Oord and R. De Vos, Leuven. Immunoelectron microscopy, × 18,400.

fixation, the vendor or other source used to obtain the antibodies and the type of label attached to the antibody for detection of the antigen. While fixation in 10% neutral formalin is acceptable for many immunohistochemical stains, some will require alternative fixatives or cryostat sections, and these factors should be considered when the biopsy specimen is initially processed.

In routine diagnostic work immunohistochemistry is helpful in four major areas:

1. *To ascertain the histogenesis of malignant tumours in the liver.* In distinguishing metastatic carcinoma from primary hepatocellular carcinoma, the former usually stains positively for epithelial membrane antigen and with the pooled monoclonal anti-keratin antibody AE1/AE3. α-Fetoprotein staining gives disappointing results in many hepatocellular carcinomas but is usually positive in hepatoblastomas.

2. *Staining for α_1-antitrypsin* (Fig. 13.14, p. 207) is important in confirming the identity of diastase-resistant, PAS-positive periportal granules in chronic hepatitis, cirrhosis and in neonatal hepatitis.

3. *Identification of bile-duct epithelium.* Biopsy specimens which show an apparent paucity of interlobular bile ducts may benefit from specific staining for biliary cytokeratins 7, 8, 18 and 19 of the catalogue of Moll.[48] Biliary epithelium that may be obscured by inflammatory cell infiltrates in drug-related hepatitis or liver transplant rejection can thereby be identified. Residual duct epithelium in segments of atretic ducts resected at the time of Kasai surgery for extrahepatic biliary atresia can also be demonstrated. Unusual patterns of bile ductular proliferation or remnants of the·bile-duct plate (Fig. 13.5, p. 199) can be studied with cytokeratin stains. AE1/AE3 pooled antibody generally gives good staining results.

4. *Localization of hepatitis B virus core and surface antigens and hepatitis D antigen.* Immunohistochemical demonstration of hepatitis B surface antigen is more sensitive than the orcein method. In addition, assessment of the distribution of core and surface antigens

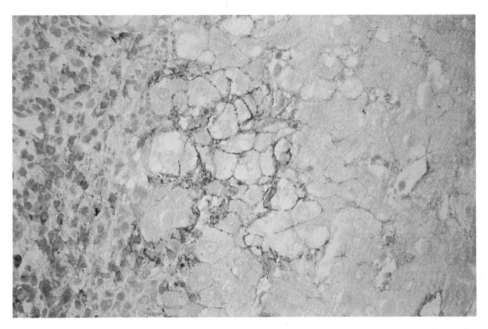

Figure 17.12. *Intercellular adhesion molecule-1 (ICAM-1) expression on hepatocytes.* Brown immunoreaction product to ICAM-1 is seen on periportal hepatocyte membranes in a case of chronic hepatitis. An inflamed portal tract is seen at left. The section was stained with monoclonal antibody 84H10 directed against ICAM-1. Illustration kindly provided by Drs V.J. Desmet, R. Volpes, J. Van den Oord and R. De Vos, Leuven.

when correlated with serum markers of viral replication and biopsy features on light microscopy usually provides a more comprehensive perspective regarding viral liver disease in any given patient. In some patients, demonstration of hepatitis D antigen by immunohistochemistry is the first evidence of delta virus infection or recurrence. Preliminary experiences with immunohistochemical staining of hepatitis C virus antigens are encouraging.[49,50]

Scientific questions of a more basic nature concerning the interaction of the immune system with the liver in various forms of injury, the composition of the extracellular matrix and factors involved in hepatocellular proliferation can be addressed with immunohistochemistry. For example, expression of **intercellular adhesion molecules** on the surfaces of hepatocytes for binding lymphocytes is of fundamental importance in piecemeal necrosis associated with chronic viral hepatitis[38] (Fig. 17.12). A histological index of liver-cell proliferation in acute and chronic liver disease can be obtained by staining for **proliferating cell nuclear antigen (PCNA)**, an intranuclear auxiliary protein of DNA polymerase-δ[51–54] (Fig. 17.13). Table 17.2 provides a basic resource list of some of the currently available antibodies for immunohistochemistry.[34,51–83]

IN SITU HYBRIDIZATION

In this technique, radioactively labelled probes for specific RNA or DNA sequences are applied to cryostat tissue sections. Biotinylated probes can also be used on formalin-fixed, paraffin-embedded sections.[84] Probes are prepared by cloning of genetic material and sub-cloning into plasmids. After preparation of the tissue sections, the probe is applied directly and hybridized. Slides treated with radiolabelled probes are then exposed to photographic

Figure 17.13. *Proliferating cell nuclear antigen (PCNA).* Liver biopsy from a patient with hepatitis C virus-related chronic hepatitis shows inflamed portal tracts at upper left and lower right. Nuclei of midzonal hepatocytes, stained with an antibody to PCNA, show brown immunoreaction product. Needle biopsy, specific immunoperoxidase.

emulsion for 1–2 weeks, resulting in a distribution of silver grains over cells containing the target RNA or DNA sequences. *In situ* hybridization is widely used in research laboratories to localize gene sequences encoding hepatic secretory proteins such as albumin and extracellular matrix proteins. One of its major applications is in the identification of viral sequences, including cytomegalovirus[84] (Fig. 1.9, p. 7), hepatitis B virus and hepatitis C virus.[85,86] The sensitivity of *in situ* hybridization can be improved by combination with **polymerase chain reaction**[87–89] (overpage).

FLOW CYTOMETRY OF LYMPHOCYTES FROM LIVER BIOPSIES

In order to immunotype lymphocytes present in liver biopsy specimens, fresh samples of liver tissue are treated with enzymatic digestion and gradient centrifugation.[90] This technique has been used to analyse lymphocyte subpopulations in various forms of liver disease, including chronic hepatitis, primary biliary cirrhosis and alcoholic liver disease.[91,92]

CONFOCAL LASER SCANNING MICROSCOPY

The confocal laser scanning microscope has been referred to as an "opto-digital microtome"[93] because of its capacity to obtain two-dimensional images from very thin optical sections of tissues or cells and to process them into three-dimensional data with digitized computer software. The primary advantages of this form of microscopy are its

Table 17.2. Antibodies Available for Studies of Liver Disease

Antibody	Reference(s)
Cell structure, synthetic products and proliferation	
Albumin	55
α-Fetoprotein	55,56
α$_1$-Antitrypsin	56
AE1/AE3 for epithelial cytokeratin	57
Cytokeratins 8 and 18 (liver-cell)	58
Cytokeratins 7 and 19 (bile-duct cell)	58
Desmin	55
Vimentin	55
Nuclear lamins	59
Proliferating cell nuclear antigen	51–54
Immune network	
Histocompatibility antigens	60–62
Lymphocyte function-associated antigen 3	63
Vascular adhesion molecules	64, 65
Tumour necrosis factor	66
Heat shock protein	67
T-lymphocyte markers	68
Growth factors	
Transforming growth factor-β	69, 70
Hepatocyte growth factor	71
Extracellular matrix and blood vessels	
Collagen type I, III, IV	34, 72, 73, 73a, 73b
Collagen type VI	74
Integrins	75, 76
Tenascin	79
Laminin	80
Factor VIII-related antigen	81
Ulex europaeus lectin	81
QBEnd10	81
Lewis blood group-related antigens	83

high resolution and **enhanced contrast**. These two advantages are obtained by using a very thin plane of focus provided by a laser light source (usually argon ion) filtered through several dichroic mirrors. The light emanating from a focal point in the specimen is imaged by back projection onto a detector pinhole aperture; the emanating light and the imaged light are in common focus, hence the name "confocal".

Following specimen fixation (usually by an aldehyde agent), one or more fluorescent reagents are used to label the specific antigen(s) under investigation. A series of two-dimensional images in a thin focal plane of approximately 0.6–1.5 μm are obtained through the confocal laser scanning microscope. These images are then aligned pixel by pixel using specific software image processing in order to generate three-dimensional data. Elements to be considered in planning confocal microscopy include the wavelength of light which the laser source can provide for excitation of the fluorochrome, appropriate stability of the antigen in tissue after fixation, mounting medium used, and type(s) of fluorochrome to be utilized.[93] Dyes with widely separated excitation and emission wavelengths are optimal, such as fluorescein (FITC) or acridine orange for simultaneous DNA and RNA staining.

This technique is versatile; one can examine protein traffic in cells, DNA of individual chromosomes and ploidy status of tumours. *In situ* hybridization can also be performed. The method has been used to localize desmin and other intermediate filament proteins in fetal rat livers.[94] An example of the application of confocal microscopy to the study of chemical hepatotoxicity is shown in Figure 17.14, from the work of Pompella and

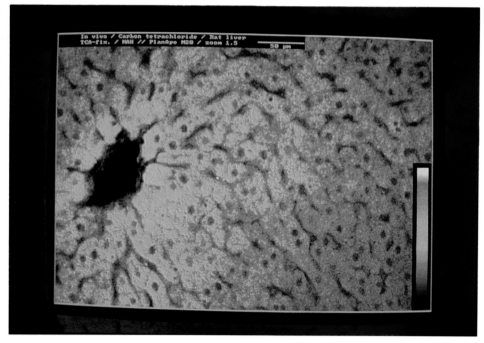

Figure 17.14. *Confocal laser scanning microscopy.* Rat liver following exposure to carbon tetrachloride. Acinar zone 3 hepatocytes at left (surrounding a terminal hepatic venule) show bright fluorescence of carbonyl species after naphthoic acid hydrazide staining. Illustration kindly provided by Dr Alfonso Pompella, Siena, Italy.

Comporti.[95] Sprague–Dawley rats were treated with intragastric carbon tetrachloride to induce acinar zone 3 (perivenular) lipid peroxidation. Degeneration of cell membrane phospholipids in affected zone 3 hepatocytes produced carbonyl species. These carbonyls were stained with naphthoic acid hydrazide, a fluorochrome, which demonstrated specific perivenular fluorescence with higher sensitivity than that available with other more routine immunohistochemical staining procedures.

POLYMERASE CHAIN REACTION (PCR)

This is an *in vitro* method of nucleic acid synthesis by which small targeted segments of DNA (or RNA) can be amplified from biological samples. The ingredients for this method include two oligonucleotide primers that complement opposite ends of each strand in the target sequence, thermostable *Taq* DNA polymerase (or reverse transcriptase, in detecting RNA) and four deoxynucleotide triphosphates (dNTPs) in a buffered solution. The DNA strands are first separated by boiling. The oligonucleotide primers are then annealed to the target DNA, after which the primers are extended by *Taq* DNA polymerase. These extension products or daughter strands are complementary to and can bind the two primers, thereby allowing repeated cycles of denaturation and amplification and an exponential (2^n) production of the target segment.[96–99]

Liver samples for polymerase chain reaction must be frozen in most instances.[100] However, extraction of nucleic acids from formalin-fixed, paraffin-embedded sections is feasible, although with far lower yield than frozen tissue.[101] PCR has wide applications in identifying hepatitis virus nucleic acids in liver tissue and in serum.

APPENDIX: FIXATION AND PROCESSING FOR TRANSMISSION ELECTRON MICROSCOPY

The tissue should preferably be processed at the time of biopsy. Optimal results are obtained by immediate immersion of fresh tissue in cold fixative of correct osmolality.[102] Results of resin embedding of tissue initially fixed in formalin are sometimes surprisingly good. It is possible to re-process material which has been embedded in paraffin for light microscopy, but structural deterioration makes interpretation more difficult.

Glutaraldehyde is currently the most widely used fixative. After primary fixation in the aldehyde, osmium tetroxide is used to achieve better membrane visualization. For immunohistochemical and many enzyme histochemical procedures, the tissue should be snap-frozen or fixed in a specialized mixture appropriate to the particular examination.

Suggested Method for the Processing of Liver Biopsies

A piece approximately 5 mm long (or several smaller pieces if sampling problems are expected) should be cut from the needle biopsy specimen and immersed in ice-cold fixative solution (solution A, below) on a sheet of dental wax. The tissue is then divided into small cubes less than 1 mm across and transferred to a larger volume of fixative. Great care must be taken not to compress the tissue, as this will cause artefacts.

The pieces should be fixed for 2–24 h at 0–4°C, and washed in at least two changes of buffer solution (solution B) for 1 h or more at 0–4°C. If the specimen is to be sent to another laboratory for processing, it is advisable to use the buffer solution as a transport medium because the tissue can be kept at this stage for many days. Dry ice or freezing mixtures should never be used because these cause unnecessary freezing artefacts. Finally, the tissue should be post-fixed in osmium tetroxide solution (solution C) for 1 h at 1–4°C before dehydration and embedding. Processing normally takes 2–3 days but the time can be reduced for urgent specimens.

Solutions for Fixation

A. *3% Glutaraldehyde Fixative*

25% purified glutaraldehyde (EM grade)	12 ml
2 M sodium cacodylate, stock solution	5 ml
2 M sucrose, stock solution	5 ml
Distilled water	70 ml
Adjust pH to 7.2 with 2 M HCl	
Distilled water	to 100 ml

This fixative will keep in the refrigerator for 1–2 weeks.   The stock solutions keep longer.

B. *Buffer Solution for Washing*

2 M sodium cacodylate, stock solution	5 ml
2 M sucrose, stock solution	5 ml
Distilled water	to 70 ml

Adjust pH to 7.2 with 2 M HCl
Distilled water $\qquad$ to 100 ml

This can be kept in the refrigerator for 1–2 weeks.

C. 1% Osmium Tetroxide Fixative

2% w/v osmium tetroxide in water
s-Collidine buffer (solution D)

Mix equal volumes immediately before fixation.

D. s-Collidine Buffer

2,4,6-Collidine	2.7 ml
Distilled water	50 ml
1 M HCl	8 ml
Adjust pH to 7.4	
Distilled water	to 100 ml

REFERENCES

1. Burt AD, Le Bail B, Balabaud C, Bioulac-Sage P. Morphologic investigation of sinusoidal cells. *Semin Liver Dis* 1993; **13**: 21–38.
2. Rieder H, Meyer zum Büschenfelde K-H, Ramadori G. Functional spectrum of sinusoidal endothelial liver cells. Filtration, endocytosis, synthetic capacities and intercellular communication. *J Hepatol* 1992; **15**: 237–250.
3. Nagore N, Howe S, Boxer L, Scheuer PJ. Liver cell rosettes: structural differences in cholestasis and hepatitis. *Liver* 1989; **9**: 43–51.
4. Nagore N, Howe S, Scheuer PJ. The three-dimensional liver. In Popper H, Schaffner F (eds): Progress in Liver Diseases, Vol. IX. Philadelphia: WB Saunders, 1989, pp 1–10.
5. Jones S, Chapman SK, Crocker PR, Carson G, Levison DA. Combined light and electron microscope in routine histopathology. *J Clin Pathol* 1982; **35**: 425–429.
6. Spycher MA. Electron microscopy: a method for the diagnosis of inherited metabolic storage diseases. Electron microscopy in diagnosis. *Path Res Prac* 1980; **167**: 118–135.
7. Ishak KG, Sharp HL. Metabolic errors and liver disease. In MacSween RNM, Anthony PP, Scheuer PJ, Portmann BC, Burt AD (eds): Pathology of the Liver, 3rd edn. Edinburgh: Churchill Livingstone, 1994.
8. Toker C, Trevino N. Hepatic ultrastructure in chronic idiopathic jaundice. *Arch Pathol* 1965; **80**: 453–460.
9. Miller SE. Detection and identification of viruses by electron microscopy. *J Electron Micro Tech* 1986; **4**: 265–301.
10. Phillips MJ, Poucell S, Patterson J, Valencia P. The Liver. An Atlas and Text of Ultrastructural Pathology. New York: Raven Press, 1987.
11. Phillips MJ, Blendis LM, Poucell S et al. Syncytial giant-cell hepatitis. Sporadic hepatitis with distinctive pathologic features, a severe clinical course, and paramyxoviral features. *N Engl J Med* 1991; **324**: 455–460.
12. Pessayre D, Bichara M, Degott C, Potet F, Benhamou JP, Feldmann G. Perhexiline maleate-induced cirrhosis. *Gastroenterology* 1979; **76**: 170–177.
13. Poucell S, Ireton J, Valencia-Mayoral P et al. Amiodarone-associated phospholipidosis and fibrosis of the liver. Light, immunohistochemical, and electron microscopic studies. *Gastroenterology* 1984; **86**: 926–936.
14. Simon JB, Manley PN, Brien JF, Armstrong PW. Amiodarone hepatotoxicity simulating alcoholic liver disease. *N Engl J Med* 1984; **311**: 167–172.
15. Pirovino M, Müller O, Zysset T, Honegger U. Amiodarone-induced hepatic phospholipidosis: correlation of morphological and biochemical findings in an animal model. *Hepatology* 1988; **8**: 591–598.
16. Lewis JH, Ranard RC, Caruso A et al. Amiodarone hepatotoxicity: prevalence and clinicopathologic correlations among 104 patients. *Hepatology* 1989; **9**: 679–685.
17. Rohr HP, Lüthy J, Gudat F et al. Stereology: a new supplement to the study of human liver biopsy specimens. In Popper H, Schaffner F (eds): Progress in Liver Diseases, Vol. V. New York: Grune and Stratton, 1976, pp 24–34.
18. Uchida T, Kronborg I, Peters RL. Alcoholic hyalin-containing hepatocytes – a characteristic morphologic appearance. *Liver* 1984; **4**: 233–243.

19. Chedid A, Jao W, Port J. Megamitochondria in hepatic and renal disease. *Am J Gastroenterol* 1980; **73**: 319–324.

20. Feldmann G, Maurice M, Husson JM, Fiessinger JN, Camilleri JP, Housset E. Hepatocyte giant mitochondria: an almost constant lesion in systemic scleroderma. *Virchows Archiv A Pathol Anat Histol* 1977; **374**: 215–227.

21. Sternlieb I. Evolution of the hepatic lesion in Wilson's disease (hepatolenticular degeneration). In Popper H, Schaffner F (eds): Progress in Liver Diseases, Vol. IV. New York: Grune and Stratton, 1972, pp 511–525.

22. Scheinberg IH, Sternlieb I. Wilson's Disease. Major Problems in Internal Medicine XXIII. Philadelphia: WB Saunders, 1984.

23. Sternlieb I. Fraternal concordance of types of abnormal hepatocellular mitochondria in Wilson's disease. *Hepatology* 1992; **16**: 728–732.

24. Tonsgard JH. Effect of Reye's syndrome serum on the ultrastructure of isolated liver mitochondria. *Lab Invest* 1989; **60**: 568–573.

25. Mooi WJ, Dingemans KP, Van Den Bergh Weerman MA, Jöbsis AC, Heymans HSA, Barth PG. Ultrastructure of the liver in cerebrohepatorenal syndrome of Zellweger. *Ultrastruc Pathol* 1983; **5**: 135–144.

26. De Craemer D, Kerckaert I, Roels F. Hepatocellular peroxisomes in human alcoholic and drug-induced hepatitis: a quantitative study. *Hepatology* 1991; **14**: 811–817.

27. Sternlieb I, Quintana N. The peroxisomes of human hepatocytes. *Lab Invest* 1977; **36**: 140–149.

28. De Craemer D, Pauwels M, Roels F. Peroxisomes in cirrhosis of the human liver: a cytochemical, ultrastructural and quantitative study. *Hepatology* 1993; **17**: 404–410.

29. Arias IM, Che M, Gatmaitan Z, Leveille C, Nishida T, St Pierre M. The biology of the bile canaliculus, 1993. *Hepatology* 1993; **17**: 318–329.

30. Horn T, Lyon H, Christoffersen P. The blood hepatocytic barrier: a light microscopical, transmission and scanning electron microscopic study. *Liver* 1986; **6**: 233–245.

31. Bardadin KA, Scheuer PJ. Endothelial cell changes in acute hepatitis. A light and electron microscopic study. *J Pathol* 1984; **144**: 213–220.

32. Schaff Z, Hoofnagle JH, Grimley PM. Hepatic inclusions during interferon therapy in chronic viral hepatitis. *Hepatology* 1986; **6**: 966–970.

33. Luu J, Bockus D, Remington F, Bean MA, Hammar SP. Tubuloreticular structures and cylindrical confronting cisternae: a review. *Hum Pathol* 1989; **20**: 617–627.

34. Friedman SL. The cellular basis of hepatic fibrosis. *N Engl J Med* 1993; **328**: 1828–1835.

35. Bouwens L, Wisse E. Pit cells in the liver. *Liver* 1992; **12**: 3–9.

36. De Vos R, De Wolf-Peeters C, van den Oord JJ, Desmet VJ. A recommended procedure for ultrastructural immunohistochemistry on small human tissue samples. *J Histochem Cytochem* 1985; **33**: 959–964.

37. Elias JM. Immunohistopathology. A Practical Approach to Diagnosis. Chicago: ASCP Press, 1990.

38. Volpes R, van den Oord JJ, Desmet VJ. Can hepatocytes serve as "activated" immunomodulating cells in the immune response? *J Hepatol* 1992; **16**: 228–240.

39. Horiike N, Onji M, Kumon I, Kanaoka M, Michitaka K, Ohta Y. Intercellular adhesion molecule-1 expression on the hepatocyte membrane of patients with chronic hepatitis B and C. *Liver* 1993; **13**: 10–14.

40. Volpes R, van den Oord JJ, De Vos R, Depla E, De Ley M, Desmet VJ. Expression of interferon-gamma receptor in normal and pathological human liver tissue. *J Hepatol* 1991; **12**: 195–202.

41. Volpes R, van den Oord JJ, De Vos R, Desmet VJ. Hepatic expression of type A and type B receptors for tumor necrosis factor. *J Hepatol* 1992; **14**: 361–369.

42. Vonnahme F-J. The Human Liver. A Scanning Electron Microscopic Atlas. Basel and Freiburg: Karger, 1993.

43. Ishak KG. Applications of scanning electron microscopy to the study of liver disease. In Popper H, Schaffner F (eds): Progress in Liver Diseases, Vol. VIII. Orlando: Grune and Stratton, 1986, pp 1–32.

44. Haratake J, Hisaoka M, Furuta A, Horie A, Yamamoto O. A scanning electron microscopic study of postnatal development of rat peribiliary plexus. *Hepatology* 1991; **14**: 1196–1200.

45. Haratake J, Hisaoka M, Yamamoto O, Horie A. Morphological changes of hepatic microcirculation in experimental rat cirrhosis: a scanning electron microscopic study. *Hepatology* 1991; **13**: 952–956.

46. Gaudio E, Pannarale L, Onori P, Riggio O. A scanning electron microscopic study of liver microcirculation disarrangement in experimental rat cirrhosis. *Hepatology* 1993; **17**: 477–485.

47. Terada T, Ishida F, Nakanuma Y. Vascular plexus around intrahepatic bile ducts in normal livers and portal hypertension. *J Hepatol* 1989; **8**: 139–149.

48. Moll R, Franke WW, Schiller D, Geiger B, Krepler R. The catalog of human cytokeratins: pattern of expression in normal epithelia, tumors and cultured cells. *Cell* 1982; **31**: 11–24.

49. Krawczynski K, Beach MJ, Bradley DW et al. Hepatitis C virus antigen in hepatocytes: immunomorphologic detection and identification. *Gastroenterology* 1992; **103**: 622–629.

50. Hiramatsu N, Hayashi N, Haruna Y et al. Immunohistochemical detection of hepatitis C virus-infected hepatocytes in chronic liver disease with monoclonal antibodies to core, envelope and NS3 regions of the hepatitis C virus genome. *Hepatology* 1992; **16**: 306–311.

51. Wolf HK, Michalopoulos GK. Hepatocyte regeneration in acute fulminant and nonfulminant hepatitis: a study of proliferating cell nuclear antigen expression. *Hepatology* 1992; **15**: 707–713.

52. Kayano K, Yasunaga M, Kubota M, et al. Detection of proliferating hepatocytes by immunohistochemical staining for proliferating cell nuclear antigen (PCNA) in patients with acute hepatic failure. *Liver* 1992; **12**: 132–136.

53. Kawakita N, Seki S, Sakaguchi H et al. Analysis of proliferating hepatocytes using a monoclonal antibody against proliferating cell nuclear antigen/cyclin in embedded tissues from various liver diseases fixed in formaldehyde. *Am J Pathol* 1992; **140**: 513–520.

54. Siitonen SM, Kallioniemi O-P, Isola JJ. Proliferating cell nuclear antigen immunohistochemistry using monoclonal antibody 19A2 and a new antigen retrieval technique has prognostic impact in archival paraffin-embedded node-negative breast cancer. *Am J Pathol* 1993; **142**: 1081–1089.

55. Foschini MP, Van Eyken P, Brock PR et al. Malignant rhabdoid tumour of the liver. A case report. *Histopathology* 1992; **20**: 157–165.

56. Thung SN, Gerber MA, Sarno E, Popper H. Distribution of five antigens in hepatocellular carcinoma. *Lab Invest* 1979; **41**: 101–105.

57. Lai Y-S, Thung SN, Gerber MA, Chen M-L, Schaffner F. Expression of cytokeratins in normal and diseased livers and in primary liver carcinomas. *Arch Pathol Lab Med* 1989; **113**: 134–138.

58. Van Eyken P, Desmet VJ. Cytokeratins and the liver. *Liver* 1993; **13**: 113–122.

59. Hytiroglou P, Choi SW, Theise ND, Chaudhary N, Worman HJ, Thung SN. The expression of nuclear lamins in human liver: an immunohistochemical study. *Hum Pathol* 1993; **24**: 169–172.

60. Hayata T, Nakano Y, Yoshizawa K, Sodeyama T, Kiyosawa K. Effects of interferon on intrahepatic human leukocyte antigens and lymphocyte subsets in patients with chronic hepatitis B and C. *Hepatology* 1991; **13**: 1022–1028.

61. Saidman SL, Duquesnoy RJ, Zeevi A, Fung JJ, Starzl TE, Demetris AJ. Recognition of major histocompatibility complex antigens on cultured human biliary epithelial cells by alloreactive lymphocytes. *Hepatology* 1991; **13**: 239–246.

62. Krawitt EL, Zannier A, Chossegros P et al. Expression of HLA antigens and T cell infiltrates in chronic viral hepatitis. *J Hepatol* 1991; **12**: 190–194.

63. Autschbach F, Meuer SC, Moebius U et al. Hepatocellular expression of lymphocyte function-associated antigen 3 in chronic hepatitis. *Hepatology* 1991; **14**: 223–230.

64. Adams DH, Hubscher SG, Shaw J et al. Increased expression of intercellular adhesion molecule 1 on bile ducts in primary biliary cirrhosis and primary sclerosing cholangitis. *Hepatology* 1991; **14**: 426–431.

65. Volpes R, van den Oord JJ, Desmet VJ. Vascular adhesion molecules in acute and chronic liver inflammation. *Hepatology* 1992; **15**: 269–275.

66. Feingold KR, Barker ME, Jones AL, Grunfeld C. Localization of tumor necrosis factor-stimulated DNA synthesis in the liver. *Hepatology* 1991; **13**: 773–779.

67. Omar R, Pappolla M, Saran B. Immunocytochemical detection of the 70-kd heat shock protein in alcoholic liver disease. *Arch Pathol Lab Med* 1990; **114**: 589–592.

68. Volpes R, van den Oord JJ, Desmet VJ. Memory T cells represent the predominant lymphocyte subset in acute and chronic liver inflammation. *Hepatology* 1991; **13**: 826–829.

69. Nagy P, Schaff Z, Lapis K. Immunohistochemical detection of transforming growth factor-β1 in fibrotic liver diseases. *Hepatology* 1991; **14**: 269–273.

70. Milani S, Herbst H, Schuppan D, Stein H, Surrenti C. Transforming growth factors β1 and β2 are differentially expressed in fibrotic liver disease. *Am J Pathol* 1991; **139**: 1221–1229.

71. Wolf HK, Zarnegar R, Michalopoulos GK. Localization of hepatocyte growth factor in human and rat tissues: an immunohistochemical study. *Hepatology* 1991; **14**: 488–494.

72. Martinez-Hernandez A. The hepatic extracellular matrix. I. Electron immunohistochemical studies in normal rat liver. *Lab Invest* 1984; **51**: 57–74.

73. Martinez-Hernandez A. The hepatic extracellular matrix. II. Electron immunohistochemical studies in rats with CCl4-induced cirrhosis. *Lab Invest* 1985; **53**: 166–186.

73a. Martinez-Hernandez A, Amenta PS. The hepatic extracellular matrix. I. Components and distribution in normal liver. *Virchows Arch A Pathol Anat* 1993; **423**: 1–11.

73b. Martinez-Hernandez A, Amenta PS. The hepatic extracellular matrix. II. Ontogenesis, regeneration and cirrhosis. *Virchows Arch A Pathol Anat* 1993; **423**: 77–84.

74. Griffiths MR, Shepherd M, Ferrier R, Schuppan D, James OFW, Burt AD. Light microscopic and ultrastructural distribution of type VI collagen in human liver: alterations in chronic biliary disease. *Histopathology* 1992; **21**: 335–344.

75. Volpes R, van den Oord JJ, Desmet VJ. Distribution of the VLA family of integrins in normal and pathological human liver tissue. *Gastroenterology* 1991; **101**: 200–206.

76. Koretz K, Schlag P, Boumsell L, Möller P. Expression of VLA-α2, VLA-α6, and VLA-β1 chains in normal mucosa and adenomas of the colon, and in colon carcinomas and their liver metastases. *Am J Pathol* 1991; **138**: 741–750.

77. Seki K, Minami Y, Nishikawa M, et al. "Nonalcoholic steatohepatitis" induced by massive doses of synthetic estrogen. *Gastroenterol Japon* 1983; **18**: 197–203.

78. Roncalli M, Borzio M, De Biagi G, Ferrari AR, Macchi R, Tombesi VM. Liver cell dysplasia in cirrhosis. A serologic and immunohistochemical study. *Cancer* 1986; **57**: 1515–1521.

79. Yamada S, Ichida T, Matsuda Y et al. Tenascin expression in human chronic liver disease and in hepatocellular carcinoma. *Liver* 1992; **12**: 10–16.

80. Grigioni WF, Garbisa S, D'Errico A et al. Evaluation of hepatocellular carcinoma aggressiveness by a panel of extracellular matrix antigens. *Am J Pathol* 1991; **138**: 647–654.

81. Dhillon AP, Colombari R, Savage K, Scheuer PJ. An immunohistochemical study of the blood vessels within primary hepatocellular tumours. *Liver* 1992; **12**: 311–318.

82. Van Eyken P, Sciot R, Paterson A, Callea F, Kew MC, Desmet VJ. Cytokeratin expression in hepatocellular carcinoma: an immunohistochemical study. *Hum Pathol* 1988; **19**: 562–568.

83. Jovanovic R, Jagirdar J, Thung SN, Paronetto F. Blood-group-related antigen Lewis-X and Lewis-Y in the differential diagnosis of cholangiocarcinoma and hepatocellular carcinoma. *Arch Pathol Lab Med* 1989; **113**: 139–142.

84. Naoumov NV, Alexander GJM, O'Grady JG, Aldis P, Portmann BC, Williams R. Rapid diagnosis of cytomegalovirus infection by in-situ hybridisation in liver grafts. *Lancet* 1988; **1**: 1361–1364.

85. Lamas E, Baccarini P, Housset C, Kremsdorf D, Bréchot C. Detection of hepatitis C virus (HCV) RNA sequences in liver tissue by in situ hybridization. *J Hepatol* 1992; **16**: 219–223.

86. Tanaka Y, Enomoto N, Kojima S et al. Detection of hepatitis C virus RNA in the liver by in situ hybridization. *Liver* 1993; **13**: 203–208.

87. Nuovo GJ, Lidonnici K, MacConnell P, Lane B. Intracellular localization of polymerase chain reaction (PCR)-amplified hepatitis C cDNA. *Am J Surg Pathol* 1993; **17**: 683–690.

88. Komminoth P, Long AA, Ray R, Wolfe HJ. In situ polymerase chain reaction detection of viral DNA, single-copy genes, and gene rearrangements in cell suspensions and cytospins. *Diagn Mol Pathol* 1992; **1**: 85–97.

89. Ray R, et al. Detection of cytomegalovirus by combined in situ hybridization and polymerase chain reaction. *Diagn Mol Pathol* 1994 (in press).

90. Hata K, Zhang XR, Iwatsuki S, Van Thiel DH, Herberman RB, Whiteside TL. Isolation, phenotyping and functional analysis of lymphocytes from human liver. *Clin Immunol Immunopathol* 1990; **56**: 401–419.

91. Hata K, Van Thiel DH, Herberman RB, Whiteside TL. Phenotypic and functional characteristics of lymphocytes isolated from liver biopsy specimens from patients with active liver disease. *Hepatology* 1992; **15**: 816–823.

92. Li X, Jeffers LJ, Reddy KR et al. Immunophenotyping of lymphocytes in liver tissue of patients with chronic liver diseases by flow cytometry. *Hepatology* 1991; **14**: 121–127.

93. Neri LM, Martelli AM, Previati M, Valmori A, Capitani S. From two dimensional (2D) to three dimensional (3D) analysis by confocal microscopy. *Liver* 1992; **12**: 268–279.

94. Vassy J, Rigaut JP, Briane D, Kraemer M. Confocal microscopy immunofluorescence localization of desmin and other intermediate filament proteins in fetal rat livers. *Hepatology* 1993; **17**: 293–300.

95. Pompella A, Comporti M. Imaging of oxidative stress at subcellular level by confocal laser scanning microscopy after fluorescent derivatization of cellular carbonyls. *Am J Pathol* 1993; **142**: 1353–1357.

96. Berk PD, Worman HJ. An introduction to molecular biology and recombinant DNA technology for the hepatologist. *Semin Liver Dis* 1992; **12**: 227–245.

97. Rose EA. Applications of the polymerase chain reaction to genome analysis. *FASEB J* 1991; **5**: 46–54.

98. Mullis KB. The unusual origin of the polymerase chain reaction. *Sci Am* 1990; **262**: 56–65.

99. Eisenstein BI. The polymerase chain reaction. A new mothod of using molecular genetics for medical diagnosis. *N Engl J Med* 1990; **322**: 178–183.

100. Shieh YSC, Shim K-S, Lampertico P et al. Detection of hepatitis C virus sequences in liver tissue by the polymerase chain reaction. *Lab Invest* 1991; **65**: 408–411.

101. Akyol G, Dash S, Shieh YSC, Malter JS, Gerber MA. Detection of hepatitis C virus RNA sequences by polymerase chain reaction in fixed liver tissue. *Modern Pathol* 1992; **5**: 501–504.

102. Arborgh B, Bell P, Brunk U, Collins VP. The osmotic effect of glutaraldehyde during fixation. A transmission electron microscopy, scanning electron microscopy and cytochemical study. *J Ultrastruc Res* 1976; **56**: 339–350.

GENERAL READING

Berk PD, Worman HJ. An introduction to molecular biology and recombinant DNA technology for the hepatologist. *Sem Liv Dis* 1992; **12**: 227–245.

Elias JM. Immunohistopathology. A Practical Approach to Diagnosis. Chicago: ASCP Press, 1990.

Phillips MJ, Poucell S, Patterson J, Valencia P. The Liver. An Atlas and Text of Ultrastructural Pathology. New York: Raven Press, 1987.

Vonnahme F-J. The Human Liver. A Scanning Electron Microscopic Atlas. Basel, Freiburg: Karger, 1993.

Watson JD, Gilman M, Witkowski J, Zoller M. Recombinant DNA, 2nd edn. New York: Scientific American Books, 1992.

Glossary

Acidophil body (Fig. 6.2) A rounded, deeply stained and refractile structure derived from a hepatocyte by apoptosis. Some acidophil bodies are the shrunken remains of entire hepatocytes while others represent fragments. They are found in increased numbers in hepatitis, in other conditions with hepatocellular damage, and when liver-cell turnover is increased.

Acinus (Fig. 3.1) An anatomical unit based on blood supply, its three parenchymal zones containing successively less oxygenated blood. Zone 1 is nearest to the terminal portal vessels in a small portal tract.

Activity (Figs 10.19 and 10.20) In histological terms, an expression of the degree of hepatocellular damage and associated inflammation. Especially used in chronic hepatitis and cirrhosis.

Apoptosis (Fig. 6.2) Shrinkage and fragmentation of cells, seen in the liver in the form ·of acidophil bodies.

Autoimmune hepatitis A form of hepatitis usually associated with high titres of abnormal serum antibodies, and responding to immunosuppressive therapy.

Ballooning degeneration Swelling and rounding of hepatocytes, with loss of their normal polygonal shape. Different forms of ballooning are seen in viral hepatitis (Fig. 6.1) and alcoholic hepatitis (Fig. 7.11).

Bile canaliculus (Fig. 5.1) The tubular space formed between the biliary poles of two or three hepatocytes, or more in diseased liver. The canaliculus has no separate epithelial lining of its own.

Bile duct (Figs 3.2 and 3.3) The smallest ducts, interlobular bile ducts, are centrally located in small portal tracts and are accompanied by blood vessels. In practice they are sometimes difficult to distinguish from bile ductules, the transition being gradual.

Bile ductule and canal of Hering (Fig. 3.4) At the portal–parenchymal interface the canalicular system drains into the canals of Hering which are partly lined by hepatocytes and partly by biliary epithelium. These in turn connect with bile ductules, fully lined by biliary epithelium. Both are difficult to find in normal liver. Proliferated ductules in disease may lack regular lumens ("atypical ductules").

Bile extravasate (Fig. 5.9) Leakage of bile from a duct into the connective tissue of the portal tract, occasionally seen in large bile-duct obstruction.

Bile infarct (Figs 5.3 and 5.4) An area of liver-cell death in a cholestatic liver; often periportal whereas canalicular cholestasis is mainly perivenular. Bile staining is variable and may be absent. Bile infarcts are easily mistaken for accumulations of foamy macrophages.

Bile lake An accumulation of bile outside a liver-cell plate.

Bile thrombus (Fig. 5.1) Synonymous with bile plug: the accumulation of visible bile in a canaliculus.

Bilirubinostasis See Cholestasis.

Bridging fibrosis (Fig. 7.16) As for bridging necrosis (below), but with laying down of new collagen.

Bridging necrosis (Fig. 6.11) Confluent hepatocellular necrosis and collapse linking vascular structures; usually and preferably confined to linking of portal tracts to terminal venules (zone 3 bridging).

Ceroid pigment (Fig. 6.2) Brown pigment in macrophages, found after hepatocellular injury; rich in oxidized lipids and PAS-positive after diastase digestion (Fig. 6.4). Distinct from lipofuscin (see below).

Cholate stasis (Fig. 5.10) A term sometimes used for chronic cholestasis, on the assumption that the hepatocellular changes result from the accumulation of toxic bile salts. Also known as precholestasis.

Cholestasis (Fig. 5.1) In morphological terms, bilirubinostasis or visible bile in a section of liver. Also defined as failure of bile to reach the duodenum, and biochemically as a type of jaundice with dark urine, pale stools, conjugated hyperbilirubinaemia and raised serum alkaline phosphatase.

Collapse (Fig. 4.1) Condensation of pre-existing reticulin framework as a result of necrosis. May be followed by fibrosis.

Confluent necrosis (Fig. 8.3) Death of groups of adjacent hepatocytes.

Disse space (Fig. 17.4) The space between the sinusoidal endothelium and hepatocytes; contents include extracellular matrix and lipocytes.

Ductopenia (Fig. 16.4) Loss of significant numbers of interlobular bile ducts, principally as a result of immunological attack. Causes include rejection of liver grafts, graft-versus-host disease, primary biliary cirrhosis, primary sclerosing cholangitis and drug injury. In the latter direct toxicity may be responsible.

Dysplasia (Figs 10.8 and 10.9) A change in the size, nuclear–cytoplasmic ratio and/or nuclear appearances of hepatocytes, usually in chronic hepatitis and cirrhosis. Large-cell and small-cell types are described.

Fat-storing cells see Lipocytes.

Feathery degeneration (Fig. 5.2) A type of liver-cell injury in cholestasis, attributed to toxic effects of bile salts. Affected hepatocytes, often single cells lying within normal parenchyma, are swollen and have pale-staining feathery cytoplasm.

Fibrosis Formation of new collagen fibres. It may follow collapse of pre-existing connective tissue framework or arise *de novo*.

Focal necrosis (Fig. 15.25) Death of hepatocytes, singly or in small groups. Because of the rapid disappearance of the dead cells, focal necrosis is usually recognized by the presence of inflammatory cells and by a break in continuity of a liver-cell plate rather than by the presence of necrotic tissue.

Follicle See Lymphoid follicle.

Glycogen vacuolation See Nuclear vacuolation.

Granuloma (Fig. 15.1) A focal accumulation of epithelioid cells, which are modified macrophages with abundant cytoplasm and often curved, elongated nuclei. To be distinguished from simple accumulations of macrophages.

Ground-glass hepatocytes (Fig. 9.11) Hepatocytes with a well-defined, lightly eosinophilic homogeneous area occupying much of the cytoplasm. One form is seen in patients infected with the hepatitis B virus.

Haemochromatosis (see also under Siderosis) A disease in which hepatic fibrosis and cirrhosis ultimately develop as a result of iron overload.

Hepatocytes Liver cells.

Interface hepatitis (Figs 9.3 and 9.4) An alternative term for piecemeal necrosis (see below).

Ito cells See Lipocytes.

Kupffer cells The resident macrophages of the liver, straddling the sinusoidal lumens.

Limiting plate The layer of hepatocytes next to a portal tract.

Lipocytes (Fig. 17.4) Cells containing vacuoles rich in vitamin A, lying within the space of Disse. They have the potential to produce collagens. Synonyms include fat-storing cells, Ito cells, parasinusoidal cells, perisinusoidal cells and stellate cells.

Lipofuscin (Figs 3.7 and 3.8) Pigmented granular material in hepatocytes, of lysosomal origin and most abundant at the biliary poles of the cells. Found in normal liver in greatly varying amounts.

Liver-cell plates (Fig. 3.5) Interconnecting walls of hepatocytes, one cell thick in adults. Thicker plates are found in children and in regenerating liver.

Lobule (Fig. 3.1) An anatomical unit with an efferent (centrilobular) vein at its centre and portal tracts peripherally.

Lupoid hepatitis An old term for autoimmune hepatitis, no longer in use.

Lymphoid follicle (Fig. 9.13) A structured accumulation of lymphocytes resembling the follicles of normal lymph nodes.

Mallory bodies (Fig. 7.11) Irregular, dense cytoplasmic inclusions with a cytokeratin component, often in the form of strands or garlands. Electron microscopy reveals a filamentous structure.

Massive necrosis (Fig. 6.14) Multiacinar necrosis (see below) involving a substantial part of the whole liver. This usually leads to severe liver insufficiency.

Multiacinar necrosis (Fig. 6.14) Confluent necrosis involving the whole of several adjacent acini. The clinical effects are variable, depending on the extent of the lesion.

Nuclear vacuolation (Fig. 7.9) Empty hepatocyte nuclei in paraffin sections. May be due to glycogen accumulation, lipid or invagination of cytoplasm. Glycogen nuclei, common in the young, the obese and the diabetic, are typically enlarged and have prominent nuclear membranes. The glycogen may be demonstrable histochemically but is often lost during processing.

Panacinar necrosis (Fig. 6.14) Necrosis of an entire acinus.

Parasinusoidal cells See Lipocytes.

Parenchyma The specialized tissue of the liver, as opposed to the connective tissue. Sometimes used loosely to describe the contents of the acini as opposed to the portal tracts.

Periportal Used in this book for the part of the hepatic acinus next to a small portal tract (acinar zone 1), but occasionally used elsewhere for the area within a portal tract immediately around a portal-vein branch.

Perisinusoidal cells See Lipocytes.

Piecemeal necrosis (Figs 9.3 and 9.4) Death of hepatocytes at the junction of connective tissue and parenchyma in chronic liver disease.

Polyploidy (Fig. 3.10) The coexistence of different classes of nuclei containing multiple sets of chromosomes (e.g. quadriploid, octaploid); a normal state in adult human liver.

Portal triad (Fig. 3.2) Another term for the portal tract, containing the triad of artery, vein and bile duct.

Pseudoacini Rosettes (see below).

Regeneration (Fig. 10.6) Loosely used to describe hepatocellular hyperplasia following injury or loss. Not easily recognized in conventional sections because of low mitotic rate; the most reliable marker in such sections is increase in the thickness of the cell plates. Immunohistochemical methods for assessing cell proliferation are available.

Rosettes (Figs 4.3 and 9.9) In liver pathology this term refers to a change of the normal plate pattern of hepatocytes to glandular structures formed by several hepatocytes. Different types of rosette formation are seen in cholestasis and in chronic hepatitis.

Septa (Fig. 10.16) Walls of fibrous tissue, seen in two-dimensional sections as lines or bands. Septa may be formed by collapse ("passive septa"), by new fibre formation ("active septa") or by both.

Siderosis (Fig. 14.6) The presence of stainable iron in any component of liver tissue. The many causes of siderosis include several diseases under the heading of haemochromatosis, in which progressive iron accumulation leads to fibrosis and cirrhosis. However, at an early stage of genetic haemochromatosis there is iron deposition without fibrosis.

Spotty necrosis (Fig. 6.3) Widespread but patchy hepatocellular necrosis, typical of acute hepatitis.

Stellate cells See Lipocytes.

Index

Bold numbers denote main entries